Idiopathic Pulmonary Fibrosis

Edited by
Ulrich Costabel, Bruno Crestani
and Athol U. Wells

Editor in Chief
Robert Bals

This book is one in a series of *ERS Monographs*. Each individual issue provides a comprehensive overview of one specific clinical area of respiratory health, communicating information about the most advanced techniques and systems required for its investigation. It provides factual and useful scientific detail, drawing on specific case studies and looking into the diagnosis and management of individual patients. Previously published titles in this series are listed at the back of this *Monograph*.

ERS Monographs are available online at www.erspublications.com and print copies are available from www.ersbookshop.com

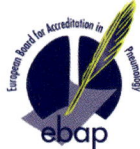

Continuing medical education (CME) credits are available through many issues of the *ERS Monograph*. Following evaluation, successful *Monographs* are accredited by the European Board for Accreditation in Pneumology (EBAP) for 5 CME credits. To earn CME credits, read the book of your choice (it is clearly indicated on the online table of contents whether CME credits are available) then complete the CME question form that is available at www.ers-education.org/e-learning/cme-tests.aspx

Editorial Board: Antonio Anzueto (San Antonio, TX, USA), Leif Bjermer (Lund, Sweden), John R. Hurst (London, UK) and Carlos Robalo Cordeiro (Coimbra, Portugal).

Managing Editor: Rachel White
European Respiratory Society, 442 Glossop Road, Sheffield, S10 2PX, UK
Tel: 44 114 2672860 | E-mail: Monograph@ersj.org.uk

Published by European Respiratory Society ©2016
March 2016
Print ISBN: 978-1-84984-067-5
Online ISBN: 978-1-84984-068-2
Print ISSN: 2312-508X
Online ISSN: 2312-5098
Printed by Latimer Trend and Company Limited, Plymouth, UK

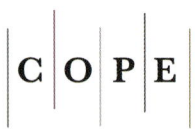
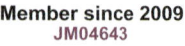

This journal is a member of and subscribes to the principles of the Committee on Publication Ethics

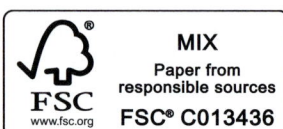

MIX
Paper from responsible sources
FSC® C013436

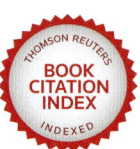

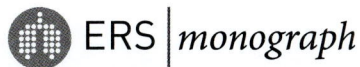

Contents

Idiopathic Pulmonary Fibrosis

Number 71
March 2016

Preface

Robert Bals

The field of ILD has gone through several years of change. Many old views on these diseases have been challenged and replaced by more convincing concepts. A good example is the change IPF therapy has undergone during recent years.

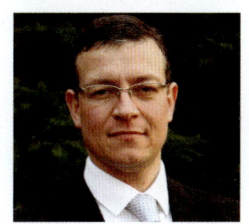

According to the US philosopher Thomas S. Kuhn (1922–1996), progress in science often undergoes paradigmatic shifts rather than continuous progress. In clinical medicine, however, many examples show that continuous progress results in improved diagnosis or therapy. The field of ILD and IPF is somehow a mixture of both paradigm shift and continuous progress. Ongoing research in recent decades provided insight into disease mechanisms and underscored the heterogeneity and complexity of these diseases. A chance paradigmatic shift in IPF therapy followed the "crisis" finding that classical therapy with immunosuppressants was more dangerous than beneficial. In parallel, novel drugs were approved after their efficacy has been demonstrated in clinical trials.

IPF is also a good example of a rare disease that needs special attention in the diagnostic process. However, if IPF is taken together with other ILDs, quite a high number of patients suffer from these conditions, meaning the whole disease area goes far beyond "rare" status. Interestingly, this field also gained much more attention when novel drugs became available; pharmaceutical advertisements in this field certainly increased.

The diagnosis and treatment of IPF is multidisciplinary, a fact that is well represented by the content and authors of this book. The book comprises chapters on molecular mechanisms, diagnosis, imaging, pathology and various aspects of therapy. It also reviews the fast developments in drug development. The critical use of data from clinical trials provides new ways to think about IPF and related diseases, and the shifted paradigms of recent years. The Guest Editors, Ulrich Costabel, Bruno Crestani and Athol U. Wells, have worked hard and very successfully to select these topics and to integrate these aspects into a comprehensive book on the current knowledge about IPF and other ILDs.

I thank the Guest Editors and all authors for their work on this excellent book. I hope the reader finds this book useful in their clinical practice.

Guest Editors

Ulrich Costabel

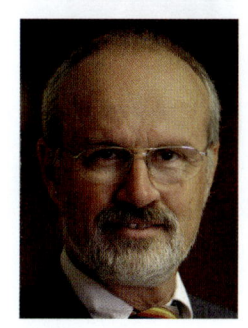

Ulrich Costabel is Professor of Medicine at the University of Duisburg-Essen (Essen, Germany) and Senior Consultant in Interstitial and Rare Lung Diseases at the Ruhrlandklinik (Essen, Germany). He was previously Chief of the Division of Pneumology and Allergology at the Ruhrlandklinik. He received his undergraduate training and his MD magna cum laude at the University of Freiburg (Freiburg, Germany). In 1992–1993, he spent a 6-month sabbatical with Professor Takateru Izumi at the Chest Disease Research Institute of the University of Kyoto in Japan (Kyoto, Japan).

Ulrich Costabel's research interests lie in clinical and immunological studies in ILDs, with a specific focus on clinical and research applications of BAL. In recent years, he has acted as principal investigator for major clinical trials in IPF. He is Past President of the World Association of Sarcoidosis and Other Granulomatous Disorders (WASOG) and organised the World Congress on Sarcoidosis in Essen in 1997. He has been Chairman of the European BAL Group since 1998 and has co-organised several international conferences on BAL.

Ulrich Costabel has been actively involved with the European Respiratory Society (ERS) since its inception, having been Chair of the Occupational and Environmental Health Group and Secretary of the Occupation and Epidemiology Assembly, and later Chair of the Bronchoalveolar Lavage Group. From 2002–2005, he was Head of the Clinical Assembly and a member of the Executive Committee of the ERS and, in 2006, he was Chairman of the ERS Congress in Munich (Germany).

Since 1990 he has served on the Editorial Board of the *European Respiratory Journal* (*ERJ*), from 1994–1999 as the Chief Editor. He was Editor of the German journal *Pneumologie* from 2001–2005, has co-edited the *ERS Monograph* on Sarcoidosis, and is currently on the board of *Sarcoidosis*, *Seminars in Respiratory and Critical Care Medicine* and *Current Opinion in Pulmonary Medicine*, among others. He is the recipient of several honours and awards, including the Sarcoidosis Research Prize presented by the German Sarcoidosis Association and the World Sarcoidosis Person of the Year Award from the Irish Sarcoidosis Charity.

Bruno Crestani

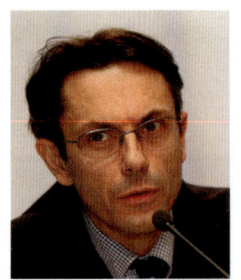

Bruno Crestani is Head of the Pneumology Department at the Bichat Hospital, Assistance Publique-Hôpitaux de Paris (AP-HP) in Paris (France). He is also a Professor of Pneumology at the Paris Diderot University School of Medicine (Paris, France). He is Director of the Lung Inflammation and Fibrosis research unit in INSERM 1152. In recent years, his team has focused on elucidating the pathophysiological mechanisms of IPF, including genetics.

Bruno Crestani is a founding member of the European IPF Network (eurIPFnet) and Head of the Fibrosis, Inflammation and REmodelling (DHU FIRE) university department at the Paris Diderot University School of Medicine. He is also an Associate Editor of the *European Respiratory Journal*.

Athol U. Wells

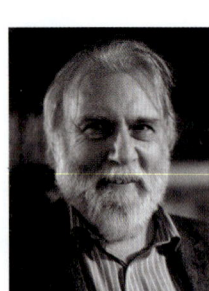

Athol U. Wells is a Professor of Respiratory Medicine, Senior Consultant and the Academic Lead of the Interstitial Lung Diseases Unit at the Royal Brompton Hospital (London, UK). He completed his undergraduate training at Otago University (Dunedin, New Zealand) where he was later awarded his MD with distinction. He trained as a post-graduate and later practised as a respiratory physician in New Zealand. From 1989 to 1994, he was a research fellow at the Royal Brompton Hospital. After returning to New Zealand for 5 years, he took up his current post at Royal Brompton Hospital in 1999.

Athol Wells has research interests in clinical and translational science with the unifying theme being studies of CT and PFT, both in staging disease and in the examination of disease behaviour (for clinical purposes and in studies of pathogenesis). He was a chair of the British Thoracic Society guidelines (BTS) for ILD, a co-chair in the recent (2013) American Thoracic Society (ATS)/European Respiratory Society (ERS) update of the classification of the IIPs, and a participant in a number of ATS/ERS expert groups. He created and developed the Disease Behaviour Classification, which was endorsed in the 2013 classification of the IIPs. He is the author/co-author of over 230 peer reviewed articles and over 100 editorials, chapters and review articles. He currently serves on the Editorial Board of the *American Journal of Respiratory and Critical Care Medicine*.

Athol Wells believes strongly in the need for an independent European voice in the field of ILD (to complement international consensus initiatives) and has led or co-led four European perspectives in recent years, including the current *ERS Monograph*. He is currently the Chair of European consensus statements on IPF and on lung disease associated with connective tissue disease.

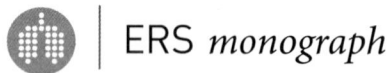
Introduction

Ulrich Costabel[1], Bruno Crestani[2] and Athol U. Wells[3]

IPF is a serious, chronic, steadily progressive and ultimately fatal disease of unknown origin, occurring predominantly in the elderly male smoker or exsmoker. Survival is worse than in many malignancies. IPF is the most dreaded and also the most frequent of the IIPs. The morphological hallmark is the UIP pattern, either on HRCT or biopsy, but it is not specific for IPF. It is crucial to differentiate this distinct entity from other ILDs with different prognoses and treatment approaches, especially from chronic extrinsic allergic alveolitis, idiopathic fibrotic NSIP and interstitial pneumonias with autoimmune features.

Recent years have seen a number of advances and changes in our understanding of the pathogenesis, diagnosis and management of IPF. It became evident that diagnostic security could be sharpened by multidisciplinary discussion and that bronchoscopic lung cryobiopsy is probably as informative as surgical lung biopsy in this setting. Many patients do not undergo surgical lung biopsy because the procedure is too risky in patients with severe disease and marked comorbidities. A number of statements and guidelines have been published but the question of how to handle a patient with probable or possible IPF compared to definite IPF has never been addressed.

After decades of therapeutic disappointment, two antifibrotic drugs are now available, which have the potential to slow disease progression by preventing ~50% of the decline in FVC. In this context, early diagnosis, which requires the recognition of velcro-like crackles on auscultation in the elderly, deserves the highest attention in the new era of IPF as a treatable disorder. There are many open questions related to antifibrotic therapy: when should we start and stop treatment? Which drug should be used first? Will the future lie in sequential or combination therapy?

This *ERS Monograph* aims to broadly describe the new achievements associated with IPF. Beginning with epidemiology, genectis and pathogenesis, the key diagnostic issues and major contributors to diagnosis, such as imaging and histopathology/BAL, are covered. This is followed by a section on how to evaluate/stage the disease for prognosis and how to monitor progression, including a discussion on the potential value of biomarkers. Several chapters are devoted to complications and comorbidities and their impact on management, such as acute exacerbation, PH, lung cancer, emphysema, cardiovascular disease and GERD. The treatment chapters cover antifibrotic drug therapy, symptom control, rehabilitation,

[1]Interstitial and Rare Lung Disease Unit, Ruhrlandklinik, University Hospital, University of Duisburg-Essen, Essen, Germany. [2]Service de Pneumologie A, Centre de Compétences Maladies Rares Pulmonaires, Hôpital Bichat, APHP, INSERM, Unité 1152, Paris, France. [3]Interstitial Lung Disease Unit, Royal Brompton Hospital, London, UK.

Correspondence: Ulrich Costabel, Ruhrlandklinik, Tüschener Weg 40, D-45239 Essen, Germany.
E-mail: ulrich.costabel@ruhrlandklinik.uk-essen.de

palliative care and transplantation. Finally, the book considers unmet patient needs, ongoing issues in clinical trials and perspectives for the future.

As editors we believe that this new *Monograph* is timely, given the numerous developments in this field. We hope that this book will be of interest to all those who are engaged as clinicians or researchers in this evolving topic of respiratory medicine.

List of abbreviations

6MWD	6 min walk distance
6MWT	6 min walk test
BAL	bronchoalveolar lavage
BALF	bronchoalveolar lavage fluid
COPD	chronic obstructive pulmonary disease
CPFE	combined pulmonary fibrosis and emphysema
CT	computed tomography
D_{LCO}	diffusing capacity of the lung for carbon monoxide
FEV_1	forced expiratory volume in 1 s
FVC	forced vital capacity
GAP	gender, age and physiology
GERD	gastro-oesophageal reflux disease
HRCT	high-resolution computed tomography
IIP	idiopathic interstitial pneumonia
ILD	interstitial lung disease
IPF	idiopathic pulmonary fibrosis
miRNA	micro RNAs
NAC	*N*-acetylcysteine
NSIP	nonspecific interstitial pneumonia
PFT	pulmonary function test
PH	pulmonary hypertension
QoL	quality of life
TGF	transforming growth factor
TLC	total lung capacity
UIP	usual interstitial pneumonia
VEGF	vascular endothelial growth factor

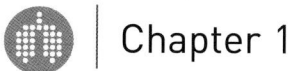

Chapter 1

Epidemiology

Vidya Navaratnam[1], Doug L. Forrester[2] and Richard B. Hubbard[1]

The precise global incidence and prevalence of IPF remain unclear, with incidence estimates ranging from 1.2 to 9.6 per 100 000 person-years. In this chapter, we summarise studies of the incidence and prevalence of IPF before discussing risk factors and comorbid illnesses. Many studies have evaluated risk factors for IPF including smoking, environmental factors, gastro-oesophageal reflux, diabetes mellitus, clotting dysfunction and genetics. Through epidemiological studies there has been considerable progress in identifying factors that are likely to be aetiologically important, and further research into the causes and progression of IPF is vital to identify biomarkers and targets for treatments. The most common cause of death in people with IPF is respiratory failure secondary to lung fibrosis. However, the incidence of comorbidities such as cardiovascular disease and lung cancer is increased in people with IPF. The association between these comorbidities may be important in helping understand the pathogenesis of IPF and the need for a holistic approach to the care of patients.

The first IPF cases were described as acute interstitial fibrosis of the lungs by HAMMAN and RICH [1]. IPF usually presents insidiously with progressive exertional breathlessness and a dry cough, with most patients complaining of a 6-month history of breathlessness prior to presentation. Physical examination commonly reveals finger clubbing [2] and over 80% of patients will have end-inspiratory crepitations at the lung bases on chest auscultation [3–5]. Cyanosis, cor pulmonale, right ventricular heave and peripheral oedema may occur in the later phases [6]. The incidence of IPF increases with older age, with mean age of presentation occurring in the seventh decade, and has been shown to be more common in men than women [7, 8].

Incidence and prevalence of IPF

Epidemiological studies have demonstrated that IPF is the most common type of ILD [9]. Overall global incidence and prevalence remain unclear, with incidence ranging from 1.2 to 90.6 per 100 000 person-years. It is also unclear how much of the variation in incidence is due to demographic and/or geographical differences, or due to sensitivity and specificity of the case definition. Most large studies estimating incidence and prevalence of IPF have used routinely collected clinical data. It is important to recognise that the definition of IPF in

[1]Division of Epidemiology and Public Health, University of Nottingham, Nottingham, UK. [2]Division of Respiratory Medicine, University of Nottingham, Nottingham, UK.

Correspondence: Vidya Navaratnam, Nottingham Respiratory Research Unit, Clinical Sciences Building, Nottingham City Hospital, Hucknall Road, Nottingham NG5 1PB, UK. E-mail: vidya.navaratnam@nottingham.ac.uk

Copyright ©ERS 2016. Print ISBN: 978-1-84984-067-5. Online ISBN: 978-1-84984-068-2. Print ISSN: 2312-508X. Online ISSN: 2312-5098.

Table 1. Incidence and prevalence of IPF by geographical region

Region	First author [ref.]	Study period	Data source	Case definition	Incidence per 100 000 person-years	Prevalence per 100 000 person-years
USA	Coultas [9]	1988–1990	Population-based registry	ICD-9 516.3, 515	10.7 [male] 7.4 [female]	20.2 [male] 13.2 [female]
	Mannino [10]	1979–1991	Registered death certificates	ICD-9 516.3, 515	3.2 (1979) 3.65 (1991)	
	Raghu [8]	1996–2000	Healthcare claim data	ICD-9 516.3	16.3 [broad] 6.8 [narrow]	42.7 [broad] 14.0 [narrow]
	Olson [19]	1992–2003	Registered death certificates	ICD-9 516.3, 515 ICD-10 J84.1	5.08	
	Fernandez-Perez [20]	1997–2005	Population-based registry	ATS/ERS 2002 criteria	17.4 [broad] 8.8 [narrow]	63 [broad] 27.9 [narrow]
	Raghu [11]	2001–2011	Medicare database, 5% random sample	ICD-9 CM 516.3, 515	92.4 (2001) 90.6 (2011)	202.2 (2001) 494.5 (2011)
	Esposito [21]	2006–2012	Healthcare claim data	ICD-9 CM 516.3, 515	14.6 [adjusted for PPV]	58.7 [adjusted for PPV]
Europe	Johnston [12]	1979–1987	Registered death certificates; review of case notes	ICD-9 516.3, 515; clinical criteria	Data displayed graphically	
	Navaratnam [15]	1968–2008	Registered death certificates	ICD-8 517, ICD-9 516.3, 515 ICD-10 J84.1	5.10 [2005–2008]	
	Gribbin [7]	1991–2003	Primary care data	Read codes for CFA, IFA	4.6	
	Kornum [22]	1995–2000	National registry	ICD-10 J84.1	4.17 [1995–2000] 2.91 [2001–2005]	
	Navaratnam [15]	2000–2008	Primary care data	Read codes for IFA/CFA/PF	7.44	
	Hyldgaard [23]	2003–2009	Hospital registry	ICD-10 codes; ATS/ERS 2011 criteria	1.3	
	Agabiti [24]	2005–2009	Regional hospital and mortality data	ICD-9 C 516.3; ATS/ERS 2011 criteria	7.5 [ICD codes] 9.3 [case review]	25.6 [2009]
	Von Plessen [16]	1984–1998	Hospital register	ICD-8 517; ICD-9 516.3, 515	4.3	23.9 [1998]

Continued

Table 1. Continued

Region	First author [ref.]	Study period	Data source	Case definition	Incidence per 100 000 person-years	Prevalence per 100 000 person-years
Rest of the world	Lᴀɪ [18]	1997–2007	Health insurance data/government records	ICD-9 516.3	1.4 [broad] 1.2 [narrow]	6.4 [broad] 4.9 [narrow]
	Oʜɴᴏ [17]	2005	Medical benefits data	ATS/ERS 2002 criteria	1.2	1.7
Multicentre	Hᴜʙʙᴀʀᴅ [13]	1979–1992	Registered death certificates	ICD-9 516.3, 515	Data displayed graphically	
	Hᴜᴛᴄʜɪɴsᴏɴ [14]	1999–2012	Registered death certificates	ICD-10 J84.1	8.28 [England and Wales, UK; 2012] 5.08 [Australia, 2011] 6.38 [Canada, 2011] 4.64 [Spain, 2011] 6.16 [USA, 2010]	

ICD: International Classification of Diseases; ATS: American Thoracic Society; ERS: European Respiratory Society; CM: Clinical Modification; CFA: cryptogenic fibrosing alveolitis; IFA: idiopathic fibrosing alveolitis; PF: pulmonary fibrosis; PPV: positive predictive value.

these epidemiological studies may be simpler than diagnostic criteria currently used in clinical practice and may not depend on histological confirmation. For clarity, we have grouped incidence and prevalence studies by three large regions: the USA, Europe and the rest of the world (table 1). What follows is an overview of selected studies.

The largest studies in the USA have used either multiple-cause mortality data or health insurance claim records. MANNINO et al. [10] used multiple-cause mortality data to show that the frequency with which lung fibrosis was listed as the underlying cause of death had increased from 1979 to 1991. Using insurance claim data, RAGHU et al. [8] set out broad and narrow criteria for the diagnosis of IPF, and estimated that the age-adjusted incidence extrapolated to the overall US population was 6.8 per 100 000 person-years (narrow definition) or 16.3 per 100 000 person-years (broad definition). A more recent study using Medicare data described an overall incidence of 93.7 per 100 000 person-years [11]. However, the study population was restricted to people ⩾65 years of age; hence, direct comparisons with other studies are limited. This study also reported that incidence remained stable over the 10-year study period, with an increasing annual cumulative prevalence [11].

One of the earliest studies in the UK using routine mortality data was by JOHNSTON et al. [12], which showed that when the diagnosis was present, the accuracy of registered death certificates of cryptogenic fibrosing alveolitis (CFA) was high but was likely to underestimate the true number of deaths from the disease. Similarly, studies by HUBBARD et al. [13] and more recently HUTCHINSON et al. [14] used registered death certificate data from different countries, and found that mortality from IPF is increasing. Similar trends have been demonstrated using UK primary care data. Studies by GRIBBIN et al. [7] as well as NAVARATNAM et al. [15] have found that the number of incident diagnoses of IPF in primary care records has continued to rise. Both studies also demonstrated regional differences in incidence of IPF in the UK [7, 15], although the underlying reasons for this are unclear. Using local hospital records in Norway, VON PLESSEN et al. [16] found the overall incidence of IPF was 4.3 per 100 000 person-years, which is broadly similar to the estimates from GRIBBIN et al. [7] using primary care data during a similar period.

There are limited data on incidence and prevalence of IPF outside the USA and Europe. A Japanese study used medical benefit data to estimate the incidence of IIP, of which 86% were IPF. [17] The estimated incidence of IPF in this population was approximately 1.2 per 100 000 person-years, whilst the prevalence was 1.7 per 100 000 person-years [17]. These estimates are similar to a study from Taiwan [18] that applied broad and narrow case definitions similar to RAGHU et al. [8]. Using the narrow definition, the incidence and prevalence of IPF in Taiwan was 1.2 and 4.9 per 100 000 person-years, respectively [18]. It needs to be highlighted that in both of studies from Japan and Taiwan, survival was lower than other studies, suggesting that only severe cases were captured [17, 18].

Clinical course and survival

The natural history of IPF is one of progressive breathlessness and decline in pulmonary function. Whilst the majority of individuals with IPF experience a slow gradual decline over many years, others experience an accelerated progression of their disease (figure 1) [25]. Unfortunately, the clinical course in people with IPF is unpredictable at the time of diagnosis. Current best estimates suggest that median survival from time of diagnosis is 2–3 years, [7, 15, 20, 26–28] although a recent study suggests that median survival has

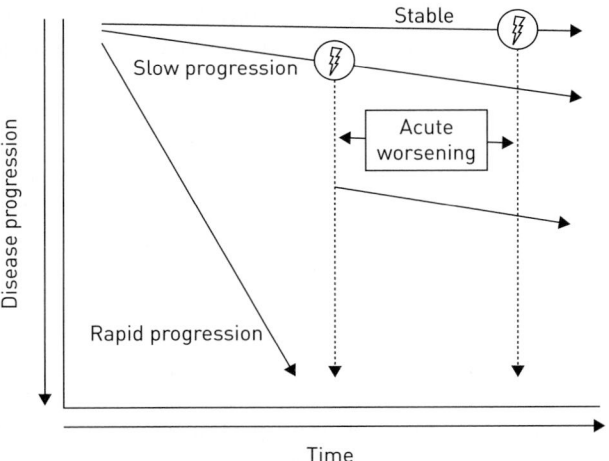

Figure 1. Natural history of IPF. There appear to be several possible natural histories for patients with IPF. The majority of patients experience a slow but steady worsening of their disease (slow progression). Some patients remain stable, while others have an accelerated decline (rapid progression). A minority of patients may experience unpredictable acute worsening of their disease (lightning bolt), either from a secondary complication such as pneumonia, or for unrecognised reasons. This event may be fatal or may leave patients with substantially worsened disease. The relative frequency of each of these natural histories is unknown. Reproduced and modified from [25] with permission from the publisher.

improved over time [11]. Studies have also consistently shown that male sex [7, 29–31], increasing age [15, 30] and impaired lung function [29, 30, 32, 33] are strong predictors of increased mortality in IPF.

Risk factors

Although IPF remains a disease of unknown aetiology, a number of studies have described potential aetiological factors. These include environmental exposures, smoking, clotting dysfunction and comorbid illnesses (such as cardiovascular disease, diabetes mellitus and gastro-oesophageal reflux disease). Large studies investigating possible risk factors for IPF are important, as increasing understanding of aetiology and pathogenesis may lead to novel treatments.

Smoking

A number of studies have demonstrated the association between cigarette smoke and IPF [34–37]. This appears to have a cumulative component, with the risk of IPF also appearing to increase with pack-years of smoking [38, 39]. However, most studies investigating the association between smoking and IPF have been case–control studies, which are limited by potential selection and recall bias. Hence, results of these studies need to be interpreted with caution. In the USA, a multicentre, case–control study found that cases with IPF were more likely to be ever-smokers or former smokers [39]. More recently, case–control studies in Mexico [37], the UK [40] and Sweden [41] have demonstrated that cases with IPF were more likely to be ever- or ex-smokers than general population controls. Using data collected as part of the Million Women Study, PIRIE et al. [42] investigated the effects of prolonged smoking and smoking cessation on mortality amongst women in the UK. This study found that current smokers had 1.5 times the mortality rate from IPF compared to nonsmokers [42].

Studies investigating the impact of smoking on survival in people with IPF have reported mixed results. Early studies by TURNER-WARWICK et al. [2] and DE CREMOUX et al. [43] reported that smoking habit did not influence survival. Similarly, studies in the 1990s in the USA and UK have demonstrated that smoking habit was not associated with greater decline in lung function [44] or survival [28, 45] in IPF, but there was some evidence the increased pack-years of cigarette smoking was associated with greater longitudinal decline in gas transfer [44]. Since then, studies have suggested that people with IPF who were current smokers had a longer median survival compared to never- or former smokers [5]. These findings contrast with a more recent study that found improved survival in individuals with IPF who were nonsmokers, even after adjusting for disease severity [46], raising speculation that studies describing improved survival in current smokers with IPF may be due to the "healthy smoker" effect [47].

Environmental factors

Various environmental exposures have been linked to an increased risk of developing IPF. A small case–control study of environmental exposures in Nottingham, UK, demonstrated that people with CFA were more likely to have been exposed to metal dust or wood dust [48]. These associations were also present in a larger case–control study by HUBBARD et al. [38], which also showed that people with CFA were more likely to have been exposed to metal or wood dust, and estimated that the aetiological component that could be ascribed to the exposure was approximately 20%. Similarly, a case–control study in Japan found that people with IPF were more likely to have been metal production workers and miners [34], consistent with the findings of a more recent, hospital-based case–control study in Japan [35].

In the USA, a large case–control study of 248 cases of IPF and 491 controls found that occupational factors associated with IPF included farming, metal dust, stone cutting or polishing, and animal or vegetable dust [49]. Using mortality data from USA, PINHEIRO et al. [50] found that industry categories with exposures recognised to be risk factors for IPF were wood buildings and mobile homes, metal mining, and fabricating structural metal products. A recent meta-analysis of six occupational case–control studies concluded that exposures that were strongly associated with IPF were agriculture or farming (OR 1.65, 95% CI 1.20–2.26), livestock (OR 2.17, 95% CI 1.28–3.68), wood dust (OR 1.94, 95% CI 1.34–2.81), metal dust (OR 2.44, 95% CI 1.74–3.40) and stone or sand dust (OR 1.94, 95% CI 1.09–3.55) [36]. GUSTAFASON et al. [51] conducted an extensive postal questionnaire completed by 140 patients with IPF and 757 controls, and found that exposure to birch and hardwood dust were more common in people with IPF. Most recently, a study in Egypt found that amongst men, IPF was associated with occupations in chemical industries, carpentry and wood working, whilst an association between IPF and farming was found amongst women [52].

Gastro-oesophageal reflux

An increasing number of studies have suggested that GERD is more common in people with IPF than in the general population [53–56], raising the possibility that chronic reflux or microaspiration is a possible initiator and/or propagator of lung injury. The prevalence of abnormal gastro-oesophageal reflux is shown to be high in people with IPF [53, 54]; however, the majority of patients with IPF do not report symptoms of reflux [54, 57]. A study by Noth et al. [58] found that the presence of hiatus hernia on CT scans was more also common in people with IPF compared to individuals with other chronic lung diseases. Using routine primary care data, Gribbin et al. [55] demonstrated that cases with IPF were more likely to have a recorded diagnosis of GERD and prescription of antireflux medication than general-population controls before the diagnosis of IPF was established. In the USA, a retrospective review of medical records revealed that the use of gastro-oesophageal reflux medication was an independent predictor of increased survival [57]. More recently, pooled data from the placebo arms of three randomised controlled trials in IPF showed that reported use of antireflux medication at enrolment into the trial was associated with a slower decline in FVC and reduced frequency of acute exacerbations, but not with survival [59]. It still remains unclear whether poor lung compliance from IPF leads to raised intrathoracic pressures and subsequent reflux, or if IPF is the end result of chronic microaspiration from gastro-oesophageal reflux. Despite lack of robust evidence from randomised clinical trials, antireflux medication has been recommended in the updated American Thoracic Society/ European Respiratory Society clinical practice guidelines for treatment of IPF [60], based on a possible improvement in survival and the cost-effectiveness of treatment.

Diabetes mellitus

Another potential risk factor for IPF that has been investigated, with varying results, is diabetes mellitus. In a study of 65 Japanese patients with IPF and 184 hospital controls, Enomoto et al. [61] found that the odds of having diabetes were four times greater in people with IPF than controls. However, a case–control study also conducted in Japan found no association between diabetes and IPF [62]. Recent case–control studies using UK longitudinal computerised primary care data found an increased recorded diagnosis of diabetes and increased prescription of antidiabetic medications in people with IPF compared to the general population [55, 63], even after excluding individuals that had been prescribed corticosteroids [55]. A national Korean survey of patients with IPF found that 17.8% had co-existent diabetes mellitus, and patients with IPF and diabetes were more likely to have typical radiological features of UIP on HRCT [64]. Using electronic records from a large American health plan, Ehrlich et al. [65] showed that the age-adjusted incidence of pulmonary fibrosis was substantially higher in diabetics. More recently, a Danish study of 121 individuals with IPF found that 11% of the cohort had a co-existing diabetes mellitus and the presence of diabetes at enrolment into the study was associated with a 2.5-fold increased risk of death [66]. It needs to be noted that most studies investigating the association between IPF and diabetes mellitus were conducted when individuals with IPF were treated with corticosteroids and immunosuppressive drugs, which may be a potential confounder in the association seen.

Clotting dysfunction

Laboratory studies have shown ex vivo that fibrinolytic activity is suppressed within the lungs of people with IPF, resulting in deposition of fibrin in the interstitial and alveolar spaces [67]. Further evidence comes from studies that have demonstrated high levels of tissue factor in bronchoalveolar lavage fluid of people with IPF [68] and overexpression of plasminogen activator inhibitor-1 in type 2 pneumocytes that line the honeycomb lesions typical of IPF [69], both of which may result in increased local fibrin deposition. Fibrin is thought to influence tissue repair and promote fibrosis by acting in combination with fibronectin to produce a matrix augmented by collagen deposition derived from fibroblasts [70]. Furthermore, *in vivo* studies have demonstrated that the extent of bleomycin-induced pulmonary fibrosis in the most commonly used murine model of IPF is increased in mice genetically modified to decrease the activity of the serine protease plasmin, whilst the opposite effect occurs in mice with increased plasmin activity [71]. Patient studies and animal models in fibrotic lung disease also support the role of thrombin (which plays a central role in the final common pathway of the clotting cascade) in activating protease-activated receptor type 1 (PAR-1) found in lung tissue. Studies have demonstrated that PAR-1 is highly expressed in the lung parenchyma of people with IPF [72, 73], suggesting that this receptor plays an important role in the pathogenic process. Activation of PAR-1 receptors on alveolar epithelial cells leads to the induction and release of potent pro-inflammatory mediators [74], whilst activation of the same receptors on fibroblasts induces differentiation of fibroblasts to myofibroblasts [75] and promotes extracellular matrix protein production [76].

Using a large primary care database representative of the UK population, HUBBARD *et al.* [77] found that people with IPF were almost twice as likely to have had a venous-thromboembolic event (VTE) before a diagnosis of pulmonary fibrosis, and DALLEYWATER *et al.* [78] demonstrated that incidence rates of deep vein thrombosis and pulmonary emboli were higher in people with IPF. A study using data from a large Danish registry showed that individuals with a previous VTE were at increased risk of developing IIP [79] and this risk was highest in the subset of individuals with a VTE who had never received anticoagulation treatment [79]. A study using registered death certificates from the USA also demonstrated that risk of a VTE was substantially higher in individuals with IPF compared to general population controls, and individuals with COPD or lung cancer [80]. This study also found that people with pulmonary fibrosis and VTE died at a younger age than those with pulmonary fibrosis alone [80]. Further evidence that coagulation dysfunction plays an important part in the aetiology and natural history of IPF comes from a general-population case–control study in England and Wales, UK, which showed that incident cases of IPF were almost five times more likely to have one or more clotting defects present compared to the general population and abnormal clotting was associated with increased short-term mortality in people with IPF [40].

Anticoagulation with warfarin as a possible treatment option in IPF has been explored by two randomised clinical trials. A small clinical trial of anticoagulation with warfarin or heparin in Japan raised the possibility that anticoagulation treatment improved survival in IPF [81]. However, a larger randomised controlled trial of warfarin in IPF was terminated early due to excessive deaths in the participants receiving warfarin, which were not due to complications of anticoagulation [82]. Observational studies have demonstrated that people with IPF are more likely to be anticoagulated with warfarin for other indications [40, 77, 78] and a recent Danish study reported that people with IPF on anticoagulation for other indications had substantially higher mortality than those who were not anticoagulated [83].

Genetic predisposition

IPF usually occurs sporadically, although familial forms of IPF account for approximately 5% of cases [84]. IPF that occurs in two or more first-degree relatives is usually considered a familial form [25], and has clinical features and a natural history that are similar to nonfamilial IPF [85]. Among individuals with familial IPF, studies have suggested an association between telomerase-related genes, which shorten the length of telomeres [86, 87].

Genes associated with surfactant proteins have also been linked with familial IPF [88, 89]. More recently, a single-nucleotide polymorphism in the promoter region of a mucin gene (*MUC5B*) was found to be present in 38% of sporadic cases of IPF and 9% of controls [90]. However, among people with IPF, this polymorphism has been shown to improve survival [91]. Genome-wide association studies have identified polymorphisms in the Toll-interacting protein gene (*TOLLIP*) and signal peptide peptidase-like 2C gene (*SPPL2C*) [92]. An analysis of participants in the randomised trial of NAC for IPF revealed that individuals with the TT *TOLLIP* genotype responded favourably to treatment with NAC, whilst those with the CC *TOLLIP* genotype did not [93]. This raises the possibility that participants of future clinical trials should be stratified by genotype.

Comorbid illnesses in IPF

The most common cause of death in people with IPF is respiratory failure secondary to progression of their lung fibrosis. However, the incidence of comorbidities such as cardiovascular disease and lung cancer has been shown to be increased in people with IPF. The association between these comorbidities may be important in helping understand the pathogenesis of IPF, but more importantly, it highlights the need for a holistic approach to the care of these individuals. With the availability of new therapies for IPF that may improve survival [94], the burden of these comorbid illnesses on morbidity and mortality in people with IPF is likely to increase.

Cardiovascular disease

Numerous studies have demonstrated that cardiovascular comorbidities are strongly associated with IPF. Ischaemic heart disease was the most frequently observed comorbid illness, with prevalence estimates ranging from 3.2% for myocardial infarction identified from US insurance claims [95], 6% for recorded diagnosis of angina within UK primary care records [77], 21% in autopsy studies [96] and 65.8% in individuals with IPF being assessed for lung transplantation [97].

Within autopsy studies, PANOS *et al.* [96] suggested that ischaemic heart disease and heart failure were the underlying cause of deaths in almost one in four people with IPF. These estimates were similar to the autopsy findings on 42 people with IPF in the Mayo Clinic (Rochester, MN, USA) [98]. In a large, cross-sectional study of patients referred for lung transplantation evaluation, KIZER *et al.* [99] found an increased prevalence of angiographic coronary artery disease in patients with fibrotic lung diseases, which is similar to the findings of another study in lung transplant candidates that found that angiographic evidence of coronary artery disease was more common in people with lung fibrosis than those with COPD, despite the smoking prevalence being much higher in people with COPD [100]. The most recent study of 73 IPF and 56 COPD patients being assessed for lung transplantation found two-thirds of people with IPF had coronary artery disease, with more severe disease also being more common [97]. Studies have also shown that individuals with IPF and coronary artery disease also appeared to have a worse survival [66, 97]. More recently, studies have suggested that moderate-to-severe coronary artery calcification seen on standard-care HRCT is a strong predictor of ischaemic heart disease in people with IPF [101], and raises the possibility of screening for coronary heart disease as part of routine care in these patients.

Using primary-care data in the UK, HUBBARD *et al.* [77] demonstrated that people with IPF were almost twice as likely to have recorded diagnoses of either angina or acute coronary syndrome than the general population in the period before the diagnosis of IPF was made, and the risk of incident acute coronary syndrome events increased three-fold in people with IPF after the diagnosis of IPF was established. More recently, DALLEYWATER *et al.* [63] demonstrated that certain cardiovascular risk factors and prescription of medications commonly used to treat cardiovascular disease were higher in people with IPF than in the general population, and after controlling for these risk factors, IPF was independently associated with an increased risk of incident cardiovascular events.

Lung cancer

The association between IPF and lung cancer has also been studied with varying results [102–104]. A study from Japan in 99 patients with IPF showed that approximately a third also had lung cancer, with squamous cell carcinoma being the most common histological type. This study also found that smokers with IPF were at the greatest risk of developing lung cancer. AUBRY *et al.* [105] compared characteristics of 24 patients with biopsy-proven IPF with and without lung cancer. This study also found that squamous cell carcinoma was the most common histological type, with men, older patients and smokers being highest at risk of developing lung cancer [105]. Contrary to this, a study using multiple cause of death mortality data from the USA found that lung cancer occurred less frequently in people with lung fibrosis (4.8%) than in people with COPD (10.1%) or asbestosis (26.6%), or the general population (6.5%) [103]. Using primary-care data from the UK, HUBBARD *et al.* [104] and LE JEUNE *et al.* [106] found that the incidence of lung cancer was substantially higher in patients with pulmonary fibrosis than in general-population controls, independent of smoking habit. The British Thoracic Society study of cryptogenic fibrosing alveolitis and lung cancer concluded that despite evidence of an association between lung cancer and pulmonary fibrosis, the relationship was strongly confounded by smoking habit [107]. Within this cohort, individuals who died from lung cancer were predominantly male and ever-smokers [107]. Unsurprisingly, mortality in people with IPF and lung cancer has been shown to be significantly higher compared to those with IPF alone. A recent Italian study has suggested that median survival in people with IPF and lung cancer is reduced by approximately 2 years [108]. Despite this increased risk, it is unclear if individuals with IPF will benefit from lung cancer screening. Poor prognosis in terms of median survival coupled with increased risk of mortality following thoracic surgery, chemotherapy or radiotherapy also limits possible treatment options. It is possible, however, that lung cancer screening programmes could be used for early identification of individuals with IPF. A recent lung cancer screening trial found that 2.1% of participants had fibrotic interstitial lung changes at baseline and 37% of individuals with fibrotic interstitial changes had radiological progression after 2 years of follow-up [109]. With emerging evidence that pirfenidone [110] and nintedanib [111] are efficacious in people with IPF and preserved lung function, this increases support for earlier diagnosis and initiation of treatment.

Conclusion

In summary, the overall global trend suggests that the incidence of IPF is steadily increasing. Current estimates suggest that in the UK, 5000 new cases and 5000 deaths occur annually [15], whilst in Europe and the USA, up to 65 000 and 17 000 deaths, respectively, occur from

IPF each year [14]. In the USA, this approximates the mortality burden similar to that of renal cancer and lymphoma. The improvement in diagnosis and treatment has resulted in a decrease in annual mortality of these two malignancies over recent years compared to the paucity of treatment options and insidious increase in mortality associated with IPF. Although accurate figures are difficult to obtain, it is tempting to speculate that a lack of funding in IPF research may be partly responsible for the lack of progress. Although the underlying aetiology of IPF remains unclear, there has been considerable progress in identifying potential factors that are likely to be aetiologically important, and further research into improving our understanding of the causes and progression of IPF is vital to identify biomarkers and targets for future treatments.

References

1. Hamman L, Rich AR. Fulminating diffuse interstitial fibrosis of the lungs. *Trans Am Clin Climatol Assoc* 1935; 51: 154–163.
2. Turner-Warwick M, Burrows B, Johnson A. Cryptogenic fibrosing alveolitis: clinical features and their influence on survival. *Thorax* 1980; 35: 171–180.
3. Scadding JG. Chronic diffuse interstitial fibrosis of the lungs. *Br Med J* 1960; 1: 443–450.
4. Douglas WW, Ryu JH, Bjoraker JA, *et al.* Colchicine *versus* prednisone as treatment of usual interstitial pneumonia. *Mayo Clin Proc* 1997; 72: 201–209.
5. King TE Jr, Tooze JA, Schwarz MI, *et al.* Predicting survival in idiopathic pulmonary fibrosis: scoring system and survival model. *Am J Respir Crit Care Med* 2001; 164: 1171–1181.
6. Panos RJ, Mortenson RL, Niccoli SA Jr, *et al.* Clinical deterioration in patients with idiopathic pulmonary fibrosis: causes and assessment. *Am J Med* 1990; 88: 396–404.
7. Gribbin J, Hubbard RB, Le Jeune I, *et al.* Incidence and mortality of idiopathic pulmonary fibrosis and sarcoidosis in the UK. *Thorax* 2006; 61: 980–985.
8. Raghu G, Weycker D, Edelsberg J, *et al.* Incidence and prevalence of idiopathic pulmonary fibrosis. *Am J Respir Crit Care Med* 2006; 174: 810–816.
9. Coultas DB, Zumwalt RE, Black WC, *et al.* The epidemiology of interstitial lung diseases. *Am J Respir Crit Care Med* 1994; 150: 967–972.
10. Mannino DM, Etzel RA, Parrish RG. Pulmonary fibrosis deaths in the United States, 1979–1991. An analysis of multiple-cause mortality data. *Am J Respir Crit Care Med* 1996; 153: 1548–1552.
11. Raghu G, Chen SY, Yeh WS, *et al.* Idiopathic pulmonary fibrosis in US Medicare beneficiaries aged 65 years and older: incidence, prevalence, and survival, 2001–11. *Lancet Respir Med* 2014; 2: 566–572.
12. Johnston I, Britton J, Kinnear W, *et al.* Rising mortality from cryptogenic fibrosing alveolitis. *BMJ* 1990; 301: 1017–1021.
13. Hubbard R, Johnston I, Coultas DB, *et al.* Mortality rates from cryptogenic fibrosing alveolitis in seven countries. *Thorax* 1996; 51: 711–716.
14. Hutchinson JP, McKeever TM, Fogarty AW, *et al.* Increasing global mortality from idiopathic pulmonary fibrosis in the twenty-first century. *Ann Am Thorac Soc* 2014; 11: 1176–1185.
15. Navaratnam V, Fleming KM, West J, *et al.* The rising incidence of idiopathic pulmonary fibrosis in the U.K. *Thorax* 2011; 66: 462–467.
16. von Plessen C, Grinde O, Gulsvik A. Incidence and prevalence of cryptogenic fibrosing alveolitis in a Norwegian community. *Respir Med* 2003; 97: 428–435.
17. Ohno S, Nakaya T, Bando M, *et al.* Idiopathic pulmonary fibrosis – results from a Japanese nationwide epidemiological survey using individual clinical records. *Respirology* 2008; 13: 926–928.
18. Lai C-C, Wang C-Y, Lu H-M, *et al.* Idiopathic pulmonary fibrosis in Taiwan – a population-based study. *Respir Med* 2012; 106: 1566–1574.
19. Olson AL, Swigris JJ, Lezotte DC, *et al.* Mortality from pulmonary fibrosis increased in the United States from 1992 to 2003. *Am J Respir Crit Care Med* 2007; 176: 277–284.
20. Fernandez Perez ER, Daniels CE, Schroeder DR, *et al.* Incidence, prevalence, and clinical course of idiopathic pulmonary fibrosis: a population-based study. *Chest* 2010; 137: 129–137.
21. Esposito DB, Lanes S, Donneyong M, *et al.* Idiopathic pulmonary fibrosis in US automated claims. Incidence, prevalence and algorithm validation. *Am J Respir Crit Care Med* 2015; 192: 1200–1207.
22. Kornum JB, Christensen S, Grijota M, *et al.* The incidence of interstitial lung disease 1995-2005: a Danish nationwide population-based study. *BMC Pulm Med* 2008; 8: 24.

23. Hyldgaard C, Hilberg O, Muller A, *et al.* A cohort study of interstitial lung diseases in central Denmark. *Respir Med* 2014; 108: 793–799.

24. Agabiti N, Porretta MA, Bauleo L, *et al.* Idiopathic Pulmonary Fibrosis (IPF) incidence and prevalence in Italy. *Sarcoidosis Vasc Diffuse Lung Dis* 2014; 31: 191–197.

25. Raghu G, Collard HR, Egan JJ, *et al.* An official ATS/ERS/JRS/ALAT statement: idiopathic pulmonary fibrosis: evidence-based guidelines for diagnosis and management. *Am J Respir Crit Care Med* 2011; 183: 788–824.

26. Flaherty KR, Toews GB, Travis WD, *et al.* Clinical significance of histological classification of idiopathic interstitial pneumonia. *Eur Respir J* 2002; 19: 275–283.

27. King TE Jr, Schwarz MI, Brown K, *et al.* Idiopathic pulmonary fibrosis: relationship between histopathologic features and mortality. *Am J Respir Crit Care Med* 2001; 164: 1025–1032.

28. Hubbard R, Johnston I, Britton J. Survival in patients with cryptogenic fibrosing alveolitis: a population-based cohort study. *Chest* 1998; 113: 396–400.

29. du Bois RM, Weycker D, Albera C, *et al.* Ascertainment of individual risk of mortality for patients with idiopathic pulmonary fibrosis. *Am J Respir Crit Care Med* 2011; 184: 459–466.

30. Ley B, Collard HR. Risk prediction in idiopathic pulmonary fibrosis. *Am J Respir Crit Care Med* 2012; 185: 6–7.

31. Navaratnam V, Fleming KM, West J, *et al.* The rising incidence of idiopathic pulmonary fibrosis in the UK. *Thorax* 2011; 66: 462–467.

32. Ley B, Bradford WZ, Weycker D, *et al.* Unified baseline and longitudinal mortality prediction in idiopathic pulmonary fibrosis. *Eur Respir J* 2015; 45: 1374–1381.

33. Nathan SD, Shlobin OA, Weir N, *et al.* Long-term course and prognosis of idiopathic pulmonary fibrosis in the new millennium. *Chest* 2011; 140: 221–229.

34. Iwai K, Mori T, Yamada N, *et al.* Idiopathic pulmonary fibrosis. Epidemiologic approaches to occupational exposure. *Am J Respir Crit Care Med* 1994; 150: 670–675.

35. Miyake Y, Sasaki S, Yokoyama T, *et al.* Occupational and environmental factors and idiopathic pulmonary fibrosis in Japan. *Ann Occup Hyg* 2005; 49: 259–265.

36. Taskar VS, Coultas DB. Is idiopathic pulmonary fibrosis an environmental disease? *Proc Am Thorac Soc* 2006; 3: 293–298.

37. Garcia-Sancho Figueroa MC, Carrillo G, Perez-Padilla R, *et al.* Risk factors for idiopathic pulmonary fibrosis in a Mexican population. A case–control study. *Respir Med* 2010; 104: 305–309.

38. Hubbard R, Lewis S, Richards K, *et al.* Occupational exposure to metal or wood dust and aetiology of cryptogenic fibrosing alveolitis. *Lancet* 1996; 347: 284–289.

39. Baumgartner KB, Samet JM, Stidley CA, *et al.* Cigarette smoking: a risk factor for idiopathic pulmonary fibrosis. *Am J Respir Crit Care Med* 1997; 155: 242–248.

40. Navaratnam V, Fogarty AW, McKeever T, *et al.* Presence of a prothrombotic state in people with idiopathic pulmonary fibrosis: a population-based case-control study. *Thorax* 2014; 69: 207–215.

41. Ekstrom M, Gustafson T, Boman K, *et al.* Effects of smoking, gender and occupational exposure on the risk of severe pulmonary fibrosis: a population-based case-control study. *BMJ Open* 2014; 4: e004018.

42. Pirie K, Peto R, Reeves GK, *et al.* The 21st century hazards of smoking and benefits of stopping: a prospective study of one million women in the UK. *Lancet* 2013; 381: 133–141.

43. de Cremoux H, Bernaudin JF, Laurent P, *et al.* Interactions between cigarette smoking and the natural history of idiopathic pulmonary fibrosis. *Chest* 1990; 98: 71–76.

44. Schwartz DA, Van Fossen DS, Davis CS, *et al.* Determinants of progression in idiopathic pulmonary fibrosis. *Am J Respir Crit Care Med* 1994; 149: 444–449.

45. Schwartz DA, Helmers RA, Galvin JR, *et al.* Determinants of survival in idiopathic pulmonary fibrosis. *Am J Respir Crit Care Med* 1994; 149: 450–454.

46. Antoniou KM, Hansell DM, Rubens MB, *et al.* Idiopathic pulmonary fibrosis: outcome in relation to smoking status. *Am J Respir Crit Care Med* 2008; 177: 190–194.

47. Becklake MR, Lalloo U. The 'healthy smoker': a phenomenon of health selection? *Respiration* 1990; 57: 137–144.

48. Scott J, Johnston I, Britton J. What causes cryptogenic fibrosing alveolitis? A case-control study of environmental exposure to dust. *BMJ* 1990; 301: 1015–1017.

49. Baumgartner KB, Samet JM, Coultas DB, *et al.* Occupational and environmental risk factors for idiopathic pulmonary fibrosis: a multicenter case-control study. *Am J Epidemiol* 2000; 152: 307–315.

50. Pinheiro GA, Antao VC, Wood JM, *et al.* Occupational risks for idiopathic pulmonary fibrosis mortality in the United States. *Int J Occup Environ Health* 2008; 14: 117–123.

51. Gustafson T, Dahlman-Hoglund A, Nilsson K, *et al.* Occupational exposure and severe pulmonary fibrosis. *Respir Med* 2007; 101: 2207–2212.

52. Awadalla NJ, Hegazy A, Elmetwally RA, *et al.* Occupational and environmental risk factors for idiopathic pulmonary fibrosis in Egypt: a multicenter case-control study. *Int J Occup Environ Med* 2012; 3: 107–116.

53. Tobin RW, Pope CE II, Pellegrini CA, *et al.* Increased prevalence of gastroesophageal reflux in patients with idiopathic pulmonary fibrosis. *Am J Respir Crit Care Med* 1998; 158: 1804–1808.

54. Raghu G, Freudenberger TD, Yang S, *et al.* High prevalence of abnormal acid gastro-oesophageal reflux in idiopathic pulmonary fibrosis. *Eur Respir J* 2006; 27: 136–142.

55. Gribbin J, Hubbard R, Smith C. Role of diabetes mellitus and gastro-oesophageal reflux in the aetiology of idiopathic pulmonary fibrosis. *Respir Med* 2009; 103: 927–931.

56. Patti MG, Tedesco P, Golden J, *et al.* Idiopathic pulmonary fibrosis: how often is it really idiopathic? *J Gastrointest Surg* 2005; 9: 1053–1056.

57. Lee JS, Ryu JH, Elicker BM, *et al.* Gastroesophageal reflux therapy is associated with longer survival in patients with idiopathic pulmonary fibrosis. *Am J Respir Crit Care Med* 2011; 184: 1390–1394.

58. Noth I, Zangan SM, Soares RV, *et al.* Prevalence of hiatal hernia by blinded multidetector CT in patients with idiopathic pulmonary fibrosis. *Eur Respir J* 2012; 39: 344–351.

59. Lee JS, Collard HR, Anstrom KJ, *et al.* Anti-acid treatment and disease progression in idiopathic pulmonary fibrosis: an analysis of data from three randomised controlled trials. *Lancet Respir Med* 2013; 1: 369–376.

60. Raghu G, Rochwerg B, Zhang Y, *et al.* An Official ATS/ERS/JRS/ALAT Clinical Practice Guideline: Treatment of Idiopathic Pulmonary Fibrosis. An Update of the 2011 Clinical Practice Guideline. *Am J Respir Crit Care Med* 2015; 192: e3–19.

61. Enomoto T, Usuki J, Azuma A, *et al.* Diabetes mellitus may increase risk for idiopathic pulmonary fibrosis. *Chest* 2003; 123: 2007–2011.

62. Miyake Y, Sasaki S, Yokoyama T, *et al.* Case-control study of medical history and idiopathic pulmonary fibrosis in Japan. *Respirology* 2005; 10: 504–509.

63. Dalleywater W, Powell HA, Hubbard RB, *et al.* Risk factors for cardiovascular disease in people with idiopathic pulmonary fibrosis: a population-based study. *Chest* 2015; 147: 150–156.

64. Kim YJ, Park JW, Kyung SY, *et al.* Clinical characteristics of idiopathic pulmonary fibrosis patients with diabetes mellitus: the national survey in Korea from 2003 to 2007. *J Korean Med Sci* 2012; 27: 756–760.

65. Ehrlich SF, Quesenberry CP, Van Den Eeden SK, *et al.* Patients diagnosed with diabetes are at increased risk for asthma, chronic obstructive pulmonary disease, pulmonary fibrosis, and pneumonia but not lung cancer. *Diabetes Care* 2010; 33: 55–60.

66. Hyldgaard C, Hilberg O, Bendstrup E. How does comorbidity influence survival in idiopathic pulmonary fibrosis? *Respir Med* 2014; 108: 647–653.

67. Chapman HA, Allen CL, Stone OL. Abnormalities in pathways of alveolar fibrin turnover among patients with interstitial lung disease. *Am Rev Respir Dis* 1986; 133: 437–443.

68. Kotani I, Sato A, Hayakawa H, *et al.* Increased procoagulant and antifibrinolytic activities in the lungs with idiopathic pulmonary fibrosis. *Thromb Res* 1995; 77: 493–504.

69. Senoo T, Hattori N, Tanimoto T, *et al.* Suppression of plasminogen activator inhibitor-1 by RNA interference attenuates pulmonary fibrosis. *Thorax* 2010; 65: 334–340.

70. Howell DC, Laurent GJ, Chambers RC. Role of thrombin and its major cellular receptor, protease-activated receptor-1, in pulmonary fibrosis. *Biochem Soc Trans* 2002; 30: 211–216.

71. Chambers RC. Role of coagulation cascade proteases in lung repair and fibrosis. *Eur Respir J* 2003; 22: Suppl. 44, 33s–35s.

72. Howell DC, Goldsack NR, Marshall RP, *et al.* Direct thrombin inhibition reduces lung collagen, accumulation, and connective tissue growth factor mRNA levels in bleomycin-induced pulmonary fibrosis. *Am J Pathol* 2001; 159: 1383–1395.

73. Mercer PF, Johns RH, Scotton CJ, *et al.* Pulmonary epithelium is a prominent source of proteinase-activated receptor-1-inducible CCL2 in pulmonary fibrosis. *Am J Respir Crit Care Med* 2009; 179: 414–425.

74. Chambers RC. Abnormal wound healing responses in pulmonary fibrosis: focus on coagulation signalling. *Eur Respir Rev* 2008; 17: 130–137.

75. Bogatkevich GS, Gustilo E, Oates JC, *et al.* Distinct PKC isoforms mediate cell survival and DNA synthesis in thrombin-induced myofibroblasts. *Am J Physiol Lung Cell Mol Physiol* 2005; 288: L190–L201.

76. Chambers RC, Dabbagh K, McAnulty RJ, *et al.* Thrombin stimulates fibroblast procollagen production via proteolytic activation of protease-activated receptor 1. *Biochem J* 1998; 333: 121–127.

77. Hubbard RB, Smith C, Le Jeune I, *et al.* The association between idiopathic pulmonary fibrosis and vascular disease: a population-based study. *Am J Respir Crit Care Med* 2008; 178: 1257–1261.

78. Dalleywater W, Powell HA, Fogarty AW, *et al.* Venous thromboembolism in people with idiopathic pulmonary fibrosis: a population-based study. *Eur Respir J* 2014; 44: 1714–1715.

79. Sode BF, Dahl M, Nielsen SF, *et al.* Venous thromboembolism and risk of idiopathic interstitial pneumonia: a nationwide study. *Am J Respir Crit Care Med* 2010; 181: 1085–1092.

80. Sprunger DB, Olson AL, Huie TJ, *et al.* Pulmonary fibrosis is associated with an elevated risk of thromboembolic disease. *Eur Respir J* 2012; 39: 125–132.

81. Kubo H, Nakayama K, Yanai M, *et al.* Anticoagulant therapy for idiopathic pulmonary fibrosis. *Chest* 2005; 128: 1475–1482.

82. Noth I, Anstrom KJ, Calvert SB, *et al.* A placebo-controlled randomized trial of warfarin in idiopathic pulmonary fibrosis. *Am J Respir Crit Care Med* 2012; 186: 88–95.

83. Hyldgaard C, Hilberg O, Bendstrup E. How does comorbidity influence survival in idiopathic pulmonary fibrosis? *Respir Med* 2014; 108: 647–653.

84. Marshall RP, Puddicombe A, Cookson WO, *et al.* Adult familial cryptogenic fibrosing alveolitis in the United Kingdom. *Thorax* 2000; 55: 143–146.

85. Lee HL, Ryu JH, Wittmer MH, *et al.* Familial idiopathic pulmonary fibrosis: clinical features and outcome. *Chest* 2005; 127: 2034–2041.

86. Mushiroda T, Wattanapokayakit S, Takahashi A, *et al.* A genome-wide association study identifies an association of a common variant in TERT with susceptibility to idiopathic pulmonary fibrosis. *J Med Genet* 2008; 45: 654–656.

87. Armanios MY, Chen JJ, Cogan JD, *et al.* Telomerase mutations in families with idiopathic pulmonary fibrosis. *N Engl J Med* 2007; 356: 1317–1326.

88. Thomas AQ, Lane K, Phillips J III, *et al.* Heterozygosity for a surfactant protein C gene mutation associated with usual interstitial pneumonitis and cellular nonspecific interstitial pneumonitis in one kindred. *Am J Respir Crit Care Med* 2002; 165: 1322–1328.

89. van Moorsel CH, van Oosterhout MF, Barlo NP, *et al.* Surfactant protein C mutations are the basis of a significant portion of adult familial pulmonary fibrosis in a dutch cohort. *Am J Respir Crit Care Med* 2010; 182: 1419–1425.

90. Seibold MA, Wise AL, Speer MC, *et al.* A common *MUC5B* promoter polymorphism and pulmonary fibrosis. *N Engl J Med* 2011; 364: 1503–1512.

91. Peljto AL, Zhang Y, Fingerlin TE, *et al.* Association between the *MUC5B* promoter polymorphism and survival in patients with idiopathic pulmonary fibrosis. *JAMA* 2013; 309: 2232–2239.

92. Noth I, Zhang Y, Ma SF, *et al.* Genetic variants associated with idiopathic pulmonary fibrosis susceptibility and mortality: a genome-wide association study. *Lancet Respir Med* 2013; 1: 309–317.

93. Oldham JM, Ma SF, Martinez FJ, *et al.* TOLLIP, MUC5B and the response to *N*-acetylcysteine among individuals with idiopathic pulmonary fibrosis. *Am J Respir Crit Care Med* 2015; 192: 1475–1482.

94. King TE Jr, Bradford WZ, Castro-Bernardini S, *et al.* A phase 3 trial of pirfenidone in patients with idiopathic pulmonary fibrosis. *N Engl J Med* 2014; 370: 2083–2092.

95. Collard HR, Ward AJ, Lanes S, *et al.* Burden of illness in idiopathic pulmonary fibrosis. *J Med Econ* 2012; 15: 829–835.

96. Panos RJ, Mortenson RL, Niccoli SA, *et al.* Clinical deterioration in patients with idiopathic pulmonary fibrosis: causes and assessment. *Am J Med* 1990; 88: 396–404.

97. Nathan SD, Basavaraj A, Reichner C, *et al.* Prevalence and impact of coronary artery disease in idiopathic pulmonary fibrosis. *Respir Med* 2010; 104: 1035–1041.

98. Daniels CE, Yi ES, Ryu JH. Autopsy findings in 42 consecutive patients with idiopathic pulmonary fibrosis. *Eur Respir J* 2008; 32: 170–174.

99. Kizer JR, Zisman DA, Blumenthal NP, *et al.* Association between pulmonary fibrosis and coronary artery disease. *Arch Intern Med* 2004; 164: 551–556.

100. Izbicki G, Ben-Dor I, Shitrit D, *et al.* The prevalence of coronary artery disease in end-stage pulmonary disease: is pulmonary fibrosis a risk factor? *Respir Med* 2009; 103: 1346–1349.

101. Nathan SD, Weir N, Shlobin OA, *et al.* The value of computed tomography scanning for the detection of coronary artery disease in patients with idiopathic pulmonary fibrosis. *Respirology* 2011; 16: 481–486.

102. Turner-Warwick M, Lebowitz M, Burrows B, *et al.* Cryptogenic fibrosing alveolitis and lung cancer. *Thorax* 1980; 35: 496–499.

103. Wells C, Mannino DM. Pulmonary fibrosis and lung cancer in the United States: analysis of the multiple cause of death mortality data, 1979 through 1991. *South Med J* 1996; 89: 505–510.

104. Hubbard R, Venn A, Lewis S, *et al.* Lung cancer and cryptogenic fibrosing alveolitis. A population-based cohort study. *Am J Respir Crit Care Med* 2000; 161: 5–8.

105. Aubry MC, Myers JL, Douglas WW, *et al.* Primary pulmonary carcinoma in patients with idiopathic pulmonary fibrosis. *Mayo Clin Proc* 2002; 77: 763–770.

106. Le Jeune I, Gribbin J, West J, *et al.* The incidence of cancer in patients with idiopathic pulmonary fibrosis and sarcoidosis in the UK. *Respir Med* 2007; 101: 2534–2540.

107. Harris JM, Johnston ID, Rudd R, *et al.* Cryptogenic fibrosing alveolitis and lung cancer: the BTS study. *Thorax* 2010; 65: 70–76.

108. Tomassetti S, Gurioli C, Ryu JH, *et al.* The impact of lung cancer on survival of idiopathic pulmonary fibrosis. *Chest* 2015; 147: 157–164.

109. Jin GY, Lynch D, Chawla A, *et al.* Interstitial lung abnormalities in a CT lung cancer screening population: prevalence and progression rate. *Radiology* 2013; 268: 563–571.

110. Noble P, Albera C, Bradford W, *et al.* Safety of pirfenidone in patients with idiopathic pulmonary fibrosis (IPF): integrated analysis of cumulative data from 5 clinical trials. *Thorax* 2015; 70: Suppl. 3, A80–A81.

111. Costabel U, Inoue Y, Richeldi L, *et al.* Efficacy of nintedanib in idiopathic pulmonary fibrosis across prespecified subgroups in INPULSIS. *Am J Respir Crit Care Med* 2015; 193: 178–185.

Support statement: V. Navaratnam is funded by a UK National Institute for Health Research Academic Clinical Fellowship. D.L. Forrester is funded by a Wellcome Trust Clinical Training Fellowship (grant number WT088614). R.B. Hubbard is the GlaxoSmithKline/British Lung Foundation Chair of Epidemiological Respiratory Research.

Disclosures: None declared

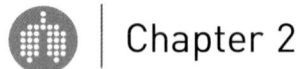

Chapter 2

Genetics

Raphael Borie[1], Caroline Kannengiesser[2,3], Nadia Nathan[4,5] and Bruno Crestani[1,3]

The occurrence of pulmonary fibrosis in numerous individuals from the same family suggests a genetic cause for the disease. During the last 10 years, mutations involving proteins from the telomerase complex and from the surfactant system have been identified in association with pulmonary fibrosis. Mutations of *TERT*, the gene encoding the telomerase reverse transcriptase, are the most frequently identified and are present in 15% of cases of familial pulmonary fibrosis. More recently, mutations in *RTEL1* and *PARN* have each been described in 5–10% of cases. Other mutations (*TERC*, surfactant proteins genes) are only rarely found in adults. Patients with mutations involving the telomerase complex may present with pulmonary fibrosis or haematological, cutaneous or hepatic diseases. Rare syndromes including pulmonary fibrosis have recently been characterised on a genetic level involving original pathways. Evidence for mutations associated with the development of pulmonary fibrosis raises numerous clinical questions, from establishing a diagnosis and providing counselling to deciding on therapy, and requires specific studies. Other genetic variations, such as a polymorphism in the promoter of *MUC5B*, have also been described in pulmonary fibrosis, and may be considered to be part of a polygenic transmission. From a pathophysiological point of view, the function of the genes involved highlights the central role of alveolar epithelium and ageing in fibrogenesis.

The pathophysiology of pulmonary fibrosis is incompletely understood. However, there is now a consensus that pulmonary fibrosis development could be linked to three principal factors: 1) a genetic predisposition; 2) repeated pulmonary injury in relation, for example, to environmental exposures; and 3) a time factor that explains why pulmonary fibrosis most often develops in older adults. These different factors can be of variable importance depending on the patient.

In contrast to sporadic pulmonary fibrosis, familial pulmonary fibrosis is defined by the presence of at least two cases of pulmonary fibrosis, either idiopathic or nonidiopathic, in a first-degree family member [1].

Genetic variants are distinguished by their overall frequency and their overall effect size. In general, common variants have small effect sizes and rare variants have larger effect sizes

[1]Service de Pneumologie A, Centre de Compétences Maladies Rares Pulmonaires, Hôpital Bichat, APHP, INSERM, Unité 1152, Paris, France. [2]Service de Génétique, Hôpital Bichat, APHP, Paris, France. [3]Université Paris Diderot, Sorbonne Paris Cité, Paris, France. [4]Service de Pneumologie Pédiatrique, Hôpital Armand Trousseau, APHP, Centre National de Référence des Maladies Respiratoires Rares, Paris, France. [5]INSERM UMRS933, Université Pierre et Marie Curie (Paris 6), Sorbonne Universités, Paris, France.

Correspondence: Bruno Crestani, Service de Pneumologie, Hôpital Bichat, 46 Rue Henri Huchard, Paris, 75018, France. E-mail: bruno.crestani@aphp.fr

ERS Monogr 2016; 71: 16–34. DOI: 10.1183/2312508X.10004715

(figure 1). Single-nucleotide polymorphisms are DNA sequence variations occurring commonly within a population (*e.g.* in 1%) in which a single nucleotide differs. Rare variants are much less common and can be so rare that they have never been found in any other individual. An example of a common variant with clinical significance is the Factor V Leiden polymorphism (R506Q, rs6025) with an allele frequency of 2.2%, which gives rise to an increased risk of thrombosis. In contrast, in cystic fibrosis, the *CFTR* G551D mutation (rs75527207) is rare, with an allele frequency of <0.1% [2].

The main genetic diseases associated with pulmonary fibrosis are presented in table 1. This chapter will present the common characteristics of the familial forms of pulmonary fibrosis, and pulmonary fibrosis in which mutation of a major gene is implicated will then be specifically considered: the telomerase complex ("telomere syndrome"), surfactant proteins and rare syndromes characterised on a genetic level. Finally, we will discuss polymorphisms, and genetic diagnosis and counselling.

General characteristics of familial pulmonary fibrosis

Epidemiology and risk factors

Whereas the prevalence of IPF is estimated to be 1 in 5000, the prevalence of ILD in a first-degree relative of a patient with IPF is 2–20%, indicating a familial linkage of cases [3–6]. The pedigree indicates an autosomal dominant transmission in 80% of cases, with the presence of cases in several successive generations (vertical transmission) without known consanguinity [1]. In a case–control Mexican study, the presence of a family history of pulmonary fibrosis was the most important risk factor for IPF with an OR of 6.1 (95% CI 2.3–15.9) [6]. There is also an increased risk of death with pulmonary fibrosis in first-degree (relative risk 4.7) and second-degree (relative risk 1.92) relatives [7]. Interestingly, there is also

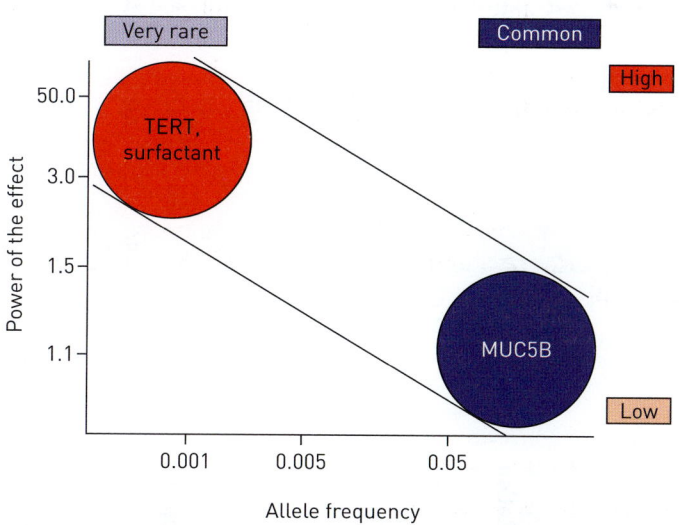

Figure 1. Significance of the principal genetic variants associated with familial fibrosis according to their strength and frequency. For example, *TERT* mutations are rare but have a powerful effect with great penetrance. In contrast, the polymorphism of the *MUC5B* promoter is frequent but with a weaker effect. Reproduced and modified from [113, 114] with permission from the publisher.

Table 1. Main genes associated with pulmonary fibrosis

Function	Gene	Transmission	Age of onset of pulmonary manifestation	Associated signs
Telomerase	TERT, TERC	AD	Adults, average 55 years	Telomere syndrome, CPFE
	TINF2	AD	Children; rarely in adults <50 years	Telomere syndrome
	DKC1	X	Children; rarely in adults <50 years	Telomere syndrome
Helicase	RTEL1	AD	Adults 35–60 years	Telomere syndrome? (to be confirmed)
mRNA regulation	PARN	AD	Adults 47–81 years	Pulmonary granulomatosis, telomere syndrome? (to be confirmed) [25]
Surfactant	SFTPA2	AD	Adults 35–72 years	Lung cancer
	SFTPB	AR	Newborn	
	SFTPC	AD	Children; rarely in adults <50 years	CPFE
	ABCA3	AR	Children; rarely in adults <50 years	CPFE
	NKX-2.1 (TITF1)	AD	Children; rarely in adults <50 years	Chorea, hypothyroidism [92]
Tumour suppressor	NF-1	AD	Adults	Type 1 neurofibromatosis [115]
Lysosome	HPS-1-8/AP-3B1	AR	Adults	Hermansky-Pudlak syndrome [88]
Stimulation of interferon synthesis	TMEM173	AD	Children; rarely in adults <50 years	Recurrent fever, alopecia, skin rash, antinuclear antibodies, vasculitis [93, 94]
Endoplasmic reticulum stress	COPA	AD	Children; rarely in adults <25 years	Arthritis, antinuclear antibodies and antineutrophil cytoplasmic antibodies [95]
Unknown	FAM111B	AD	7–30 years	Myopathy, poikiloderma [96]
Mucin	MUC5B	Polymorphism	Adults >50 years	[63]

AD: autosomal dominant; X: X-linked; AR: autosomal recessive.

an increased risk of developing hypersensitivity pneumonitis (HP) in the same family. In a retrospective Japanese study involving 114 patients with chronic HP, 17.5% of them gave a family history of pulmonary fibrosis [8]. Genetic factors could explain such a clustering of cases, associated with common environmental factors. Thus, familial fibrosis is not always idiopathic. One should not exclude a possible diagnosis of a monogenic form of pulmonary fibrosis in nonidiopathic conditions.

Two series of familial pulmonary fibrosis have revealed that, in these families, the presence of ILD was more frequent in men (55% in the ILD group *versus* 37% in the group without ILD), in smokers (45–67 in smokers *versus* 34% in nonsmokers) and in older subjects (mean age 68 years in patients with ILD *versus* 53 years without ILD) [1]. Autoimmunity is possible in familial fibrosis. In a small series, antinuclear antibodies were found in seven out of 16 (44%) patients and rheumatoid factors in five out of 15 (33%) patients after exclusion of definite connective tissue disorders [9].

Radiographic pattern

In a retrospective series of 309 patients from 111 families, all presenting with familial ILD, chest CT evoked a UIP pattern in 80% of the cases, an NSIP pattern in 6.4% of the cases and, more rarely, an organising pneumonia pattern in 1% of cases. In 12% of the cases, the CT pattern was unclassifiable [1]. However, in a recent series of 289 patients, CT could be classified in approximately half of the cases only, the predominant aspects being UIP (22%) and NSIP (12%). An HP pattern (6%) or an organising pneumonia (2%) pattern was much rarer [10].

Pathological pattern

Pathologically, UIP is the most frequent pattern described in familial fibrosis: 11 out of 21 cases in one series [10]. A pattern of NSIP, HP or organising pneumonia may be observed. However, in a series of 30 biopsies re-evaluated by three pathologists, the histological pattern was considered as unclassifiable in 17 out of 30 cases, while a UIP pattern was observed in 25–50% of the cases [11].

Evolution

Familial pulmonary fibrosis may be diagnosed earlier than sporadic pulmonary fibrosis [12]. Mean survival after diagnosis in patients with familial IPF did not appear to be different from that of sporadic IPF [9]. However, the main limiting factor of these series was the absence of a correlation with genetic analysis. In most series, the evolution of familial pulmonary fibrosis is comparable to that of the sporadic forms, with age and the causes of death being similar to those observed in the sporadic forms [9, 12, 13]. As observed in sporadic pulmonary fibrosis, a definite UIP pattern, on CT or on lung biopsy, is associated with a poorer prognosis in familial pulmonary fibrosis [1, 11]. However, although specific genetic abnormalities could influence prognosis, genetic testing was not known in these cohorts. Indeed, the presence of one polymorphism in the promoter of *MUC5B* increases the risk of IPF but is associated with better survival, and the presence of one polymorphism in *TOLLIP*, encoding the Toll-interacting protein, could be associated with the response to NAC [14–16].

Asymptomatic involvement

Systematic chest HRCT in asymptomatic members of families with familial pulmonary fibrosis has revealed asymptomatic ILD in 14–25% [1, 17, 18]. The most commonly observed anomalies were: thickening of septal lines, peribronchovascular thickening, reticular opacities and ground-glass opacities.

KROPSKI et al. [17] performed chest CT on 75 asymptomatic first-degree relatives of familial pulmonary fibrosis patients. At a mean age of 50.8 years, 11 (14.7%) relatives had evidence of early ILD: interlobular reticular opacities (n=11, 14.7%), irregular septal thickening (n=9, 12%), ground-glass opacities (n=3, 4%), traction bronchiectasis (n=2, 2.6%) or honeycombing (n=1, 1.3%). Whereas BAL was reported previously to show an increased lymphocyte percentage (mean±SD 13±2%) [18], no differences were detected in BAL cell counts compared with normal control subjects [17]. Transbronchial biopsies, performed in 71 subjects, were abnormal in 26 (36.6%) and showed: interstitial fibrosis (n=12, 16.9%), peribronchiolar fibrosis (n=15, 21.1%), chronic inflammation (n=10, 14.1%), respiratory bronchiolitis (n=2, 2.8%) or granulomas (n=6, 8.5%).

PFTs most often show normal results in relatives and should not be used as a screening tool owing to the low sensitivity of the procedures [17, 18].

Description of familial pulmonary fibrosis according to underlying genetic abnormalities

Telomerase complex mutations

Genetic mutations
The telomerase complex catalyses the addition of repeated DNA sequences in the telomere region, thereby protecting the chromosomes from loss of material during mitoses [19]. The activity of the telomerase complex requires the activity of several proteins, including telomerase reverse transcriptase (encoded by the *TERT* gene), dyskerin (encoded by *DKC1*) and the telomere binding protein TIN2 (encoded by *TINF2*), interacting with the telomerase repeat binding factor (TERF1) and the telomerase RNA component (TERC, encoded by *TERC*, also known as *TR*), a specialised RNA that contains a template for telomere repeat addition [19]. More recently, besides the telomerase complex, other proteins, such as a helicase called RTEL1 and a ribonuclease called PARN, have been implicated in telomere maintenance [20].

Heterozygous *TERT* mutations have been detected in approximately 15% of the cases of the familial forms of IPF, whereas heterozygous *TERC* mutations are rarer in IPF [12, 14]. *TERT* or *TERC* mutations are found in about 1–3% of sporadic IPF cases [14]. There is no frequent *TERT* mutation, and over 70 different *TERT* mutations have already been described (http://telomerase.asu.edu/diseases.html#tr). Most *TERT* mutations are missense variations and are considered pathogenic according to different arguments, such as absence or very low frequency in the variant databases, and conservation of the affected amino acid. It is sometimes difficult to conclude on the pathogenicity of certain missense variants and on the causality of these variants in the phenotype observed in the absence of *in vitro* functional tests.

Mutations in *DKC1* and *TINF2* have been described recently in association with pulmonary fibrosis [21–23]. Mutations in *TINF2* are usually described in children with severe diseases. However, somatic reversion leads to a partial loss of the germline mutation, a situation that could explain a "milder" phenotype in patients with IPF compared with "classical" patients with *TINF2* mutations [22–24].

Very recently, two other genes involved in the maintenance of telomeres have been associated with familial pulmonary fibrosis and will be described individually in later sections. Heterozygous mutations of *RTEL1* were evidenced in 5–11% of the families and heterozygous mutations of *PARN* in 6%, after exclusion of *TERT* and *TERC* mutations [25–27].

Pulmonary involvement

In an American cohort of 134 patients from 21 families with *TERT* mutations, the presence of ILD was associated with increased age [14]. Under 40 years of age, none of the mutated patients presented ILD compared with >60% over the age of 60 years. The mean age of patients with ILD was 57 years, about 10 years younger than that of patients with sporadic IPF. The male/female ratio of patients with ILD was 1.5, and men were younger (54 years) than women (63 years) at ILD diagnosis. Almost all (96%) of the patients with ILD were smokers or declared having a pneumotoxic exposure.

PFTs showed a restrictive pattern in 87% of the cases and the D_{LCO} was always decreased [14]. A typical UIP pattern was detected on chest CT in 74% of the cases and a possible UIP pattern in 13% (figure 2). Unusual features were observed in 13% of the cases, such as honeycomb lesions with an upper lung predominance, or centrolobular fibrosis. Mediastinal adenomegaly was observed in 38% of the cases [14].

TERT mutations have been associated with CPFE and with familial emphysema in female smokers [28]. In a recent study, three patients with *TERT* mutations were found in a cohort of 292 patients (1%) with severe COPD [29]. All three mutation carriers were female smokers with a mean age of 48 years at diagnosis, and only one had additional ILD. The authors further reviewed their cohort of 50 "telomere syndrome" patients with lung disease. Only 11 (22%) patients were smokers, and four (14%) patients presented emphysema, including five (10%) patients with ILD. The authors suggested that emphysema could manifest predominantly in females and could be associated with an increased risk of pneumothorax.

The presence of hypoxaemia despite no or little parenchymal disease should lead to a suspicion of hepatopulmonary syndrome (see later section on Liver involvement) [30].

Lung biopsy has been reported in a series of 29 patients [14]. All of the patients with possible or typical UIP pattern on chest CT were considered as having UIP on pathological examination. Atypical features could nevertheless be observed: the presence of inflammation in fibrotic zones (35% of cases) or non-necrotising granulomas (17% of cases). In four cases, the pattern was considered as unclassifiable pulmonary fibrosis [14].

Pulmonary fibrosis associated with *TERT* mutations is a lethal disease with a mean survival of 3 years after diagnosis [11]. The mean age at death was 57.7 years for men and 66.6 years for women. All of the patients died of respiratory causes. However, the evolution can be longer and a >30-year evolution was also described in two sisters [31].

There is no specific treatment for pulmonary fibrosis associated with *TERT* mutations and no specific guidelines. The usual recommendations for treatment of lung fibrosis should be used [32].

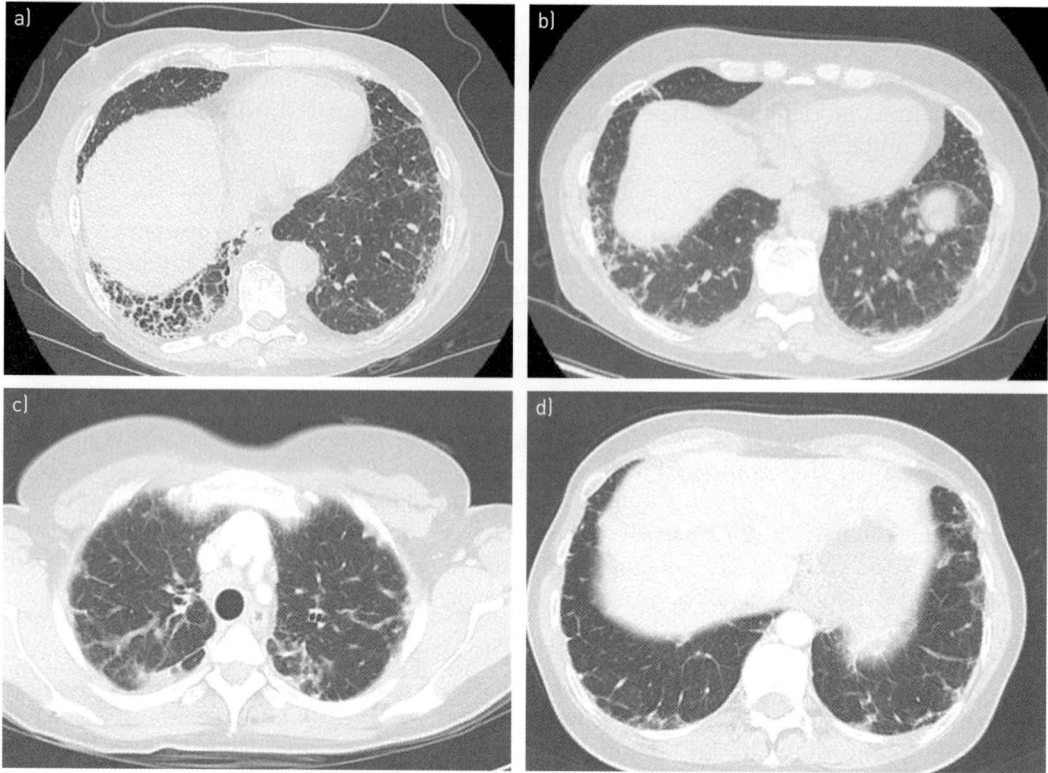

Figure 2. Representative CT scans of patients with *TERT* mutations showing a) a UIP pattern, b) a possible UIP pattern, and c and d) an inconsistent UIP pattern.

Given the young age of most of the patients, lung transplantation is often discussed. Three retrospective series recently reported the outcome of lung transplantation in patients with *TERT* or *TERC* mutations, with 26 patients mainly from France and the USA [33–35]. Almost all of the patients required an adjustment of immunosuppression. Thrombocytopenia and the need for platelet transfusion were frequent, and some patients developed myelodysplastic syndrome and/or bone marrow failure. The need for dialysis appeared to be unexpectedly high, ranging 0–50% according to each series [33]. The prevalence of infections and acute/chronic rejections did not seem to differ from historical data, but there was no control group. Unexpected elevated liver enzymes were not reported in any of these series.

Some groups suggest performing bone marrow biopsy in the evaluation before lung transplantation and adapting immunosuppression for selected patients [36]. Our current recommendation is to postpone lung transplantation in patients with established bone marrow diseases. Treatment of these patients must, in any event, be performed by a specialised team with genetic expertise.

Extrapulmonary manifestations

TERT or *TERC* mutations can be associated with certain extrarespiratory disorders that, when present in a patient with ILD or with ILD in his/her family, indicate a telomere syndrome and should prompt a search for these mutations.

Mucocutaneous involvement
Mutations in telomerase enzyme components were first identified in a rare syndrome called dyskeratosis congenita (DKC). DKC is classically defined based on a triad of mucocutaneous manifestations: reticular skin pigmentation, nail dystrophy and oral mucosal leukoplakia. The triad is present in childhood, and bone marrow failure appears between the age of 10 and 20 years. These patients develop severe pulmonary complications after haematopoietic stem-cell transplantation [37].

The classic triad of DKC is usually absent in patients with *TERT* mutations and IPF. However, in a cohort of subjects who were asymptomatic *TERT* mutation carriers, 40% presented early hair greying (before 30 years of age) compared with 5% in family members who were noncarriers [38]. Hair loss did not appear to be more frequent or to occur earlier.

Haematological involvement
TERT and *TERC* mutations have been described in patients with bone marrow failure, myelodysplasia or acute leukaemia in the absence of DKC signs [39–41]. The coexistence of pulmonary fibrosis and bone marrow failure in a given individual or in a family with autosomal dominant transmission is highly suggestive of telomerase complex mutation [42].

Anaemia without other details was described in 13% of cases in a cohort of 134 patients with *TERT* mutations [14]. In asymptomatic relatives, the presence of a *TERT* mutation was associated with an increased mean±SD globular volume (97±4 *versus* 90±5 fL) and a slightly lower platelet count ($209 \times 10^9 \pm 56 \times 10^9 \cdot L^{-1}$ *versus* $237 \times 10^9 \pm 57 \times 10^9 \cdot L^{-1}$) when compared with relatives without mutations [38]. In a French cohort of 43 probands with ILD and carriers of *TERT* or *TERC* mutations, 41.8% presented macrocytosis at diagnosis and 48.8% thrombocytopenia [43].

Liver involvement
Patients presenting a *TERT* or *TERC* mutation can also present with liver cirrhosis, which may be cryptogenic, viral or alcoholic. In a series of 134 patients with liver cirrhosis, nine (7%) presented a *TERT* mutation and one (1%) had a *TERC* mutation [44]. All 10 patients were considered to have secondary cirrhosis, due to hepatitis C (n=4), alcohol (n=3), Wilson's disease (n=1), nonalcoholic steatohepatitis (n=1) or primary biliary cirrhosis (n=1).

The presence of a mutation increases the risk of developing cirrhosis in the case of hepatitis C virus infection even where there is equivalent consumption of alcohol [45, 46]. Overall, 5–8% of patients with a *TERT* mutation present increased liver enzymes [14]. Patients with the same mutation, even in the same family, may present normal or elevated liver enzymes with variable degrees of necrosis, inflammation, fibrosis and regeneration on liver histology [45].

GORGY *et al.* [30] highlighted the high frequency of hepatopulmonary syndrome associated with telomerase complex mutation. In a retrospective series of 42 patients with dyspnoea and complex telomerase mutation, they identified nine patients with minimal or absent ILD. All nine patients presented hepatopulmonary syndrome, defined as liver disease associated with evidence of intrapulmonary vascular dilatation resulting in pulmonary gas exchange abnormalities and hypoxaemia. Genetic analysis showed mutations in *TERT* (n=4), *RTEL1* (n=1) or *DKC1* (n=1), but mutations were not found for three patients, despite a typical DKC phenotype. Among the six patients with available liver biopsy, the most common abnormality was nodular regenerative hyperplasia (n=4). The diagnosis was noncirrhotic portal hypertension. Two patients received liver transplantation and developed lung fibrosis 18 months and 12 years later, respectively.

Other manifestations

Other manifestations linked to telomeropathy have been described, such as cellular or humoral immunodeficiency, exudative retinopathies, central neurological involvement with cerebral calcifications and gastrointestinal bleeding [47, 48]. Hoyeraal–Hreidarsson syndrome is, for example, a rare and severe form of DKC. It is associated with four of the six following characteristics: microcephalia, cerebellar hypoplasia, delayed pre-natal growth, delayed development, immunodeficiency and bone marrow failure. All of these manifestations have mainly been described in children and to the best of our knowledge have not been described in association with adult pulmonary fibrosis [49].

A recent report on *TINF2* mutation associated with IPF suggested that patients with complex telomerase complex mutation may present an increased risk of infertility [23]. Further studies are needed on this topic.

Telomere length

The detection of a reduction in telomere length in patients presenting a *TERT* or *TERC* mutation is an argument for the pathogenicity of these mutations. Telomere length has been measured in circulating leukocytes or in pulmonary epithelial cells [14, 50]. Telomere length diminishes physiologically with age by approximately 20% between 20 and 80 years of age [50]. It also diminishes in the case of exposure to tobacco or pesticides and in numerous chronic illnesses [51–53]. There is no standardised technique to measure telomere length.

In a cohort of 134 patients with *TERT* mutation, 15% of the mutated patients had normal telomere measurements, whereas 85% of them presented shortened telomeres below the 10th percentile [14]. Likewise, some patients with Hoyeraal–Hreidarsson syndrome did not present short telomeres [54]. This observation is in keeping with the hypothesis of telomeropathies with a qualitative and nonquantitative defect without a reduction in telomere size [54].

Moreover, 23% of the patients with sporadic IPF presented shortened telomeres without *TERT* or *TERC* mutations [50]. Telomere shortening is not specific to IPF, as it has been detected in almost all ILDs [55] and also in COPD [56]. However, telomere shortening seems to be more important in familial fibrosis, particularly in patients with *TERT* mutations [55].

Telomeres shorten from generation to generation in patients with *TERT* mutations [14]. This could explain, on the one hand, the phenomenon of genetic anticipation in families with the mutation, characterised by an earlier onset of the disease from generation to generation and, on the other hand, an enhanced risk of pulmonary fibrosis without transmission of the mutation because of transmission of shortened telomeres in a given family [57, 58]. It is probable that telomere length has an influence on the physiopathology of IPF [57, 59, 60].

RTEL1 mutations

RTEL1 (regulator of telomere elongation helicase 1) is an adenosine triphosphate dependent DNA helicase that participates in DNA replication, genome stability, DNA repair and telomere maintenance [61]. *RTEL1* biallelic mutations were first described in Hoyeraal–Hreidarsson syndrome [49].

Using the same approach, three independent groups identified heterozygous mutations of *RTEL1* in nine (4.7%) out of 188, four (11.4%) out of 35 and five (5%) out of 99 families with familial fibrosis [25–27]. The mean age of the patients varied from 49.8 to 65.3 years. The younger ages of the second generation suggest a mechanism of anticipation. IPF was reported in 55–67% of the cases, but rheumatoid arthritis-associated ILD and sarcoidosis were also reported (figure 3). The clinical manifestations have not yet been fully described, but shortened telomere length and anticipation suggest including *RTEL1* mutations in the telomerase complex mutations.

PARN mutations

PARN encodes a polyadenylation-specific ribonuclease deadenylation nuclease. STUART *et al.* [25] identified heterozygous mutations of *PARN* in six (6%) out of 99 families with familial fibrosis. Biallelic *PARN* mutations were then identified in three families with severe DKC [62]. Individuals with biallelic *PARN* mutations exhibit reduced RNA levels for *TERC*, *DKC1*, *RTEL1* and *TERF1*. Moreover, *PARN*-deficient cells present short telomeres and early DNA damage upon ultraviolet treatment [62]. *PARN* is the first gene of the telomere complex to be initially described in familial fibrosis before haematological disease.

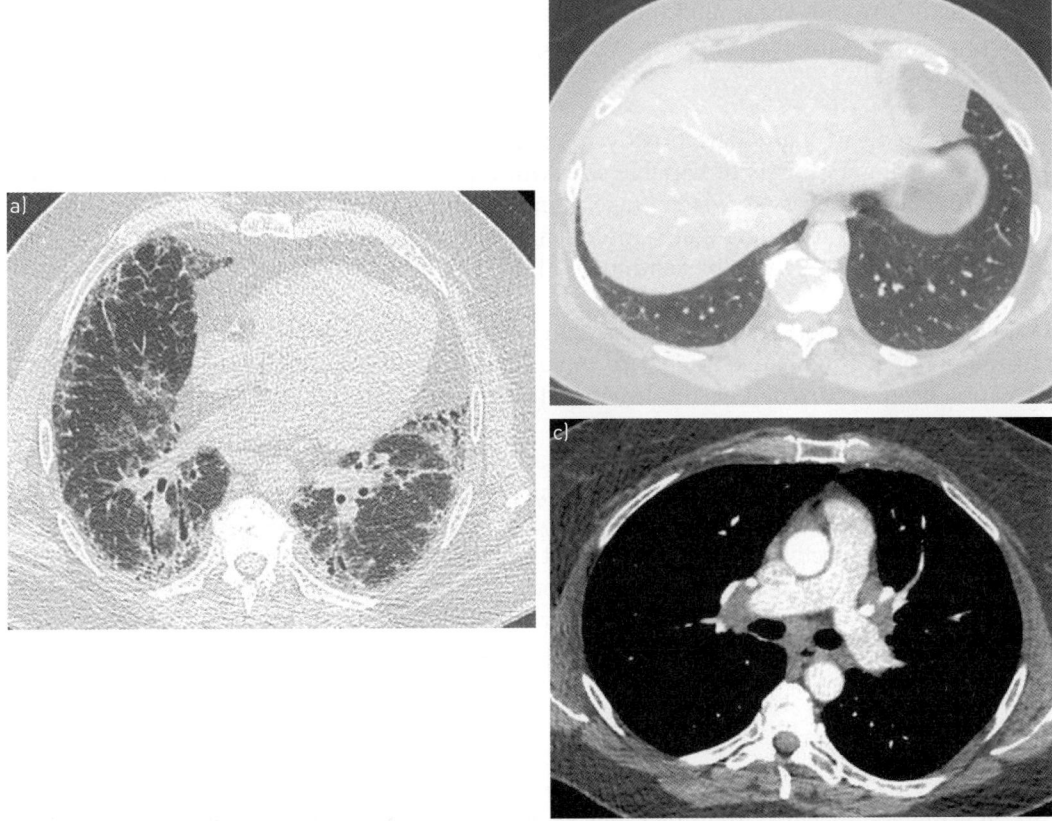

Figure 3. Representative CT scans of patients with *RTEL1* mutations with a) a UIP pattern, and b and c) ILD associated with granulomatosis. Image provided by J. Cadranel (Hôpital Tenon, Paris, France).

The clinical manifestations have not yet been fully described, but liver cirrhosis might be also a consequence of *PARN* mutation [25].

Surfactant protein mutations

Surfactant is secreted by type II epithelial alveolar cells and is composed of 90% lipids and 10% proteins. The main surfactant proteins are surfactant protein (SP)-A, SP-B, SP-C and SP-D, and the corresponding genes are called *SFTPA*, *SFTPB*, *SFTPC* and *SFTPD* [63]. The hydrophobic proteins SP-B and SP-C are transported towards the cell membrane in lamellar bodies by the ABCA3 (ATB binding cassette family A, member 3) transporter encoded by *ABCA3* [64]. Among surfactant gene mutations, *SFTPC* mutations are the most described in adult familial ILD.

SFTPC mutations

SFTPC mutations were first reported in children with ILD before being reported in adults [65, 66]. At the cellular level, *SFTPC* mutation induces endoplasmic reticulum stress and an unfolded protein response due to the altered intracellular trafficking of the abnormal protein [67–69].

Transmission of the mutation is autosomal dominant. However, neomutations are frequent and may explain as many as 50% of the cases [69]. A Dutch study detected *SFTPC* mutations in five out of the 20 families tested from a cohort of familial ILD [70]. Such a high prevalence is unique and has not been observed in other populations, where it is usually <5% [12].

The most frequent radiological pattern associates predominant ground-glass opacities, septal thickening and cysts of variable size with a predominant distribution in the superior lobes [70–72]. However, at a later stage, honeycombing can predominate (figure 4b). It is sometimes difficult to differentiate emphysema from cysts, and an *SFTPC* mutation may be suspected in a young patient presenting CPFE [73].

Histologically, the most frequently described pattern in adults is UIP, but NSIP, organising pneumonia or desquamative interstitial pneumonia can also be observed [70]. Granulomas have not been reported, but moderate inflammation and centrolobular fibrosis can be observed [70].

In children, different treatments have been reported with success: methylprednisolone, hydroxychloroquine and azithromycin [71, 74, 75]. However, these reports were clinical cases or uncontrolled retrospective series. No treatment appears to improve a patient with predominant honeycombing lesions. The effect of antifibrotic drugs, such as pirfenidone or nintedanib, is unknown. The disease does not appear to recur after pulmonary transplantation [76].

Other proteins in the surfactant system

Homozygous *SFTPB* mutations have only been associated with a neonatal respiratory distress syndrome [63].

SFTPA2 mutations have been detected in three families. Transmission was autosomal dominant with a phenotype associating early pulmonary fibrosis and lung cancer [77, 78]. *SFTPA1* and *SFTPA2* are highly homologous and sequencing requires specific methods [79].

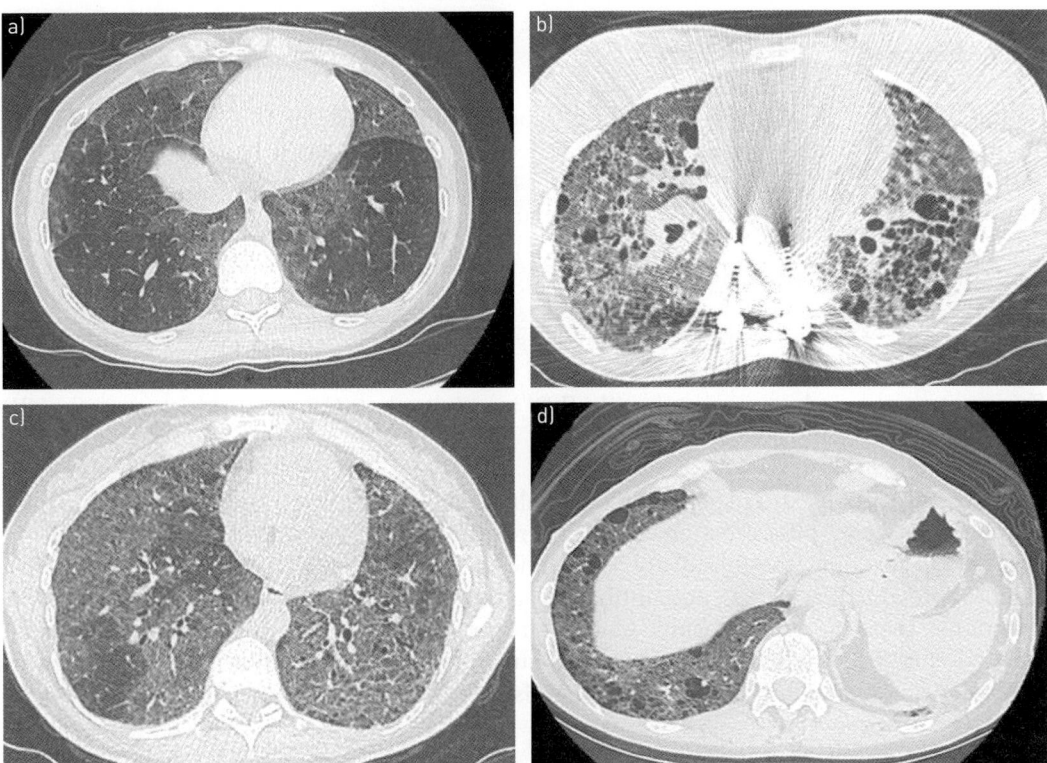

Figure 4. Representative CT scans inconsistent with UIP in patients with a) an *NFKX2.1* heterozygous mutation, b) an *SFTPC* heterozygous mutation (surgical treatment of kyphoscoliosis may be related to fibrotic lung disease during childhood), c) an *ABCA3* homozygous mutation and d) type 1 neurofibromatosis.

Biallelic *ABCA3* mutations were first reported in children with ILD [64, 80]. There is a genotype–phenotype correlation [76]. All children with biallelic frameshift and nonsense mutations presented with respiratory failure at birth. Biallelic missense, predicted splice site mutations or insertion/deletions were associated with older age of presentation and better prognosis. Indeed, a large family in which the oldest patient was a male non-smoker (57 years of age), with CPFE associated with *ABCA3* mutations, has been reported recently (figure 4c) [81, 82].

Other syndromes with pulmonary fibrosis associated with monogenic disorders

In addition to genetic disorders linked to mutations of surfactant or telomerase complex genes, pulmonary fibrosis has been described during certain rare familial syndromes (table 1). However, none of these was associated with a UIP pattern either on CT or on histology.

Hermansky–Pudlak syndrome is a genetic disorder associated with defective lysosome-related organelles [83]. Patients present oculocutaneous albinism and a pre-disposition to bleeding [84]. Depending on the mutated gene, up to 80% of patients can present pulmonary fibrosis [85]. CT shows reticulations and consolidations, while histology reveals a peribronchial fibrosis [86]. Two trials evaluated the effect of pirfenidone *versus* placebo, but contradictory results were reported [87, 88]. The first trial, with 35 patients, did not find a difference between the two groups [87]. The other, with 21 patients, reported a slowing of lung function decline in treated patients [88].

Neurofibromatosis is a dysplasia of the mesoderm and ectoderm that is characterised by the presence of neurofibromas, café au lait lesions and pigmented hamartoma of the iris [89]. A review performed in 2007, reported 64 cases of pulmonary fibrosis associated with type 1 neurofibromatosis (NF1) [90]. The association between pulmonary fibrosis and NF1 is still a matter of discussion; however, there appears to be an association between NF1 and a specific pulmonary cystic disease (figure 4d) [91].

Heterozygous *NKX-2.1* (TITF1) mutations in children are associated with ILD, hypothyroidism and neurological anomalies (hypotonia, delayed development, chorea). This mutation may be associated with ILD in adults, but CT is inconsistent with UIP (figure 4a) [92].

Very recently, 10 paediatric and young adult patients presented systemic inflammation, peripheral vascular inflammation and ILD, revealed to be associated with mutations in *TMEM173*, encoding the stimulator of interferon genes (STING) [93, 94]. Another five families presented arthritis, autoantibodies and ILD that were associated with *COPA* mutations, impairing endoplasmic–Golgi transport [95]. At least five families presented poikiloderma associated with tendon contractures and pulmonary fibrosis associated with *FAM111B* mutations [96]. In this series, CT also seemed to be inconsistent with UIP.

Genetic polymorphisms

In addition to monogenic Mendelian disease, several genetic polymorphisms have been associated with IPF. The presence of these polymorphisms increases the risk of developing IPF.

A polymorphism in the *MUC5B* promoter (rs35705950) is strongly associated with IPF in the Caucasian population, with the presence of the minor T allele being associated with IPF [97–99]. This polymorphism is present in 10% of the general population compared with 35% in the sporadic and familial forms of IPF. The relative risk of developing IPF is approximately 6 for heterozygous patients and 20 for homozygous patients. Paradoxically, the presence of this polymorphism in patients with IPF is associated with an increase in survival [15]. Patients with the increased-risk allele have increased *MUC5B* expression. MUC5B is a mucin that is normally absent in the alveolar epithelium but is expressed by the epithelial cells in the submucosal glands. MUC5B is strongly expressed by the cells that cover the honeycomb cysts [100]. The role of MUC5B in IPF is not clear, but these results highlight the importance of the bronchiolar epithelial response during the pathophysiology of IPF [101].

This polymorphism is present in <2% of the Asian general population (Korean, Chinese and Japanese) and in 3–7% of their sporadic respective IPF populations [97, 102, 103]. The presence of the rare allele is thus associated with IPF, but the association is less strong than in Caucasian patients (French, American, Mexican, English and German) [97–99, 102–104]. However, the presence of the rare allele is not associated with sarcoidosis or with systemic sclerosis ILD [98, 104].

In a prospective analysis of *MUC5B* polymorphisms, CHUNG *et al.* [105] suggested that patients homozygous for the minor T allele may specifically present a UIP pattern on CT or on histology. However, at least two out of 31 German patients with an NSIP diagnosis were also homozygous for the at-risk polymorphism [97]. Further studies are needed to evaluate the value of testing for *MUC5B* polymorphisms in the diagnosis decision algorithm of ILD.

Numerous other polymorphisms have been associated with IPF [106–108]. Genome-wide pulmonary fibrosis association studies have not only confirmed the association between IPF and *MUC5B*, *TERT* or *TERC*, but have also revealed several new locations of interest such as a polymorphism in *TOLLIP*, encoding the Toll-interacting protein [109–111]. This last polymorphism could influence the response to NAC in patients with IPF [16].

Moreover, epigenetic regulation mechanisms could contribute to certain forms of familial pulmonary fibrosis. For instance, there are methylation modifications of certain genes during IPF [112]. This subject requires a specific review [112].

Genetic diagnosis and counselling

When a genetic form of pulmonary fibrosis is suspected, there are currently no guidelines on the genes to be analysed. We suggest searching for *TERT*, *TERC*, *RTEL1* and *PARN* mutations for the telomerase complex and *SFTPA2*, *SFTPC* and *ABCA3* mutations for surfactant (table 2 and figure 5). The search for telomerase complex mutations is also performed for patients with pulmonary fibrosis and suspected telomere syndrome. Genetic analysis is not systematic in patients with sporadic IPF but can be discussed before lung transplantation [50].

A mutation of one of these genes is found in approximately 25% of families. Without any mutation identified, a more advanced genetic analysis such as exome sequencing may be considered.

In cases where a mutation is identified in the index case, the risks to relatives can be evaluated according to the type of transmission and the degree of kinship. This may be specified by molecular exploration for those relatives who request it. In any case, patients must be encouraged to avoid all toxic factors, whether respiratory, hepatic or medullar, and especially tobacco smoke, environmental toxins and cytotoxic drugs. Professional outplacement may be considered to avoid known occupational risks.

Regarding the risk of anticipation and the pleiotropic effects of telomerase complex mutations, genetic counselling has to be considered using a multidisciplinary approach and discussed case by case. For this purpose, in our hospital (Bichat Hospital), we have developed

---

Table 2. Patients for whom we propose genetic testing

Idiopathic or nonidiopathic ILD with at least one of the following:
    Familial ILD
    Idiopathic ILD at <50 years old
    Personal or familial history of:
        Bone marrow failure, thrombocytopenia or myelodysplasia
        Dyskeratosis congenita
        Cryptogenic cirrhosis

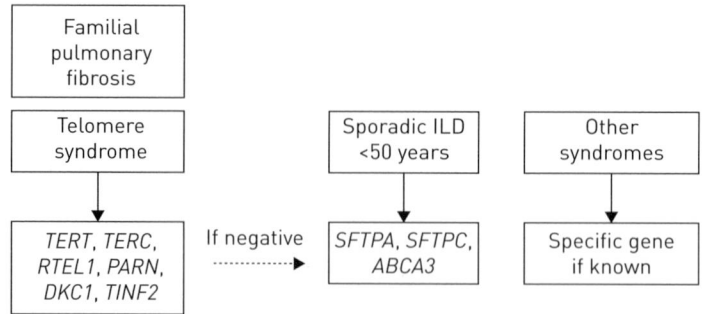

Figure 5. Proposal for genetic testing in pulmonary fibrosis. Telomerase complex gene mutations are most frequently found in familial pulmonary fibrosis. However, they are rarely found in the proband before 50 years of age. Surfactant gene mutations are most frequently found in children and may be considered in young adults. *SFTPA2* mutations may be associated with familial clustering of pulmonary fibrosis and lung cancer.

a multidisciplinary discussion involving: pulmonologists specialised in ILD and in lung transplantation, paediatricians specialised in ILD, geneticists, haematologists, hepatologists, dermatologists, immunologists and psychologists. However, some families also require advice from gynaecologists, nephrologists or rheumatologists. In practice, we always rapidly see relatives from familial fibrosis cases who ask for a specialised evaluation, as there is often a great deal of anxiety. The first evaluation is based on an explanation of the potential risks and a clinical evaluation, and, if the subject agrees, a complete blood count, liver blood test and genetic testing are performed. If the subject is asymptomatic without any abnormalities at clinical examination, we propose a chest HRCT scan in the supine position 10 years before the age of onset in the proband. If the subject is symptomatic or if the clinical evaluation is abnormal, chest HRCT and PFTs are performed. When a UIP pattern is detected, antifibrotic treatment (pirfenidone, nintedanib) is discussed.

Conclusion

Familial pulmonary fibrosis is relatively frequent and raises specific problems. Approximately 25% of families have an identified mutation and should benefit from specific genetic counselling. Current studies aim to identify new genes by complete exome sequencing techniques in order to increase this percentage and develop specific therapies.

In adults, the most frequently detected mutations are *TERT* and *RTEL1* mutations. Beyond physiopathological knowledge, detection of these mutations has practical consequence for patients. Mutations of *TERT* and *TERC* are responsible for haematological complications following lung transplantation and may require an adapted immunosuppression.

References

1. Steele MP, Speer MC, Loyd JE, *et al.* Clinical and pathologic features of familial interstitial pneumonia. *Am J Respir Crit Care Med* 2005; 172: 1146–1152.
2. Castaldo G, Polizzi A, Tomaiuolo R, *et al.* Comprehensive cystic fibrosis mutation epidemiology and haplotype characterization in a southern Italian population. *Ann Hum Genet* 2005; 69: 15–24.
3. Marshall RP, Puddicombe A, Cookson WO, *et al.* Adult familial cryptogenic fibrosing alveolitis in the United Kingdom. *Thorax* 2000; 55: 143–146.

4.   Hodgson U, Laitinen T, Tukiainen P. Nationwide prevalence of sporadic and familial idiopathic pulmonary fibrosis: evidence of founder effect among multiplex families in Finland. *Thorax* 2002; 57: 338–342.

5.   Loyd JE. Pulmonary fibrosis in families. *Am J Respir Cell Mol Biol* 2003; 29: Suppl., S47–S50.

6.   Garcia-Sancho C, Buendia-Roldan I, Fernandez-Plata MR, *et al.* Familial pulmonary fibrosis is the strongest risk factor for idiopathic pulmonary fibrosis. *Respir Med* 2011; 105: 1902–1907.

7.   Scholand MB, Coon H, Wolff R, *et al.* Use of a genealogical database demonstrates heritability of pulmonary fibrosis. *Lung* 2013; 191: 475–481.

8.   Okamoto T, Miyazaki Y, Tomita M, *et al.* A familial history of pulmonary fibrosis in patients with chronic hypersensitivity pneumonitis. *Respiration* 2013; 85: 384–390.

9.   Lee HL, Ryu JH, Wittmer MH, *et al.* Familial idiopathic pulmonary fibrosis: clinical features and outcome. *Chest* 2005; 127: 2034–2041.

10. Lee HY, Seo JB, Steele MP, *et al.* High-resolution CT scan findings in familial interstitial pneumonia do not conform to those of idiopathic interstitial pneumonia. *Chest* 2012; 142: 1577–1583.

11. Leslie KO, Cool CD, Sporn TA, *et al.* Familial idiopathic interstitial pneumonia: histopathology and survival in 30 patients. *Arch Pathol Lab Med* 2012; 136: 1366–1376.

12. Fernandez BA, Fox G, Bhatia R, *et al.* A Newfoundland cohort of familial and sporadic idiopathic pulmonary fibrosis patients: clinical and genetic features. *Respir Res* 2012; 13: 64.

13. Ravaglia C, Tomassetti S, Gurioli C, *et al.* Features and outcome of familial idiopathic pulmonary fibrosis. *Sarcoidosis Vasc Diffuse Lung Dis* 2014; 31: 28–36.

14. Diaz de Leon A, Cronkhite JT, Katzenstein AL, *et al.* Telomere lengths, pulmonary fibrosis and telomerase (*TERT*) mutations. *PLoS One* 2010; 5: e10680.

15. Peljto AL, Zhang Y, Fingerlin TE, *et al.* Association between the *MUC5B* promoter polymorphism and survival in patients with idiopathic pulmonary fibrosis. *JAMA* 2013; 309: 2232–2239.

16. Oldham JM, Ma SF, Martinez FJ, *et al.* TOLLIP, MUC5B and the response to *N*-acetylcysteine among individuals with idiopathic pulmonary fibrosis. *Am J Respir Crit Care Med* 2015; 192: 1475–1482.

17. Kropski JA, Pritchett JM, Zoz DF, *et al.* Extensive phenotyping of individuals at-risk for familial interstitial pneumonia reveals clues to the pathogenesis of interstitial lung disease. *Am J Respir Crit Care Med* 2014; 191: 417–426.

18. Rosas IO, Ren P, Avila NA, *et al.* Early interstitial lung disease in familial pulmonary fibrosis. *Am J Respir Crit Care Med* 2007; 176: 698–705.

19. Calado RT, Young NS. Telomere diseases. *N Engl J Med* 2009; 361: 2353–2365.

20. Townsley DM, Dumitriu B, Young NS. Bone marrow failure and the telomeropathies. *Blood* 2014; 124: 2775–2783.

21. Alder JK, Parry EM, Yegnasubramanian S, *et al.* Telomere phenotypes in females with heterozygous mutations in the dyskeratosis congenita 1 (*DKC1*) gene. *Hum Mutat* 2013; 34: 1481–1485.

22. Fukuhara A, Tanino Y, Ishii T, *et al.* Pulmonary fibrosis in dyskeratosis congenita with *TINF2* gene mutation. *Eur Respir J* 2013; 42: 1757–1759.

23. Alder JK, Stanley SE, Wagner CL, *et al.* Exome sequencing identifies mutant *TINF2* in a family with pulmonary fibrosis. *Chest* 2015; 147: 1361–1368.

24. Kannengiesser C, Borie R, Revy P. Pulmonary fibrosis associated with *TINF2* gene mutation: is somatic reversion required? *Eur Respir J* 2014; 44: 269–270.

25. Stuart BD, Choi J, Zaidi S, *et al.* Exome sequencing links mutations in *PARN* and *RTEL1* with familial pulmonary fibrosis and telomere shortening. *Nat Genet* 2015; 47: 512–517.

26. Cogan JD, Kropski JA, Zhao M, *et al.* Rare variants in *RTEL1* are associated with familial interstitial pneumonia. *Am J Respir Crit Care Med* 2015; 191: 646–655.

27. Kannengiesser C, Borie R, Menard C, *et al.* Heterozygous *RTEL1* mutations are associated with familial pulmonary fibrosis. *Eur Respir J* 2015; 46: 474–485.

28. Nunes H, Monnet I, Kannengiesser C, *et al.* Is telomeropathy the explanation for combined pulmonary fibrosis and emphysema syndrome?: report of a family with TERT mutation. *Am J Respir Crit Care Med* 2014; 189: 753–754.

29. Stanley SE, Chen JJ, Podlevsky JD, *et al.* Telomerase mutations in smokers with severe emphysema. *J Clin Invest* 2015; 125: 563–570.

30. Gorgy AI, Jonassaint NL, Stanley SE, *et al.* Hepatopulmonary syndrome is a frequent cause of dyspnea in the short telomere disorders. *Chest* 2015; 148: 1019–1026.

31. El-Chemaly S, Ziegler SG, Calado RT, *et al.* Natural history of pulmonary fibrosis in two subjects with the same telomerase mutation. *Chest* 2011; 139: 1203–1209.

32. Cottin V, Crestani B, Valeyre D, *et al.* [French practical guidelines for the diagnosis and management of idiopathic pulmonary fibrosis. From the National Reference and the Competence Centers for Rare Diseases and the Societe de Pneumologie de Langue Francaise]. *Rev Mal Respir* 2013; 30: 879–902.

33. Silhan LL, Shah PD, Chambers DC, *et al.* Lung transplantation in telomerase mutation carriers with pulmonary fibrosis. *Eur Respir J* 2014; 44: 178–187.

34. Borie R, Kannengiesser C, Hirschi S, *et al.* Severe hematologic complications after lung transplantation in patients with telomerase complex mutations. *J Heart Lung Transplant* 2015; 34: 538–546.

35. Tokman S, Singer JP, Devine MS, *et al.* Clinical outcomes of lung transplant recipients with telomerase mutations. *J Heart Lung Transplant* 2015; 34: 1318–1324.

36. George G, Rosas IO, Cui Y, *et al.* Short telomeres, telomeropathy, and subclinical extrapulmonary organ damage in patients with interstitial lung disease. *Chest* 2015; 147: 1549–1557.

37. Langston AA, Sanders JE, Deeg HJ, *et al.* Allogeneic marrow transplantation for aplastic anaemia associated with dyskeratosis congenita. *Br J Haematol* 1996; 92: 758–765.

38. Diaz de Leon A, Cronkhite JT, Yilmaz C, *et al.* Subclinical lung disease, macrocytosis, and premature graying in kindreds with telomerase (*TERT*) mutations. *Chest* 2011; 140: 753–763.

39. Ball SE, Gibson FM, Rizzo S, *et al.* Progressive telomere shortening in aplastic anemia. *Blood* 1998; 91: 3582–3592.

40. Yamaguchi H, Baerlocher GM, Lansdorp PM, *et al.* Mutations of the human telomerase RNA gene (*TERC*) in aplastic anemia and myelodysplastic syndrome. *Blood* 2003; 102: 916–918.

41. Yamaguchi H, Calado RT, Ly H, *et al.* Mutations in *TERT*, the gene for telomerase reverse transcriptase, in aplastic anemia. *N Engl J Med* 2005; 352: 1413–1424.

42. Parry EM, Alder JK, Qi X, *et al.* Syndrome complex of bone marrow failure and pulmonary fibrosis predicts germline defects in telomerase. *Blood* 2011; 117: 5607–5611.

43. Tabeze L, Borie R, Cottin V, *et al.* Prévalence de mutations identifiées dans les suspicions de formes génétiques de fibroses. *Rev Mal Respir* 2015; 32: A19.

44. Calado RT, Brudno J, Mehta P, *et al.* Constitutional telomerase mutations are genetic risk factors for cirrhosis. *Hepatology* 2011; 53: 1600–1607.

45. Calado RT, Regal JA, Kleiner DE, *et al.* A spectrum of severe familial liver disorders associate with telomerase mutations. *PLoS One* 2009; 4: e7926.

46. Hartmann D, Srivastava U, Thaler M, *et al.* Telomerase gene mutations are associated with cirrhosis formation. *Hepatology* 2011; 53: 1608–1617.

47. Armanios M, Price C. Telomeres and disease: an overview. *Mutat Res* 2012; 730: 1–2.

48. Dokal I. Dyskeratosis congenita. *Hematology Am Soc Hematol Educ Program* 2011; 2011: 480–486.

49. Mialou V, Leblanc T, Peffault de Latour R, *et al.* [Dyskeratosis congenita: an update]. *Arch Pediatr* 2013; 20: 299–306.

50. Cronkhite JT, Xing C, Raghu G, *et al.* Telomere shortening in familial and sporadic pulmonary fibrosis. *Am J Respir Crit Care Med* 2008; 178: 729–737.

51. Haque S, Rakieh C, Marriage F, *et al.* Shortened telomere length in patients with systemic lupus erythematosus. *Arthritis Rheum* 2013; 65: 1319–1323.

52. Hou L, Andreotti G, Baccarelli AA, *et al.* Lifetime pesticide use and telomere shortening among male pesticide applicators in the Agricultural Health Study. *Environ Health Perspect* 2013; 121: 919–924.

53. Alder JK, Guo N, Kembou F, *et al.* Telomere length is a determinant of emphysema susceptibility. *Am J Respir Crit Care Med* 2011; 184: 904–912.

54. Touzot F, Gaillard L, Vasquez N, *et al.* Heterogeneous telomere defects in patients with severe forms of dyskeratosis congenita. *J Allergy Clin Immunol* 2012; 129: 473–482.

55. Snetselaar R, van Moorsel CH, Kazemier KM, *et al.* Telomere length in interstitial lung diseases. *Chest* 2015; 148: 1011–1018.

56. Savale L, Chaouat A, Bastuji-Garin S, *et al.* Shortened telomeres in circulating leukocytes of patients with chronic obstructive pulmonary disease. *Am J Respir Crit Care Med* 2009; 179: 566–571.

57. Alder JK, Cogan JD, Brown AF, *et al.* Ancestral mutation in telomerase causes defects in repeat addition processivity and manifests as familial pulmonary fibrosis. *PLoS Genet* 2011; 7: e1001352.

58. Gansner JM, Rosas IO, Ebert BL. Pulmonary fibrosis, bone marrow failure, and telomerase mutation. *N Engl J Med* 2012; 366: 1551–1553.

59. Alder JK, Chen JJ, Lancaster L, *et al.* Short telomeres are a risk factor for idiopathic pulmonary fibrosis. *Proc Natl Acad Sci U S A* 2008; 105: 13051–13056.

60. Collopy LC, Walne AJ, Cardoso S, *et al.* Triallelic and epigenetic-like inheritance in human disorders of telomerase. *Blood* 2015; 126: 176–184.

61. Uringa EJ, Lisaingo K, Pickett HA, *et al.* RTEL1 contributes to DNA replication and repair and telomere maintenance. *Mol Biol Cell* 2012; 23: 2782–2792.

62. Tummala H, Walne A, Collopy L, *et al.* Poly(A)-specific ribonuclease deficiency impacts telomere biology and causes dyskeratosis congenita. *J Clin Invest* 2015; 125: 2151–2160.

63. Whitsett JA, Wert SE, Weaver TE. Alveolar surfactant homeostasis and the pathogenesis of pulmonary disease. *Annu Rev Med* 2010; 61: 105–119.

64. Flamein F, Riffault L, Muselet-Charlier C, *et al.* Molecular and cellular characteristics of *ABCA3* mutations associated with diffuse parenchymal lung diseases in children. *Hum Mol Genet* 2012; 21: 765–775.

65. Nogee LM, Dunbar AE III, Wert SE, *et al.* A mutation in the surfactant protein C gene associated with familial interstitial lung disease. *N Engl J Med* 2001; 344: 573–579.

66. Thomas AQ, Lane K, Phillips J III, *et al.* Heterozygosity for a surfactant protein C gene mutation associated with usual interstitial pneumonitis and cellular nonspecific interstitial pneumonitis in one kindred. *Am J Respir Crit Care Med* 2002; 165: 1322–1328.

67. Lawson WE, Crossno PF, Polosukhin VV, *et al.* Endoplasmic reticulum stress in alveolar epithelial cells is prominent in IPF: association with altered surfactant protein processing and herpesvirus infection. *Am J Physiol Lung Cell Mol Physiol* 2008; 294: L1119–L1126.

68. Mulugeta S, Nguyen V, Russo SJ, *et al.* A surfactant protein C precursor protein BRICHOS domain mutation causes endoplasmic reticulum stress, proteasome dysfunction, and caspase 3 activation. *Am J Respir Cell Mol Biol* 2005; 32: 521–530.

69. Brasch F, Griese M, Tredano M, *et al.* Interstitial lung disease in a baby with a *de novo* mutation in the SFTPC gene. *Eur Respir J* 2004; 24: 30–39.

70. van Moorsel CH, van Oosterhout MF, Barlo NP, *et al.* Surfactant protein C mutations are the basis of a significant portion of adult familial pulmonary fibrosis in a Dutch cohort. *Am J Respir Crit Care Med* 2010; 182: 1419–1425.

71. Mechri M, Epaud R, Emond S, *et al.* Surfactant protein C gene (*SFTPC*) mutation-associated lung disease: high-resolution computed tomography (HRCT) findings and its relation to histological analysis. *Pediatr Pulmonol* 2010; 45: 1021–1029.

72. Ono S, Tanaka T, Ishida M, *et al.* Surfactant protein C G100S mutation causes familial pulmonary fibrosis in Japanese kindred. *Eur Respir J* 2011; 38: 861–869.

73. Cottin V, Reix P, Khouatra C, *et al.* Combined pulmonary fibrosis and emphysema syndrome associated with familial *SFTPC* mutation. *Thorax* 2011; 66: 918–919.

74. Thouvenin G, Abou Taam R, Flamein F, *et al.* Characteristics of disorders associated with genetic mutations of surfactant protein C. *Arch Dis Child* 2010; 95: 449–454.

75. Kroner C, Reu S, Teusch V, *et al.* Genotype alone does not predict the clinical course of *SFTPC* deficiency in paediatric patients. *Eur Respir J* 2015; 46: 197–206.

76. Wambach JA, Casey AM, Fishman MP, *et al.* Genotype–phenotype correlations for infants and children with ABCA3 deficiency. *Am J Respir Crit Care Med* 2014; 189: 1538–1543.

77. Wang Y, Kuan PJ, Xing C, *et al.* Genetic defects in surfactant protein A2 are associated with pulmonary fibrosis and lung cancer. *Am J Hum Genet* 2009; 84: 52–59.

78. Coghlan MA, Shifren A, Huang HJ, *et al.* Sequencing of idiopathic pulmonary fibrosis-related genes reveals independent single gene associations. *BMJ Open Respir Res* 2014; 1: e000057.

79. Horton CJ, Mitui M, Leos NK, *et al.* Long-range PCR based sequencing of the highly homologous genes, SFTPA1 and SFTPA2. *Mol Cell Probes* 2013; 27: 115–117.

80. Thouvenin G, Nathan N, Epaud R, *et al.* Diffuse parenchymal lung disease caused by surfactant deficiency: dramatic improvement by azithromycin. *BMJ Case Rep* 2013; 2013.

81. Epaud R, Delestrain C, Louha M, *et al.* Combined pulmonary fibrosis and emphysema syndrome associated with *ABCA3* mutations. *Eur Respir J* 2014; 43: 638–641.

82. Campo I, Zorzetto M, Mariani F, *et al.* A large kindred of pulmonary fibrosis associated with a novel *ABCA3* gene variant. *Respir Res* 2014; 15: 43.

83. Huizing M, Helip-Wooley A, Westbroek W, *et al.* Disorders of lysosome-related organelle biogenesis: clinical and molecular genetics. *Annu Rev Genomics Hum Genet* 2008; 9: 359–386.

84. Santiago Borrero PJ, Rodriguez-Perez Y, Renta JY, *et al.* Genetic testing for oculocutaneous albinism type 1 and 2 and Hermansky–Pudlak syndrome type 1 and 3 mutations in Puerto Rico. *J Invest Dermatol* 2006; 126: 85–90.

85. Gahl WA, Brantly M, Kaiser-Kupfer MI, *et al.* Genetic defects and clinical characteristics of patients with a form of oculocutaneous albinism (Hermansky–Pudlak syndrome). *N Engl J Med* 1998; 338: 1258–1264.

86. Pierson DM, Ionescu D, Qing G, *et al.* Pulmonary fibrosis in Hermansky–Pudlak syndrome. A case report and review. *Respiration* 2006; 73: 382–395.

87. Gahl WA, Brantly M, Troendle J, *et al.* Effect of pirfenidone on the pulmonary fibrosis of Hermansky–Pudlak syndrome. *Mol Genet Metab* 2002; 76: 234–242.

88. O'Brien K, Troendle J, Gochuico BR, *et al.* Pirfenidone for the treatment of Hermansky–Pudlak syndrome pulmonary fibrosis. *Mol Genet Metab* 2011; 103: 128–134.

89. Riccardi VM. Von Recklinghausen neurofibromatosis. *N Engl J Med* 1981; 305: 1617–1627.

90. Zamora AC, Collard HR, Wolters PJ, *et al.* Neurofibromatosis-associated lung disease: a case series and literature review. *Eur Respir J* 2007; 29: 210–214.

91. Ryu JH, Parambil JG, McGrann PS, *et al.* Lack of evidence for an association between neurofibromatosis and pulmonary fibrosis. *Chest* 2005; 128: 2381–2386.

92. Hamvas A, Deterding RR, Wert SE, *et al.* Heterogeneous pulmonary phenotypes associated with mutations in the thyroid transcription factor gene *NKX2-1*. *Chest* 2013; 144: 794–804.

93. Liu Y, Jesus AA, Marrero B, *et al.* Activated STING in a vascular and pulmonary syndrome. *N Engl J Med* 2014; 371: 507–518.

94. Jeremiah N, Neven B, Gentili M, *et al.* Inherited STING-activating mutation underlies a familial inflammatory syndrome with lupus-like manifestations. *J Clin Invest* 2014; 124: 5516–5520.

95.   Watkin LB, Jessen B, Wiszniewski W, et al. COPA mutations impair ER–Golgi transport and cause hereditary autoimmune-mediated lung disease and arthritis. Nat Genet 2015; 47: 654–660.
96.   Mercier S, Kury S, Shaboodien G, et al. Mutations in FAM111B cause hereditary fibrosing poikiloderma with tendon contracture, myopathy, and pulmonary fibrosis. Am J Hum Genet 2013; 93: 1100–1107.
97.   Horimasu Y, Ohshimo S, Bonella F, et al. MUC5B promoter polymorphism in Japanese patients with idiopathic pulmonary fibrosis. Respirology 2015; 20: 439–444.
98.   Borie R, Crestani B, Dieude P, et al. The MUC5B variant is associated with idiopathic pulmonary fibrosis but not with systemic sclerosis interstitial lung disease in the European Caucasian population. PLoS One 2013; 8: e70621.
99.   Seibold MA, Wise AL, Speer MC, et al. A common MUC5B promoter polymorphism and pulmonary fibrosis. N Engl J Med 2011; 364: 1503–1512.
100. Plantier L, Crestani B, Wert SE, et al. Ectopic respiratory epithelial cell differentiation in bronchiolised distal airspaces in idiopathic pulmonary fibrosis. Thorax 2011; 66: 651–657.
101. Roy MG, Livraghi-Butrico A, Fletcher AA, et al. Muc5b is required for airway defence. Nature 2014; 505: 412–416.
102. Peljto AL, Selman M, Kim DS, et al. The MUC5B promoter polymorphism is associated with idiopathic pulmonary fibrosis in a Mexican cohort but is rare among Asian ancestries. Chest 2015; 147: 460–464.
103. Wang C, Zhuang Y, Guo W, et al. Mucin 5B promoter polymorphism is associated with susceptibility to interstitial lung diseases in Chinese males. PLoS One 2014; 9: e104919.
104. Stock CJ, Sato H, Fonseca C, et al. Mucin 5B promoter polymorphism is associated with idiopathic pulmonary fibrosis but not with development of lung fibrosis in systemic sclerosis or sarcoidosis. Thorax 2013; 68: 436–441.
105. Chung JH, Chawla A, Peljto AL, et al. CT scan findings of probable usual interstitial pneumonitis have a high predictive value for histologic usual interstitial pneumonitis. Chest 2015; 147: 450–459.
106. Korthagen NM, van Moorsel CH, Kazemier KM, et al. IL1RN genetic variations and risk of IPF: a meta-analysis and mRNA expression study. Immunogenetics 2012; 64: 371–377.
107. Bournazos S, Grinfeld J, Alexander KM, et al. Association of FcγRIIa R131H polymorphism with idiopathic pulmonary fibrosis severity and progression. BMC Pulm Med 2010; 10: 51.
108. Korthagen NM, van Moorsel CH, Barlo NP, et al. Association between variations in cell cycle genes and idiopathic pulmonary fibrosis. PLoS One 2012; 7: e30442.
109. Fingerlin TE, Murphy E, Zhang W, et al. Genome-wide association study identifies multiple susceptibility loci for pulmonary fibrosis. Nat Genet 2013; 45: 613–620.
110. Codd V, Nelson CP, Albrecht E, et al. Identification of seven loci affecting mean telomere length and their association with disease. Nat Genet 2013; 45: 422–427.
111. Noth I, Zhang Y, Ma S, et al. Genetic variants associated with idiopathic pulmonary fibrosis susceptibility and mortality: a genome-wide association study. Lancet Respir Med 2013; 1: 309–317.
112. Helling BA, Yang IV. Epigenetics in lung fibrosis: from pathobiology to treatment perspective. Curr Opin Pulm Med 2015; 21: 454–462.
113. Manolio TA, Collins FS, Cox NJ, et al. Finding the missing heritability of complex diseases. Nature 2009; 461: 747–753.
114. McCarthy MI, Abecasis GR, Cardon LR, et al. Genome-wide association studies for complex traits: consensus, uncertainty and challenges. Nat Rev Genet 2008; 9: 356–369.
115. Montani D, Coulet F, Girerd B, et al. Pulmonary hypertension in patients with neurofibromatosis type I. Medicine (Baltimore) 2011; 90: 201–211.

Disclosures: R. Borie reports receiving the following: personal fees and non-financial support from Intermune/Roche; personal fees and non-financial support from Actelion; non-financial support from MundiPharma; non-financial support from LVL; non-financial support from AstraZeneca; and personal fees and non-financial support from Boehringer Ingelheim. During the last 5 years, B. Crestani has received fees or funding for participation in congresses, papers, training sessions, consulting, participation in groups of experts and research from the following laboratories or firms: AstraZeneca, Boehringer Ingelheim, Intermune/Roche, LVL Medimmune and Sanofi.

Chapter 3

Pathogenesis

Benjamin Loeh[1,2], Martina Korfei[2], Poornima Mahavadi[2,3],
Roxana Wasnick[2], Daniel von der Beck[2] and Andreas Günther[1,2,3,4,5]

The pathogenesis of IPF is characterised by a defective interplay between the epithelium and mesenchyme. The early events are thought to take place in epithelial cells with an initial injury, followed by a stress response that is linked to endoplasmic reticulum stress and apoptosis. Impaired regenerative capacities lead to defective re-epithelisation. Mesenchymal cells then proliferate and form large amounts of extracellular matrix. The origin of these cells can be diverse. They can result from epithelial-to-mesenchymal transition, circulating fibrocytes or activation of resident cells by factors such as inflammatory cytokines. These alterations eventually result in a gradual exchange of normal lung parenchyma with fibrotic tissue.

The exact pathogenesis of IPF, by definition, remains unknown, although research progress made in the field of IPF, especially with regard to the genetics and epithelial homeostasis, has shed light on the key processes. As a result, there is a growing body of evidence that the disease may start in the epithelium and that defective epithelial–mesenchymal cross-talk, alongside alternatively activated immune cells, may represent the key changes.

The epithelium appears to be the initial site of injury

There are numerous changes observed in the alveolar epithelium of IPF subjects. Meanwhile, it is widely believed that recurrent microinjuries to the epithelium, followed by a defective mechanism of regeneration represent the initial event in IPF (figure 1 and table 1) [1]. This view is supported by the identification of familial IPF cases (5–10%) with mutations in surfactant specific proteins A (SFTPA) and C (SFTPC) and the telomerase/shelterin complex (TERT, TERC, PARN, RTEL1 [2, 3]), which may lead to intracellular stress (DNA damage and endoplasmic reticulum (ER) stress), premature cellular senescence and impaired re-epithelialisation. Concordantly, the incidence of IPF is age related [4]. In addition, other forms of intracellular stress, such as lysosomal stress, have been closely linked to other types of lung fibrosis that are also characterised by a UIP pattern in histopathology, such as the Hermansky–Pudlak syndrome interstitial pneumonia (figure 1) [5]. Based on the highly variable penetrance in familial cases of IPF, it also appears obvious

[1]Agaplesion Lung Clinic Waldhof Elgershausen, Greifenstein, Germany. [2]Dept of Internal Medicine, Justus-Liebig-University Giessen, Giessen, Germany. [3]Universities of Giessen and Marburg Lung Center (UGMLC), Member of the German Center for Lung Research (DZL). [4]European IPF Network. [5]Excellence Cluster Cardio-Pulmonary System (ECCPS), Giessen, Germany and European IPF Registry.

Correspondence: Andreas Günther, Dept of Internal Medicine II, Justus-Liebig-University Giessen, Klinikstrasse 36, Giessen D-35392, Germany. E-mail: Andreas.Guenther@innere.med.uni-giessen.de

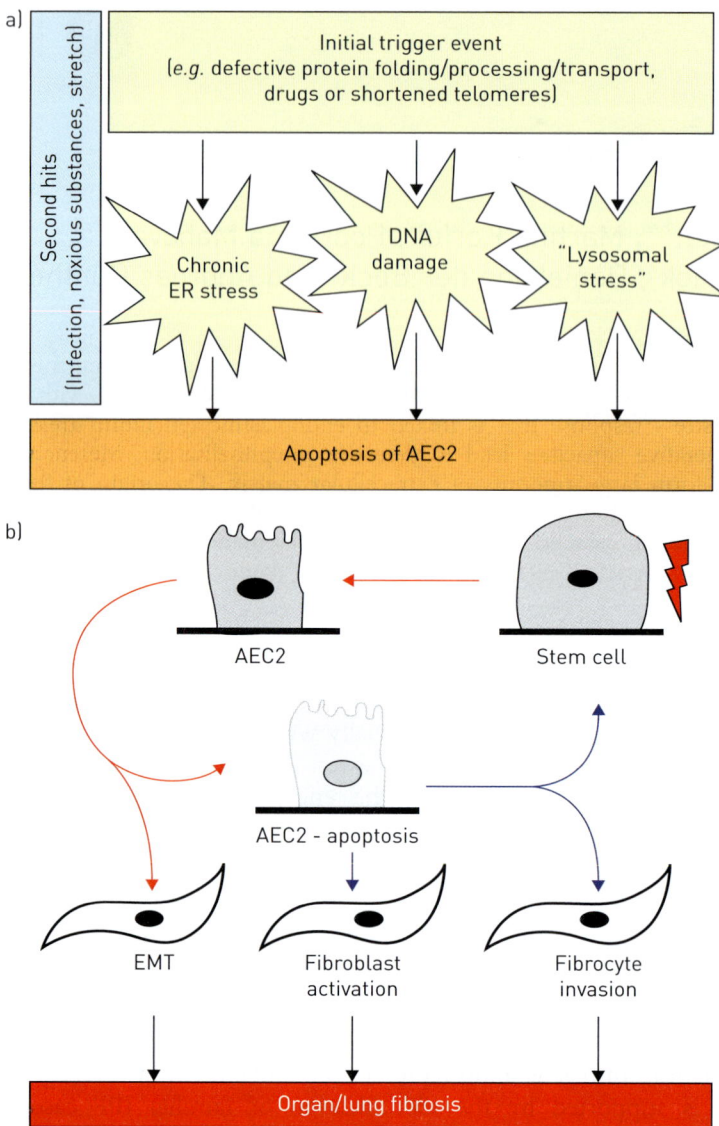

Figure 1. a) Possible mechanisms leading to apoptosis of alveolar epithelial type 2 cells (AEC2s). b) Epithelial injury can lead to fibrosis due to epithelial-to-mesenchymal transition (EMT), impaired regeneration of apoptotic AEC2s and fibroblast activation or invasion. ER: endoplasmic reticulum.

to assume an important role for secondary hits (figure 1), *e.g.* respiratory infection or environmental exposures [6]. However, with the exception of smoking, an established risk factor of IPF, this remains to be substantiated.

In general, it seems that the ability of alveolar epithelial type 2 cells (AEC2) to restore damaged alveolar epithelial type 1 (AEC1) cells is seriously impaired [7]. The structural damage to the epithelial cell layer is thought to also affect the subepithelial and endothelial basement membranes [1]. Electron microscopy studies have shown that resident mesenchymal cells are found in close vicinity between the epithelial layer and pulmonary capillaries. These might be activated by cytokines that are secreted in a paracrine fashion and migrate through the damaged basement membranes [8]. The aberrant process of

Table 1. Profibrotic conditions and mediators

Underlying alveolar type 2 cell stress and injury
  Inherited mutations [2, 3]
    Surfactant proteins (SFTPA and SFTPC)
    ABCA3
    Telomerase/shelterin complex (TERT, TERC, PARN, RTEL1)
  Pro-apoptotic endoplasmic reticulum stress
    Cleaved ATF6, PERK-mediated activation of EIF2, IRE1α-mediated XBP1 splicing, CHOP, JNK
      and caspase 4/12 activation [20, 21, 26]
    Epstein–Barr virus latent membrane protein 1 [20]
  Lysosomal stress
    Amiodarone toxicity [130]
    Hermansky–Pudlak syndrome interstitial pneumonia [5]
Excessive fibroblast activation and collagen synthesis
  "Aggressive" fibroblast phenotype, characterised by thymocyte-1 antigen [37] C1q [39],
    transdifferentiation into myofibroblasts [32, 33] and extensive epigenetic changes via HDAC [34]
  Apoptosis resistance of fibroblasts mediated by:
    STAT-3 [45]
    SPARC-expression [46] and
    Low prostaglandin E2 [42, 43] as well as
    Low FoxO3 mediated by high Akt-activity [47]
  Contribution to the fibroblast pool by circulating fibrocytes [70]
  Extensive collagen synthesis via:
    Increased LOXL2 [76]
    Predominance of synthesis and deposition [77]
    Extracellular matrix remodelling [77]
  Activation of the TGF-β pathway via:
    Thrombin [13], PARs [131, 132] and other coagulation compounds
    Sphingosine-1-phosphate [13–15]
    LPA and LPARs [15–18]
  Other profibrotic signalling pathways such as CTGF [133], FGF [134], VEGF [135], IGF-1 [136]
    and endothelin-1 [137]
Concomitant inflammatory changes and responses
  Cytokines, chemokines:
    Low interferon-γ [100], IL-4, IL-13 and TGF-β [102–105], TGF-α [138]
    IL-1β [139], CXC ligand epithelial neutrophil activating protein 78 [140], MCP-1 [141],
      TNF-α [127]
  Alternative activation of macrophages [115]

SFTPA: surfactant specific protein A; SFTPC: surfactant specific protein C; ATF6: activating transcription factor 6; PERK: protein kinase RNA-like ER kinase; EIF2: eukaryotic translation initiation factor 2; XBP1: X-box binding protein 1; HDAC: histone deacetylase; LOXL2: lysyl oxidase-like 2; PAR: protease-activated receptor; LPA: lysophosphatidic acid; LPAR: LPA receptor; CTGF: connective tissue growth factor; FGF: fibroblast growth factor; IGF-1: insulin-like growth factor 1; IL: interleukin; MCP-1: monocyte chemoattractant protein-1; TNF: tumour necrosis factor.

---

re-epithelialisation is associated with an abnormal activation of Wnt signalling. The activation of the Wnt pathway causes an accumulation of β-catenin and activation of transcription factors of the lymphoid enhancing factor/T-cell factor family [9].

There is a large amount of data indicating that altered epithelial cells are responsible for the production of pro-fibrogenic growth factors and cytokines. In this context, the Krebs von den Lungen-6 antigen glycoprotein has been widely studied as a diagnostic and prognostic biomarker. It is a mucin-like glycoprotein and is expressed on the surface of AEC2 and bronchiolar epithelial cells [10]. It is linked to migration [11], survival [12] and proliferation of fibroblasts in IPF. It has been studied in many ILDs as a nonspecific marker of fibrosis.

AECs also express the integrin αVβ6, which has been identified as an activator of TGF-β1. TGF-β1 is complexed to latency-associated peptide, which interacts with the binding motifs RGD (arginine–glycine–aspartate). The liberation and activation of TGF-β is then triggered upon release from its latent complex. This process can be caused by different stimuli such as thrombin or sphingosine-1-phosphate [13–15]. Another pathway of TGF-β activation is triggered by lysophosphatidic acid (LPA) and its receptors (LPAR). The G-protein coupled LPAR2 induces a conformational change in the β-chain of αVβ6 resulting in TGF-β liberation. The signalling molecules involved include Galphaq (Gαq) and the Rho/Rac kinase [15]. LPAR2 deficient mice show protection against bleomycin-induced lung injury and fibrosis [16]. However, other LPARs such LPAR1 also promote fibrosis [16, 17]. The production of LPA is controlled by autotaxin, a lysophospholipase that converts lysophosphatidylcholine into LPA. The local delivery of autotaxin to sites of physical stress is mediated by binding to integrins with β1 or β3-chains [18]. Taken together, these observations implicate a local and tightly controlled TGF-β activation by physical forces.

ER stress in AEC2 is a primary stress reaction in IPF

The ER is an organelle of eukaryotic cells that forms a network of membrane structures, which are responsible for protein synthesis and lipid and carbohydrate metabolism. The ER stress response (ER stress) is seen in states of protein overexpression, altered redox state, increased calcium, metabolic deprivation and viral infection [19]. This type of stress response is seen in a variety of diseases and has also been linked to both familial and sporadic IPF (figure 1) [20, 21].

ER stress leads to the activation of the unfolded protein response (UPR). In order to restore normal cellular function the UPR inhibits protein translation and targets proteins for degradation to the proteasome, while increasing the production of chaperones that are involved in protein folding. If the cell is not able to restore the homeostasis between protein production and the capacity of the ER, a terminal pathway is activated that leads to cellular apoptosis. Chronic activation of the UPR has been linked most prominently to prion-associated neurodegenerative disease [22].

Three pathways are activated in response to ER stress to activate the UPR. The first pathway is the activating transcription factor 6 (ATF6). ATF6 is a transcription factor that stimulates the transcription of chaperones. It is activated by proteolytic cleavage in the presence of misfolded proteins. The cleaved cytosolic part of ATF6 can then move to the nucleus and act as a transcription factor [23]. The second pathway involves PERK (protein kinase RNA-like ER kinase), a kinase, which phosphorylates the alpha subunit of eukaryotic translation initiation factor 2 (EIF2). This inactivates EIF2 leading to a downregulation of general protein translation with the exception of proteins such as ATF4 [24]. The third factor is IRE1α. This protein has an ATP-binding pocket that acts as a trans-autophosphorylation kinase domain and an RNase domain responsible for an endonuclease activity. If activated, IRE1α oligomerises and splices the RNA of X-box binding protein 1 (XBP1) mRNA removing an intron. The spliced XBP1 mRNA is then translated into a functional transcription factor upregulating ER chaperones and endoplasmic reticulum associated degradation (ERAD) genes [25]. ERAD designates misfolded proteins for ubiquitination and subsequent degradation by the proteasome.

All of these pathways have been found to be activated in alveolar type 2 cells in IPF. Likewise the amounts of the cleaved form of ATF6 (p50ATF6), the transcription factor CHOP (DNA damage-inducible transcript 3 or C/EBP homologous protein), IRE1α and the chaperone BiP (binding immunoglobulin protein or HSP70) are increased [20, 21, 26]. This is paralleled by an accumulation of phosphorylated XBP1 and IRE1α.

Different trigger-factors for ER stress have been described. For instance the UPR may be activated by increased synthesis of viral proteins. This is suggested by the colocalisation of ER stress markers with the latent membrane protein 1 of Epstein–Barr virus [20]. Another initiating factor might be the production of misfolded surfactant proteins. As mentioned earlier, mutations of SFTPA and SFTPC have been identified in familial cases of IPF. In an experimental model of AECs expressing either the delta-exon4 or the L188Q mutation of SFTPC, markers of ER stress can be found such as spliced XBP1, phosphorylated EIF2α and increased levels of BiP and EDEM (ER degradation-enhancing α-mannosidase-like 1) [27–29]. For the heterozygous mutation of SFTPA-2, G231V and F198S, these variants undergo degradation *via* ERAD and induce ER stress in AECs, as demonstrated by increased levels of BiP and spliced XBP1. Interestingly, total SFTPA levels in familial cases of IPF with these mutations are not decreased, suggesting a direct role of ER stress rather than a lack of these surfactant proteins in these patients with IPF [30]. Of course, the exact role of these factors remains unclear as mutations of surfactant proteins are only rarely seen in IPF and results of the detection of viruses are inconsistent [31]. Therefore, other causes of ER stress have to be identified in IPF.

Mesenchymal cells execute the fibrotic response in IPF

In response to the epithelial injury, a plethora of signalling molecules lead to the activation of pulmonary fibroblasts, myofibroblast transdifferentiation and the production of extracellular matrix (ECM). To data, at least three pathways have been described for how the fibroblast pool in IPF can be activated and expand. One is mediated by direct action of growth factors such TGF-β on fibroblasts, another involves the transformation of local epithelial cells into fibroblasts (epithelial-to-mesenchymal transition (EMT)) and the third is the invasion of the lung by circulating fibrocytes (figure 1). Especially under the influence of TGF-β, phenotypic changes appear in fibroblasts, which resemble their transdifferentiation into myofibroblasts and result in the excessive production of type I collagen [32]. These changes represent the hallmark of lung fibrosis and result in the formation of the UIP-typical fibroblast foci. Besides TGF-β, and other growth factors such as connective tissue growth factor and platelet-derived growth factor (PDGF), other factors of differentiation are essential for this process such as myoD, a factor that commits mesoderm cells to a skeletal myoblast lineage, and the absence of fibroblast growth factor (FGF) [33]. Beside these factors of the local microenvironment, other changes such as the resistance to apoptosis and the migrating phenotype even persist in *in vitro* cultures of myofibroblasts of IPF patients, which could be ascribed to epigenetic changes [34].

Fibroblasts

In IPF, there is evidence that fibroblasts consist of different subpopulations with unique properties. One subset is characterised by the expression of the thymocyte-1 antigen (Thy1).

These Thy1 negative or positive fibroblasts are distinct with respect to their morphology, expression of surface markers and antigen presentation to T-lymphocytes, ECM production and cytokine release. Even when taken into culture their specific properties remain over time. Thy1 negative fibroblasts seem to play a role in chronic inflammation, as they present antigens to T-lymphocytes *via* major histocompatibility complex (MHC)-I and MHC-II [35, 36]. Thy1 negative fibroblasts show increased TGF-β activity and downstream signalling with consecutive expression of α-smooth muscle actin (SMA) upon stimulation with PDGF, interleukin (IL)-1, IL-4 and bleomycin in contrast to Thy1 positive fibroblasts [37]. Interestingly, the different proportions of Thy1 negative and positive fibroblasts seem to be associated with different propensity towards lung fibrosis in two rat strains [38].

Another characteristic subpopulation of fibroblasts is characterised by C1q expression. C1q is part of the complement fixation of immunoglobulin on cells. There are high and low C1q expressing fibroblasts [39]. These fibroblasts also exhibit differences in cell proliferation and type I collagen synthesis.

Taken together these results indicate that there are characteristic subpopulations of fibroblasts in pulmonary fibrosis. However, it remains unclear whether the observed differences in these subpopulations are induced by local factors in response to fibrosis or have a distinct role in the initiation of fibrosis.

One of the characteristics of fibroblasts in IPF is their augmented ability to proliferate [39–41]. Certain factors have been identified to be relevant in this context. Prostaglandin E2 (PGE2) suppresses T-cell receptor signalling and is believed to play a role in the resolution of inflammation. Fibroblasts in IPF produce less PGE2 and do not induce cyclooxygenase-2 (COX-2) upon stimulation with phorbol 12-myristate 13-acetate, lipopolysaccharide or IL-1. Furthermore, fibroblasts show increased resistance to PGE2 mediated apoptosis in IPF [42, 43].

Further mechanisms of resistance to apoptosis include survivin expression [44], an activation of STAT-3 [45] and SPARC-expression [46]. Another study showed the presence of inactive FoxO3 in fibroblast foci, an effect that is mediated by high activity of Akt, a negative regulator of FoxO3 [47].

Epithelial-to-mesenchymal transition

EMT is recognised to play a role in invasive tumour growth. Characteristically, epithelial cells loose epithelial markers such as zonula occludens-1 protein through this process, which is typical for polarised cells, and E-cadherin, which inhibits cellular mobility. Likewise, the cells gain myofibroblast or fibroblast markers such as α-SMA or fibroblast specific protein 1. There are numerous growth factors which endorse EMT under conditions of cancer such as hepatocyte growth factor, TGF-β, epidermal growth factor and FGF. In lung fibrosis, the TGF-β downstream signalling involves transcription factors of the Smad-family, which activate downstream gene transcription through snail family zinc finger 2, lymphoid enhancer-binding factor 1 (lef-1) and β-catenin [48]. EMT has also been described in models of renal fibrosis [49].

Myofibroblasts

Myofibroblasts synthesise considerably larger amounts of extracellular collagen fibres than fibroblasts [50–52]. Upon completion of wound healing, myofibroblasts typically undergo apoptosis, thus stopping the production of excessive ECM [53]. The collagen fibres interact with the myofibroblasts by integrin-mediated pulling and intracellular contraction leading to a concomitant alignment of fibres [50]. In the model of bleomycin lung injury, fibroblasts and myofibroblasts proliferate and expand. However, while the amount of fibroblasts diminishes after day 14, myofibroblasts positive for α-SMA and procollagen persist [52]. Another study demonstrated the presence of vimentin- and α-SMA-positive cells, but not desmin-positive cells, in fibroblastic foci. In these cells, the actin filaments were aligned in parallel with connection to fibronectin-containing fibrils (microtendons) [54]. In another study the targeted overexpression of the hyaluronan synthase 2 resulted in a more aggressive phenotype of bleomycin-induced lung injury which could be ameliorated by blockage of the hyaluronan receptor CD44 [55].

Myofibroblasts have contractile properties that can be inhibited by anti-inflammatory lipoxin A4 [56]. There is a relationship between the proportion of myofibroblasts and the contractile properties of fibroblast-populated culture of three-dimensional collagen gels, which is regulated by TGF-β [57]. TGF-β is also important for the induction of α-SMA [58]. The alveolar epithelium also interacts with mesenchymal cells and capillaries *via* bundles of microfilaments and SMA in the physiological state [59].

miRNA are small non-coding RNA molecules containing about 22 nucleotides that function in RNA silencing and regulation of gene expression. miRNA 21 has been found to be upregulated in IPF, this miRNA-family is also associated with certain types of cancers and is believed to promote myofibroblast growth and differentiation. By contrast, the miRNA family let-7 is downregulated, which might promote EMT. miRNAs are thought to increase signalling *via* TGF-β, Wnt, p52, sonic hedgehog and VEGF [60]. Other miRNAs have been found to have either profibrotic (miR-145, miR-154, miR-199a-5p) or antifibrotic properties (miR-326, miR-17~92-cluster) [61–65]. In addition, miRNAs may also affect ECM protein production. To this end, miR-29 has been shown to downregulate ECM targets while being downregulated itself in fibroblasts grown on IPF-derived ECM. Therefore, a positive feedback loop of altered ECM, miR-29 suppression and ECM synthesis has been proposed [66]. These results suggest that there is a role of post-transcriptional gene regulation in IPF fibroblasts and that the distinct features of the fibroblast-phenotype are related to this process.

Fibrocytes

Circulating fibrocytes might contribute to IPF by direct synthesis of ECM, undergoing a phenotypic change from fibrocytes into fibroblasts or myofibroblasts, or by the production of cytokines. Circulating fibrocytes are found in peripheral blood expressing type I collagen and haematopoietic markers CD34 or CD35 indicating their bone marrow derived origin [67–69]. Their potential relevance in IPF is underlined by their prognostic impact [70]. The recruitment of circulating fibrocytes might be mediated by the chemokine receptors CCR2 and CXCR4, while the alveolar epithelium expresses the corresponding ligands CCL2 and CXCL12. The pool of fibrocytes in the lung could therefore be expanded by the interaction of circulating fibrocytes with epithelial cells *via* CXCR4/CXCL12 or CCR2/CCL2 [71]. Furthermore, fibrocytes are a potential source of lung fibroblasts [72]. However, the concept of circulating fibrocytes in IPF is still under debate, mainly because human data are largely descriptive and experimental models have not always been reproducible.

Collagen homeostasis

One of the key features of IPF is the excess of ECM, mainly collagen, which is synthesised largely by myofibroblasts. Collagen is also the main type of ECM protein in healthy lungs and has important biophysical properties such as elastic recoil. Collagen proteins are composed of a triple helix consisting of two identical alpha 1 chains and a slightly different alpha 2 chain. Collagen types I and III are predominant in human lung and represent more than 90% of all collagen. These types of collagen are found in the interstitial space, the alveolus and in proximity to bronchovascular bundles [73]. Collagen is formed after processing the precursor, procollagen. Procollagen undergoes intracellular post-translational modification by hydroxylation of proline and lysine residues. These residues are important for later glycosylation and the creation of the triple-helical structure [74]. After secretion, membrane-bound collagen peptidases process the procollagen molecule to tropocollagen by removing the ends. The final step in collagen synthesis is performed by lysyl-oxidase, an extracellular enzyme. In this step lysine and hydroxylysine residues are oxidised to aldehyde groups undergoing covalent cross-linking (aldol reaction) between tropocollagen molecules to form the final collagen fibrils [75]. Out of the four lysyl oxidase homologs, LOXL2 seems to be an attractive therapeutic target in IPF, as it is associated with disease progression [76].

In wound healing, there is an increase of both collagen production and degradation after the initial injury. Collagen degradation is important to prevent the formation of permanent scar tissue. Free collagenolytic activity is present even in the fibrotic areas of IPF lungs, hence, there seems to be an imbalance of collagen production and degradation in IPF, with a predominance of collagen synthesis and deposition [77]. There are two routes for collagen degradation, one extracellular and one intracellular. The extracellular pathway involves proteolytic enzymes such as metalloproteinases. The intracellular pathway is characterised by phagocytosis and lysosomal degradation by fibroblasts and macrophages (reviewed in [78]). In mouse models of pulmonary fibrosis, inhibition of intracellular collagen degradation leads to pronounced fibrosis [79, 80].

In IPF, there is a differential role for the types of collagen. While collagen type I is typically found in areas of later stage fibrosis, in areas of early stage fibrosis collagen type III is predominantly found [81]. Overall, the number of fibroblasts producing collagen is clearly increased in IPF. However, these fibroblasts are typically grouped in clusters forming the fibroblast foci which are located directly under the epithelial layers of the injured lung [82].

Interestingly, the increased amounts of collagen synthesis are mainly a feature of fibroblast foci. While there is increased expression of type I procollagen in these areas, other areas show normal levels of procollagen expression [83]. This might explain why isolated human lung fibroblasts from patients with IPF or systemic sclerosis show a similar rate of collagen synthesis compared with controls [84]. These results suggest that collagen production is a variable process dependent on local factors and not the product of global fibroblast activation in IPF.

In addition, the ECM is pathologically remodelled in progressive IPF and may itself affect fibroblast activation. In this regard, matrix stiffness has been described as an inducer of the "aggressive" myofibroblast phenotype, with increased α-SMA and decreased COX-2 expression [85–87].

The unresolved issue of inflammation in IPF

In IPF, obvious signs of inflammation are easily observed: enlarged mediastinal lymph nodes and modest ground-glass opacity on the HRCT as well as recruitment of inflammatory cells such as neutrophils, eosinophils, lymphocytes and macrophages into the areas of injury on a histopathological level [88]. However, due to the lack of benefit of immunosuppressive agents in IPF [89, 90], the influence of inflammation on the process of fibrosis has been under debate for some time now [91]. During wound healing, an early inflammatory response is essential for the formation of matrix. TGF-β and IL-13 are in part produced by local inflammatory cells [92–95]. However, inflammatory cells may not only promote fibrosis, but may also have a resolving function in phagocytosis of excessive ECM, inhibition of proliferation and removal of apoptotic cells. These differential roles of inflammation are important for the different stages of wound healing, with an early profibrotic phase and a late antifibrotic phase. In this late phase, macrophages assist in the removal of fibroblasts [96], while regulatory T-cells secreting IL-10 downregulate local chemokine production and TGF-β [97]. This process inhibits further proliferation of fibroblasts. Taken together, these notions might explain why there is not a uniform role of inflammation in IPF and differential regulation of inflammation could also be part of future IPF therapy.

The three main forms of T-cell response, the T-helper cell (Th)1, Th2 and Th17 response, have been linked to the pathogenesis of IPF. The Th17 response is induced by TGF-β, IL-6, IL-21 and IL-23. These cells can have anti-inflammatory properties, which are mediated by IL-6 and TGF-β inducing specific regulatory T-cells (Treg17), as well as proinflammatory properties *via* IL-23 and IL-1β [98].

The type of T-cell response has implications for further recruitment of inflammatory cells, but also for the response of the local tissue. In asthmatics for instance, the inflammatory response triggered by allergens is typically associated with an increase of Th2 cytokines (IL-4, IL-5, IL-9, IL-13 and IL-31). However, in IPF, Th1 cytokines are also produced (IL-1α, IL-1β, tumour necrosis factor (TNF)-α, TGF-β and PDGF) [99]. In contrast, the levels of interferon-γ are diminished in IPF. Interferon-γ negatively regulates fibroblast growth and ECM synthesis [100], and supresses the Th2-response. Unfortunately, subcutaneous humanised interferon γ-1b did not improve outcome in IPF [101].

Certain cytokines are generally considered profibrotic such as IL-4, IL-13, and TGF-β as they activate fibroblasts and myofibroblasts [102–105].

Levels of IL-4 are elevated in different fibrotic states such as radiation-induced pulmonary fibrosis [106], liver fibrosis associated with schistosomiasis [107] and IPF [108, 109]. There is a direct role of IL-4 signalling on pulmonary fibroblasts, which exhibit IL-4 receptors, in positively regulating ECM production. Interestingly, IL-4 is a strong promoter of fibroblast proliferation and collagen synthesis [103]. IL-4 also induces the alternative activation of macrophages, which are characterised by the expression of Fizz-1 [110], arginase [111], Ym-1 [112] and mannose receptors [113]. Alternatively activated macrophages produce profibrotic cytokines such as TGF-β and PDGF, and play a role in collagen production [114]. Alternatively activated macrophages can be isolated from BALF in IPF patients [115]. Alternatively activated macrophages induce collagen production by isolated human fibroblasts in a CCL18-dependent manner. IL-4 further promotes the Th2 type of T-cell response, promoting the production of a number of other cytokines (IL-5, IL-9, IL-13 and IL-21). These Th2 cytokines propagate a further profibrotic response. For instance, eosinophils are recruited to the lung [116], which produce TGF-β in an IL-4 dependent manner [92]. IL-5 itself increases local production of IL-13, a potent promoter of fibrosis [117]. Mast cells are recruited to the lung by IL-9 and chymase from the mast cells increases TGF-β activity [118, 119]. Mast cells also mediate fibroblast proliferation and ECM production [120]. IL-21 has been found to be a positive regulator of IL-4/IL-13 receptor expression. In a mouse model of asthma-related airway fibrosis mediated by IL-13 fibrosis is diminished in the absence of IL-21-receptors [121]. For animal models of bleomycin-induced lung injury the absence of IL-13, but not IL-4, reduced collagen deposition [122, 123] and fluorescein isothiocyanate-induced pulmonary fibrosis [124]. Another study showed an increase in TGF-β production by fibroblasts in co-culture with human epithelial cells pre-treated with IL-13 [125]. Fibroblasts isolated from IPF patients demonstrate hyperresponsiveness to IL-13 [126]. These results suggest that there is a direct role of IL-13 in ECM production by fibroblasts and an indirect role in inducing a profibrotic milieu.

Studies on TNF-α expression in IPF have demonstrated increased levels of this cytokine. TNF-α increases the production of TGF-β and activates fibroblast proliferation and promotes collagen production [127]. In a rat model of pulmonary fibrosis, exogenous TNF-α enhances the fibrotic response while activating TGF-β and myofibroblasts [128]. However, in established fibrosis TNF-α might promote a faster resolution of fibrosis [129].

Implications for therapy

IPF is now thought to be a disease of recurrent alveolar epithelial cell injury. In response, alterations of the epithelial cell layer, the mesenchyme and the epithelial–mesenchymal cross-talk are seen and result in fibrosis. However, the exact injury remains hypothetical and may be diverse among patients. The identification of these factors will be difficult, yet necessary, as it is thought that the initial injury precedes symptomatic fibrosis by a long time. This might explain the failure of anti-inflammatory therapeutic concepts in IPF, to date, even if inflammatory triggers caused fibrosis. Once the precise triggers and methods for their early detection are known, epithelial-protective strategies may represent an interesting therapeutic avenue.

Up to this point, the best conceivable and currently widely followed strategy is to modify the fibrotic response itself. Therapies that influence fibroblast growth, excessive ECM production and cytokines have been approved or are under clinical investigation. Data on whether IPF truly is an irreversible disease are awaited, or whether combinations of treatments or novel treatment modalities yet to be identified may result in reversal of fibrosis, which to our understanding should be the ultimate treatment goal for this devastating disease.

References

1.   Hecker L, Thannickal VJ. Nonresolving fibrotic disorders: idiopathic pulmonary fibrosis as a paradigm of impaired tissue regeneration. *Am J Med Sci* 2011; 341: 431–434.
2.   Stuart BD, Choi J, Zaidi S, *et al.* Exome sequencing links mutations in PARN and RTEL1 with familial pulmonary fibrosis and telomere shortening. *Nat Genet* 2015; 47: 512–517.
3.   Kannengiesser C, Borie R, Ménard C, *et al.* Heterozygous RTEL1 mutations are associated with familial pulmonary fibrosis. *Eur Respir J* 2015; 46: 474–485.
4.   Garcia CK. Idiopathic pulmonary fibrosis: update on genetic discoveries. *Proc Am Thorac Soc* 2011; 8: 158–162.

5. Mahavadi P, Korfei M, Henneke I, *et al.* Epithelial stress and apoptosis underlie Hermansky-Pudlak syndrome-associated interstitial pneumonia. *Am J Respir Crit Care Med* 2010; 182: 207–219.

6. Lee SH, Kim DS, Kim YW, *et al.* Association between occupational dust exposure and prognosis of idiopathic pulmonary fibrosis: a Korean national survey. *Chest* 2015; 147: 465–474.

7. Kasper M, Haroske G. Alterations in the alveolar epithelium after injury leading to pulmonary fibrosis. *Histol Histopathol* 1996; 11: 463–483.

8. Chilosi M, Poletti V, Zamò A, *et al.* Aberrant Wnt/beta-catenin pathway activation in idiopathic pulmonary fibrosis. *Am J Pathol* 2003; 162: 1495–1502.

9. Königshoff M, Kramer M, Balsara N, *et al.* WNT1-inducible signaling protein-1 mediates pulmonary fibrosis in mice and is upregulated in humans with idiopathic pulmonary fibrosis. *J Clin Invest* 2009; 119: 772–787.

10. Bandoh S, Fujita J, Ohtsuki Y, *et al.* Sequential changes of KL-6 in sera of patients with interstitial pneumonia associated with polymyositis/dermatomyositis. *Ann Rheum Dis* 2000; 59: 257–262.

11. Hirasawa Y, Kohno N, Yokoyama A, *et al.* KL-6, a human MUC1 mucin, is chemotactic for human fibroblasts. *Am J Respir Cell Mol Biol* 1997; 17: 501–507.

12. Ohshimo S, Yokoyama A, Hattori N, *et al.* KL-6, a human MUC1 mucin, promotes proliferation and survival of lung fibroblasts. *Biochem Biophys Res Commun* 2005; 338: 1845–1852.

13. Jenkins RG, Su X, Su G, *et al.* Ligation of protease-activated receptor 1 enhances alpha(v)beta6 integrin-dependent TGF-β activation and promotes acute lung injury. *J Clin Invest* 2006; 116: 1606–1614.

14. Giacomini MM, Travis MA, Kudo M, *et al.* Epithelial cells utilize cortical actin/myosin to activate latent TGF-β through integrin α(v)β(6)-dependent physical force. *Exp Cell Res* 2012; 318: 716–722.

15. Xu MY, Porte J, Knox AJ, *et al.* Lysophosphatidic acid induces alphavbeta6 integrin-mediated TGF-beta activation *via* the LPA2 receptor and the small G protein G alpha(q). *Am J Pathol* 2009; 174: 1264–1279.

16. Huang LS, Fu P, Patel P, *et al.* Lysophosphatidic acid receptor-2 deficiency confers protection against bleomycin-induced lung injury and fibrosis in mice. *Am J Respir Cell Mol Biol* 2013; 49: 912–922.

17. Funke M, Zhao Z, Xu Y, *et al.* The lysophosphatidic acid receptor LPA1 promotes epithelial cell apoptosis after lung injury. *Am J Respir Cell Mol Biol* 2012; 46: 355–364.

18. Tabchy A, Tigyi G, Mills GB. Location, location, location: a crystal-clear view of autotaxin saturating LPA receptors. *Nat Struct Mol Biol* 2011; 18: 117–118.

19. Xu C, Bailly-Maitre B, Reed JC. Endoplasmic reticulum stress: cell life and death decisions. *J Clin Invest* 2005; 115: 2656–2664.

20. Lawson WE, Crossno PF, Polosukhin VV, *et al.* Endoplasmic reticulum stress in alveolar epithelial cells is prominent in IPF: association with altered surfactant protein processing and herpesvirus infection. *Am J Physiol Lung Cell Mol Physiol* 2008; 294: L1119–L1126.

21. Korfei M, Ruppert C, Mahavadi P, *et al.* Epithelial endoplasmic reticulum stress and apoptosis in sporadic idiopathic pulmonary fibrosis. *Am J Respir Crit Care Med* 2008; 178: 838–846.

22. Moreno JA, Halliday M, Molloy C, *et al.* Oral treatment targeting the unfolded protein response prevents neurodegeneration and clinical disease in prion-infected mice. *Sci Transl Med* 2013; 5: 206ra138.

23. Li M, Baumeister P, Roy B, *et al.* ATF6 as a transcription activator of the endoplasmic reticulum stress element: thapsigargin stress-induced changes and synergistic interactions with NF-Y and YY1. *Mol Cell Biol* 2000; 20: 5096–5106.

24. Koumenis C, Naczki C, Koritzinsky M, *et al.* Regulation of protein synthesis by hypoxia *via* activation of the endoplasmic reticulum kinase PERK and phosphorylation of the translation initiation factor eIF2alpha. *Mol Cell Biol* 2002; 22: 7405–7416.

25. Calfon M, Zeng H, Urano F, *et al.* IRE1 couples endoplasmic reticulum load to secretory capacity by processing the XBP-1 mRNA. *Nature* 2002; 415: 92–96.

26. Cha S, Ryerson CJ, Lee JS, *et al.* Cleaved cytokeratin-18 is a mechanistically informative biomarker in idiopathic pulmonary fibrosis. *Respir Res* 2012; 13: 105.

27. Bridges JP, Xu Y, Na CL, *et al.* Adaptation and increased susceptibility to infection associated with constitutive expression of misfolded SP-C. *J Cell Biol* 2006; 172: 395–407.

28. Lawson WE, Cheng DS, Degryse AL, *et al.* Endoplasmic reticulum stress enhances fibrotic remodeling in the lungs. *Proc Natl Acad Sci USA* 2011; 108: 10562–10567.

29. Tanjore H, Cheng DS, Degryse AL, *et al.* Alveolar epithelial cells undergo epithelial-to-mesenchymal transition in response to endoplasmic reticulum stress. *J Biol Chem* 2011; 286: 30972–30980.

30. Maitra M, Wang Y, Gerard RD, *et al.* Surfactant protein A2 mutations associated with pulmonary fibrosis lead to protein instability and endoplasmic reticulum stress. *J Biol Chem* 2010; 285: 22103–22113.

31. Kropski JA, Lawson WE, Blackwell TS. Right place, right time: the evolving role of herpesvirus infection as a "second hit" in idiopathic pulmonary fibrosis. *Am J Physiol Lung Cell Mol Physiol* 2012; 302: L441–L444.

32. Nakao A, Fujii M, Matsumura R, *et al.* Transient gene transfer and expression of Smad7 prevents bleomycin-induced lung fibrosis in mice. *J Clin Invest* 1999; 104: 5–11.

33. Xaubet A, Marin-Arguedas A, Lario S, *et al.* Transforming growth factor-beta1 gene polymorphisms are associated with disease progression in idiopathic pulmonary fibrosis. *Am J Respir Crit Care Med* 2003; 168: 431–435.

34. Korfei M, Skwarna S, Henneke I, et al. Aberrant expression and activity of histone deacetylases in sporadic idiopathic pulmonary fibrosis. *Thorax* 2015; 70: 1022–1032.

35. Phipps RP, Penney DP, Keng P, et al. Characterization of two major populations of lung fibroblasts: distinguishing morphology and discordant display of Thy 1 and class II MHC. *Am J Respir Cell Mol Biol* 1989; 1: 65–74.

36. Sempowski GD, Derdak S, Phipps RP. Interleukin-4 and interferon-gamma discordantly regulate collagen biosynthesis by functionally distinct lung fibroblast subsets. *J Cell Physiol* 1996; 167: 290–296.

37. Zhou Y, Hagood JS, Murphy-Ullrich JE. Thy-1 expression regulates the ability of rat lung fibroblasts to activate transforming growth factor-beta in response to fibrogenic stimuli. *Am J Pathol* 2004; 165: 659–669.

38. McIntosh JC, Hagood JS, Richardson TL, et al. Thy1 (+) and (−) lung fibrosis subpopulations in LEW and F344 rats. *Eur Respir J* 1994; 7: 2131–2138.

39. Akamine A, Raghu G, Narayanan AS. Human lung fibroblast subpopulations with different C1q binding and functional properties. *Am J Respir Cell Mol Biol* 1992; 6: 382–389.

40. Jordana M, Schulman J, McSharry C, et al. Heterogeneous proliferative characteristics of human adult lung fibroblast lines and clonally derived fibroblasts from control and fibrotic tissue. *Am Rev Respir Dis* 1988; 137: 579–584.

41. Raghu G, Chen YY, Rusch V, et al. Differential proliferation of fibroblasts cultured from normal and fibrotic human lungs. *Am Rev Respir Dis* 1988; 138: 703–708.

42. Wilborn J, Crofford LJ, Burdick MD, et al. Cultured lung fibroblasts isolated from patients with idiopathic pulmonary fibrosis have a diminished capacity to synthesize prostaglandin E2 and to express cyclooxygenase-2. *J Clin Invest* 1995; 95: 1861–1868.

43. Maher TM, Evans IC, Bottoms SE, et al. Diminished prostaglandin E2 contributes to the apoptosis paradox in idiopathic pulmonary fibrosis. *Am J Respir Crit Care Med* 2010; 182: 73–82.

44. Sisson TH, Maher TM, Ajayi IO, et al. Increased survivin expression contributes to apoptosis-resistance in IPF fibroblasts. *Adv Biosci Biotechnol* 2012; 3: 657–664.

45. Moodley YP, Scaffidi AK, Misso NL, et al. Fibroblasts isolated from normal lungs and those with idiopathic pulmonary fibrosis differ in interleukin-6/gp130-mediated cell signaling and proliferation. *Am J Pathol* 2003; 163: 345–354.

46. Chang W, Wei K, Jacobs SS, et al. SPARC suppresses apoptosis of idiopathic pulmonary fibrosis fibroblasts through constitutive activation of beta-catenin. *J Biol Chem* 2010; 285: 8196–8206.

47. Nho RS, Hergert P, Kahm J, et al. Pathological alteration of FoxO3a activity promotes idiopathic pulmonary fibrosis fibroblast proliferation on type i collagen matrix. *Am J Pathol* 2011; 179: 2420–2430.

48. Willis BC, du Bois RM, Borok Z. Epithelial origin of myofibroblasts during fibrosis in the lung. *Proc Am Thorac Soc* 2006; 3: 377–382.

49. Iwano M, Plieth D, Danoff TM, et al. Evidence that fibroblasts derive from epithelium during tissue fibrosis. *J Clin Invest* 2002; 110: 341–350.

50. Adler KB, Low RB, Leslie KO, et al. Contractile cells in normal and fibrotic lung. *Lab Invest* 1989; 60: 473–485.

51. Gabbiani G. Evolution and clinical implications of the myofibroblast concept. *Cardiovasc Res* 1998; 38: 545–548.

52. Zhang K, Rekhter MD, Gordon D, et al. Myofibroblasts and their role in lung collagen gene expression during pulmonary fibrosis. A combined immunohistochemical and *in situ* hybridization study. *Am J Pathol* 1994; 145: 114–125.

53. Thannickal VJ, Horowitz JC. Evolving concepts of apoptosis in idiopathic pulmonary fibrosis. *Proc Am Thorac Soc* 2006; 3: 350–356.

54. Kuhn C, McDonald JA. The roles of the myofibroblast in idiopathic pulmonary fibrosis. Ultrastructural and immunohistochemical features of sites of active extracellular matrix synthesis. *Am J Pathol* 1991; 138: 1257–1265.

55. Li Y, Jiang D, Liang J, et al. Severe lung fibrosis requires an invasive fibroblast phenotype regulated by hyaluronan and CD44. *J Exp Med* 2011; 208: 1459–1471.

56. Roach KM, Feghali-Bostwick CA, Amrani Y, et al. Lipoxin A4 attenuates constitutive and TGF-β1-dependent profibrotic activity in human lung myofibroblasts. *J Immunol* 2015; 195: 2852–2860.

57. Zhang HY, Gharaee-Kermani M, Zhang K, et al. Lung fibroblast alpha-smooth muscle actin expression and contractile phenotype in bleomycin-induced pulmonary fibrosis. *Am J Pathol* 1996; 148: 527–537.

58. Mitchell JJ, Woodcock-Mitchell JL, Perry L, et al. *In vitro* expression of the alpha-smooth muscle actin isoform by rat lung mesenchymal cells: regulation by culture condition and transforming growth factor-beta. *Am J Respir Cell Mol Biol* 1993; 9: 10–18.

59. Kapanci Y, Costabella PM, Cerutti P, et al. Distribution and function of cytoskeletal proteins in lung cells with particular reference to 'contractile interstitial cells'. *Methods Achiev Exp Pathol* 1979; 9: 147–168.

60. Pandit KV, Milosevic J, Kaminski N. MicroRNAs in idiopathic pulmonary fibrosis. *Transl Res* 2011; 157: 191–199.

61. Yang S, Cui H, Xie N, et al. miR-145 regulates myofibroblast differentiation and lung fibrosis. *FASEB J* 2013; 27: 2382–2391.

62. Milosevic J, Pandit K, Magister M, et al. Profibrotic role of miR-154 in pulmonary fibrosis. *Am J Respir Cell Mol Biol* 2012; 47: 879–887.

63. Lino Cardenas CL, Henaoui IS, Courcot E, *et al.* miR-199a-5p is upregulated during fibrogenic response to tissue injury and mediates TGFβ-induced lung fibroblast activation by targeting caveolin-1. *PLoS Genet* 2013; 9: e1003291.

64. Das S, Kumar M, Negi V, *et al.* MicroRNA-326 regulates profibrotic functions of transforming growth factor-β in pulmonary fibrosis. *Am J Respir Cell Mol Biol* 2014; 50: 882–892.

65. Dakhlallah D, Batte K, Wang Y, *et al.* Epigenetic regulation of miR-17~92 contributes to the pathogenesis of pulmonary fibrosis. *Am J Respir Crit Care Med* 2013; 187: 397–405.

66. Parker MW, Rossi D, Peterson M, *et al.* Fibrotic extracellular matrix activates a profibrotic positive feedback loop. *J Clin Invest* 2014; 124: 1622–1635.

67. Bucala R, Spiegel LA, Chesney J, *et al.* Circulating fibrocytes define a new leukocyte subpopulation that mediates tissue repair. *Mol Med* 1994; 1: 71–81.

68. Strieter RM, Keeley EC, Hughes MA, *et al.* The role of circulating mesenchymal progenitor cells (fibrocytes) in the pathogenesis of pulmonary fibrosis. *J Leukoc Biol* 2009; 86: 1111–1118.

69. Mehrad B, Burdick MD, Zisman DA, *et al.* Circulating peripheral blood fibrocytes in human fibrotic interstitial lung disease. *Biochem Biophys Res Commun* 2007; 353: 104–108.

70. Moeller A, Gilpin SE, Ask K, *et al.* Circulating fibrocytes are an indicator of poor prognosis in idiopathic pulmonary fibrosis. *Am J Respir Crit Care Med* 2009; 179: 588–594.

71. Ekert JE, Murray LA, Das AM, *et al.* Chemokine (C-C motif) ligand 2 mediates direct and indirect fibrotic responses in human and murine cultured fibrocytes. *Fibrogenesis Tissue Repair* 2011; 4: 23.

72. Andersson-Sjöland A, de Alba CG, Nihlberg K, *et al.* Fibrocytes are a potential source of lung fibroblasts in idiopathic pulmonary fibrosis. *Int J Biochem Cell Biol* 2008; 40: 2129–2140.

73. McAnulty RJ, Laurent GJ. Collagen synthesis and degradation *in vivo*. Evidence for rapid rates of collagen turnover with extensive degradation of newly synthesized collagen in tissues of the adult rat. *Coll Relat Res* 1987; 7: 93–104.

74. Myllylä R, Majamaa K, Günzler V, *et al.* Ascorbate is consumed stoichiometrically in the uncoupled reactions catalyzed by prolyl 4-hydroxylase and lysyl hydroxylase. *J Biol Chem* 1984; 259: 5403–5405.

75. Csiszar K. Lysyl oxidases: a novel multifunctional amine oxidase family. *Prog Nucleic Acid Res Mol Biol* 2001; 70: 1–32.

76. Chien JW, Richards TJ, Gibson KF, *et al.* Serum lysyl oxidase-like 2 levels and idiopathic pulmonary fibrosis disease progression. *Eur Respir J* 2014; 43: 1430–1438.

77. Nkyimbeng T, Ruppert C, Shiomi T, *et al.* Pivotal role of matrix metalloproteinase 13 in extracellular matrix turnover in idiopathic pulmonary fibrosis. *PLoS One* 2013; 8: e73279.

78. McKleroy W, Lee TH, Atabai K. Always cleave up your mess: targeting collagen degradation to treat tissue fibrosis. *Am J Physiol Lung Cell Mol Physiol* 2013; 304: L709–L721.

79. Atabai K, Jame S, Azhar N, *et al.* Mfge8 diminishes the severity of tissue fibrosis in mice by binding and targeting collagen for uptake by macrophages. *J Clin Invest* 2009; 119: 3713–3722.

80. Bundesmann MM, Wagner TE, Chow YH, *et al.* Role of urokinase plasminogen activator receptor-associated protein in mouse lung. *Am J Respir Cell Mol Biol* 2012; 46: 233–239.

81. Kaarteenaho-Wiik R, Pääkkö P, Herva R, *et al.* Type I and III collagen protein precursors and mRNA in the developing human lung. *J Pathol* 2004; 203: 567–574.

82. Kuhn C, Boldt J, King TE, *et al.* An immunohistochemical study of architectural remodeling and connective tissue synthesis in pulmonary fibrosis. *Am Rev Respir Dis* 1989; 140: 1693–1703.

83. Broekelmann TJ, Limper AH, Colby TV, *et al.* Transforming growth factor beta 1 is present at sites of extracellular matrix gene expression in human pulmonary fibrosis. *Proc Natl Acad Sci USA* 1991; 88: 6642–6646.

84. Raghu G, Masta S, Meyers D, *et al.* Collagen synthesis by normal and fibrotic human lung fibroblasts and the effect of transforming growth factor-beta. *Am Rev Respir Dis* 1989; 140: 95–100.

85. Booth AJ, Hadley R, Cornett AM, *et al.* Acellular normal and fibrotic human lung matrices as a culture system for *in vitro* investigation. *Am J Respir Crit Care Med* 2012; 186: 866–876.

86. Liu F, Mih JD, Shea BS, *et al.* Feedback amplification of fibrosis through matrix stiffening and COX-2 suppression. *J Cell Biol* 2010; 190: 693–706.

87. Marinković A, Liu F, Tschumperlin DJ. Matrices of physiologic stiffness potently inactivate idiopathic pulmonary fibrosis fibroblasts. *Am J Respir Cell Mol Biol* 2013; 48: 422–430.

88. Erjefält JS, Sundler F, Persson CG. Eosinophils, neutrophils, and venular gaps in the airway mucosa at epithelial removal-restitution. *Am J Respir Crit Care Med* 1996; 153: 1666–1674.

89. Davies HR, Richeldi L, Walters EH. Immunomodulatory agents for idiopathic pulmonary fibrosis. *Cochrane Database Syst Rev* 2003; 3: CD003134.

90. Richeldi L, Davies HR, Ferrara G, *et al.* Corticosteroids for idiopathic pulmonary fibrosis. *Cochrane Database Syst Rev* 2003; 3: CD002880.

91. Bringardner BD, Baran CP, Eubank TD, *et al.* The role of inflammation in the pathogenesis of idiopathic pulmonary fibrosis. *Antioxid Redox Signal* 2008; 10: 287–301.

92. Elovic AE, Ohyama H, Sauty A, et al. IL-4-dependent regulation of TGF-alpha and TGF-beta1 expression in human eosinophils. J Immunol 1998; 160: 6121–6127.

93. Minshall EM, Leung DY, Martin RJ, et al. Eosinophil-associated TGF-beta1 mRNA expression and airways fibrosis in bronchial asthma. Am J Respir Cell Mol Biol 1997; 17: 326–333.

94. Ohno I, Nitta Y, Yamauchi K, et al. Transforming growth factor beta 1 (TGF beta 1) gene expression by eosinophils in asthmatic airway inflammation. Am J Respir Cell Mol Biol 1996; 15: 404–409.

95. Zagai U, Dadfar E, Lundahl J, et al. Eosinophil cationic protein stimulates TGF-beta1 release by human lung fibroblasts in vitro. Inflammation 2007; 30: 153–160.

96. Moodley Y, Rigby P, Bundell C, et al. Macrophage recognition and phagocytosis of apoptotic fibroblasts is critically dependent on fibroblast-derived thrombospondin 1 and CD36. Am J Pathol 2003; 162: 771–779.

97. Nakagome K, Dohi M, Okunishi K, et al. In vivo IL-10 gene delivery attenuates bleomycin induced pulmonary fibrosis by inhibiting the production and activation of TGF-beta in the lung. Thorax 2006; 61: 886–894.

98. Zambrano-Zaragoza JF, Romo-Martínez EJ, Durán-Avelar Mde J, et al. Th17 cells in autoimmune and infectious diseases. Int J Inflam 2014; 2014: 651503.

99. Agostini C, Gurrieri C. Chemokine/cytokine cocktail in idiopathic pulmonary fibrosis. Proc Am Thorac Soc 2006; 3: 357–363.

100. Eickelberg O, Pansky A, Koehler E, et al. Molecular mechanisms of TGF-(beta) antagonism by interferon (gamma) and cyclosporine A in lung fibroblasts. FASEB J 2001; 15: 797–806.

101. Raghu G, Brown KK, Bradford WZ, et al. A placebo-controlled trial of interferon gamma-1b in patients with idiopathic pulmonary fibrosis. N Engl J Med 2004; 350: 125–133.

102. Fertin C, Nicolas JF, Gillery P, et al. Interleukin-4 stimulates collagen synthesis by normal and scleroderma fibroblasts in dermal equivalents. Cell Mol Biol 1991; 37: 823–829.

103. Sempowski GD, Beckmann MP, Derdak S, et al. Subsets of murine lung fibroblasts express membrane-bound and soluble IL-4 receptors. Role of IL-4 in enhancing fibroblast proliferation and collagen synthesis. J Immunol 1994; 152: 3606–3614.

104. Strutz F, Zeisberg M, Renziehausen A, et al. TGF-beta 1 induces proliferation in human renal fibroblasts via induction of basic fibroblast growth factor (FGF-2). Kidney Int 2001; 59: 579–592.

105. Wynn TA. IL-13 effector functions. Annu Rev Immunol 2003; 21: 425–456.

106. Büttner C, Skupin A, Reimann T, et al. Local production of interleukin-4 during radiation-induced pneumonitis and pulmonary fibrosis in rats: macrophages as a prominent source of interleukin-4. Am J Respir Cell Mol Biol 1997; 17: 315–325.

107. Booth M, Mwatha JK, Joseph S, et al. Periportal fibrosis in human Schistosoma mansoni infection is associated with low IL-10, low IFN-gamma, high TNF-alpha, or low RANTES, depending on age and gender. J Immunol 2004; 172: 1295–1303.

108. Emura M, Nagai S, Takeuchi M, et al. In vitro production of B cell growth factor and B cell differentiation factor by peripheral blood mononuclear cells and bronchoalveolar lavage T lymphocytes from patients with idiopathic pulmonary fibrosis. Clin Exp Immunol 1990; 82: 133–139.

109. Wallace WA, Ramage EA, Lamb D, et al. A type 2 (Th2-like) pattern of immune response predominates in the pulmonary interstitium of patients with cryptogenic fibrosing alveolitis (CFA). Clin Exp Immunol 1995; 101: 436–441.

110. Liu T, Jin H, Ullenbruch M, et al. Regulation of found in inflammatory zone 1 expression in bleomycin-induced lung fibrosis: role of IL-4/IL-13 and mediation via STAT-6. J Immunol 2004; 173: 3425–3431.

111. Pauleau A, Rutschman R, Lang R, et al. Enhancer-mediated control of macrophage-specific arginase I expression. J Immunol 2004; 172: 7565–7573.

112. Lee E, Yook J, Haa K, et al. Induction of Ym1/2 in mouse bone marrow-derived mast cells by IL-4 and identification of Ym1/2 in connective tissue type-like mast cells derived from bone marrow cells cultured with IL-4 and stem cell factor. Immunol Cell Biol 2005; 83: 468–474.

113. Martinez-Pomares L, Reid DM, Brown GD, et al. Analysis of mannose receptor regulation by IL-4, IL-10, and proteolytic processing using novel monoclonal antibodies. J Leukoc Biol 2003; 73: 604–613.

114. Hesse M, Modolell M, La Flamme AC, et al. Differential regulation of nitric oxide synthase-2 and arginase-1 by type 1/type 2 cytokines in vivo: granulomatous pathology is shaped by the pattern of L-arginine metabolism. J Immunol 2001; 167: 6533–6544.

115. Prasse A, Pechkovsky DV, Toews GB, et al. A vicious circle of alveolar macrophages and fibroblasts perpetuates pulmonary fibrosis via CCL18. Am J Respir Crit Care Med 2006; 173: 781–792.

116. Takatsu K, Nakajima H. IL-5 and eosinophilia. Curr Opin Immunol 2008; 20: 288–294.

117. Reiman RM, Thompson RW, Feng CG, et al. Interleukin-5 (IL-5) augments the progression of liver fibrosis by regulating IL-13 activity. Infect Immun 2006; 74: 1471–1479.

118. Eklund KK, Ghildyal N, Austen KF, et al. Induction by IL-9 and suppression by IL-3 and IL-4 of the levels of chromosome 14-derived transcripts that encode late-expressed mouse mast cell proteases. J Immunol 1993; 151: 4266–4273.

119. Tomimori Y, Muto T, Saito K, *et al.* Involvement of mast cell chymase in bleomycin-induced pulmonary fibrosis in mice. *Eur J Pharmacol* 2003; 478: 179–185.

120. Garbuzenko E, Nagler A, Pickholtz D, *et al.* Human mast cells stimulate fibroblast proliferation, collagen synthesis and lattice contraction: a direct role for mast cells in skin fibrosis. *Clin Exp Allergy* 2002; 32: 237–246.

121. Fröhlich A, Marsland BJ, Sonderegger I, *et al.* IL-21 receptor signaling is integral to the development of Th2 effector responses *in vivo*. *Blood* 2007; 109: 2023–2031.

122. Belperio JA, Dy M, Burdick MD, *et al.* Interaction of IL-13 and C10 in the pathogenesis of bleomycin-induced pulmonary fibrosis. *Am J Respir Cell Mol Biol* 2002; 27: 419–427.

123. Jakubzick C, Choi ES, Joshi BH, *et al.* Therapeutic attenuation of pulmonary fibrosis *via* targeting of IL-4- and IL-13-responsive cells. *J Immunol* 2003; 171: 2684–2693.

124. Kolodsick JE, Toews GB, Jakubzick C, *et al.* Protection from fluorescein isothiocyanate-induced fibrosis in IL-13-deficient, but not IL-4-deficient, mice results from impaired collagen synthesis by fibroblasts. *J Immunol* 2004; 172: 4068–4076.

125. Malavia NK, Mih JD, Raub CB, *et al.* IL-13 induces a bronchial epithelial phenotype that is profibrotic. *Respir Res* 2008; 9: 27.

126. Murray LA, Argentieri RL, Farrell FX, *et al.* Hyper-responsiveness of IPF/UIP fibroblasts: interplay between TGFβ1, IL-13 and CCL2. *Int J Biochem Cell Biol* 2008; 40: 2174–2182.

127. Ortiz LA, Lasky J, Lungarella G, *et al.* Upregulation of the p75 but not the p55 TNF-alpha receptor mRNA after silica and bleomycin exposure and protection from lung injury in double receptor knockout mice. *Am J Respir Cell Mol Biol* 1999; 20: 825–833.

128. Sime PJ, Marr RA, Gauldie D, *et al.* Transfer of tumor necrosis factor-alpha to rat lung induces severe pulmonary inflammation and patchy interstitial fibrogenesis with induction of transforming growth factor-beta1 and myofibroblasts. *Am J Pathol* 1998; 153: 825–832.

129. Redente EF, Keith RC, Janssen W, *et al.* Tumor necrosis factor-α accelerates the resolution of established pulmonary fibrosis in mice by targeting profibrotic lung macrophages. *Am J Respir Cell Mol Biol* 2014; 50: 825–837.

130. Mahavadi P, Henneke I, Ruppert C, *et al.* Altered surfactant homeostasis and alveolar epithelial cell stress in amiodarone-induced lung fibrosis. *Toxicol Sci* 2014; 142: 285–297.

131. Bardou O, Menou A, François C, *et al.* Membrane-anchored serine protease matriptase is a trigger of pulmonary fibrogenesis. *Am J Respir Crit Care Med* 2015 [in press; DOI: 10.1164/rccm.201502-0299OC].

132. Wygrecka M, Kwapiszewska G, Jablonska E, *et al.* Role of protease-activated receptor-2 in idiopathic pulmonary fibrosis. *Am J Respir Crit Care Med* 2011; 183: 1703–1714.

133. Leask A, Abraham DJ. The role of connective tissue growth factor, a multifunctional matricellular protein, in fibroblast biology. *Biochem Cell Biol* 2003; 81: 355–363.

134. Wollin L, Wex E, Pautsch A, *et al.* Mode of action of nintedanib in the treatment of idiopathic pulmonary fibrosis. *Eur Respir J* 2015; 45: 1434–1445.

135. Ando M, Miyazaki E, Ito T, *et al.* Significance of serum vascular endothelial growth factor level in patients with idiopathic pulmonary fibrosis. *Lung* 2010; 188: 247–252.

136. Krein PM, Winston BW. Roles for insulin-like growth factor I and transforming growth factor-beta in fibrotic lung disease. *Chest* 2002; 122: 289S–293S.

137. Ross B, D'Orléans-Juste P, Giaid A. Potential role of endothelin-1 in pulmonary fibrosis: from the bench to the clinic. *Am J Respir Cell Mol Biol* 2010; 42: 16–20.

138. Madala SK, Korfhagen TR, Schmidt S, *et al.* Inhibition of the αvβ6 integrin leads to limited alteration of TGF-α-induced pulmonary fibrosis. *Am J Physiol Lung Cell Mol Physiol* 2014; 306: L726–L735.

139. Wilson MS, Madala SK, Ramalingam TR, *et al.* Bleomycin and IL-1beta-mediated pulmonary fibrosis is IL-17A dependent. *J Exp Med* 2010; 207: 535–552.

140. Keane MP, Donnelly SC, Belperio JA, *et al.* Imbalance in the expression of CXC chemokines correlates with bronchoalveolar lavage fluid angiogenic activity and procollagen levels in acute respiratory distress syndrome. *J Immunol* 2002; 169: 6515–6521.

141. Moore BB, Paine R, Christensen PJ, *et al.* Protection from pulmonary fibrosis in the absence of CCR2 signaling. *J Immunol* 2001; 167: 4368–4377.

Disclosures: B. Loeh reports personal fees from Boehringer Ingelheim, outside the submitted work. A. Günther reports personal fees from Actelion, Roche, Pfizer, Novartis and Boehringer Ingelheim for board membership and from Nycomed and Activero for consultancy; all outside the submitted work.

Chapter 4

Key diagnostic issues

Dominique Valeyre[1,2], Florence Jeny[1,2], Olivia Freynet[1] and
Hilario Nunes[1,2]

Early and accurate IPF diagnosis is essential in order to offer patients the best treatment. The 2011 guidelines significantly improved IPF diagnosis. The diagnosis relies, in a specific context, on either a UIP pattern on CT or the combination of adequate CT and pathological findings after a multidisciplinary discussion. The diagnosis may remain difficult due to: unclear honeycombing on CT; unclear pathology; discrepancies between CT and pathology; possible confusion with UIP secondary to a known cause; and surgical lung biopsy contraindicated when it is indispensable. In difficult cases the diagnosis might be supported by taking into account age, subtle CT findings, BAL, transbronchial cryobiopsy results or the observed behaviour of the disease. Advances in the near future may stem from new biomarkers, which might overhaul the diagnosis and even lead to more personalised medicine. An important challenge will be to shorten the delay between initial symptoms and confirmed IPF diagnosis.

IPF is the most frequent entity among IIPs [1]. It belongs to the "chronic fibrosing IIP" category [1]. Improvements in diagnosis have stemmed from advances in CT and pathology interpretation, and the contribution of multidisciplinary discussions involving clinicians, radiologists and pathologists. All these elements have been extensively detailed in the American Thoracic Society (ATS)/European Respiratory Society (ERS)/Japanese Respiratory Society (JRS)/Latin American Thoracic Association (ALAT) guidelines [2]. These new guidelines impacted on IPF diagnosis in a significant proportion of cases in comparison to the previous guidelines [3, 4]. Although the diagnosis of IPF or not IPF may often be confirmed with a high level of confidence, it may remain difficult to diagnose in up to 25–50% of patients for different reasons, which are the focus of this chapter and include a low level of interobserver agreement for CT or pathology, flagrant discrepancies between their findings, or a surgical lung biopsy contraindicated despite indispensable for a confident diagnosis. The agreement between multidisciplinary discussion teams has not yet been explored. Moreover, some other points may still be a subject of controversy, for example: in what context might BAL be helpful for diagnosis?; and what is the threshold below which occupational or environmental exposures can definitely be ruled out as inducing a true occupational or environmental fibrosis (a situation not uncommon in clinical practice)?

[1]Assistance publique hôpitaux de Paris, Hôpital Avicenne, Bobigny, France. [2]Université Paris 13, COMUE Université Sorbonne Paris Cité, Bobigny, France.

Correspondence: Dominique Valeyre, Assistance publique hôpitaux de Paris, Hôpital Avicenne, 125 rue de Stalingrad, 93009 Bobigny, France. E-mail: Dominique.valeyre@aphp.fr

Until 2012, the therapeutic consequences of making a correct diagnosis of IPF were limited since therapeutic options between IPF and other IIPs, mainly NSIP, were not very different. However, since 2012, an early and accurate diagnosis of IPF has been crucial due to two major findings: 1) corticosteroids and immunosuppressive drugs were shown to be harmful in IPF and have to be avoided [5]; and 2) specific antifibrotic drugs (pirfenidone and nintedanib) were shown to be efficient for slowing down IPF progression, and these drugs may be offered to treat patients with IPF [6–9].

The rapid advances in the pathogenetic knowledge and the emergence of valuable new biomarkers may radically transform diagnostic practice in the near future, allowing for more personalised medical practice [10].

In this chapter, we will mainly focus on current clinical practice and then consider possible future evolutions. After a short reminder of the diagnostic criteria according to the 2011 ATS/ERS/JRS/ALAT guidelines [2] we will consider what constitutes a grey area when a diagnosis of IPF is not definitely confirmed or excluded (figure 1). Only an initial positive diagnosis of IPF will be considered here and not the diagnostic problems that may arise during the course of IPF.

Contribution of the 2011 ATS/ERS/JRS/ALAT guidelines

The 2011 guidelines significantly improved the way a diagnosis of IPF is made as the criteria were simplified [2, 4]. The diagnosis of IPF relies, in a specific clinical context, on either a UIP pattern on CT or, in patients without a UIP pattern on CT, the conjunction of adequate CT and pathological findings after a multidisciplinary discussion. CT and pathological signs were pedagogically included in boxes, thus classifying presentations from high probability (UIP pattern including all typical signs) to low probability (inconsistent with UIP pattern with signs suggesting an alternative diagnosis). Then, for patients needing both CT and pathology, the guidelines included a table combining the probabilities for UIP on CT and pathology, and proposed a final IPF diagnosis probability [2]. A multidisciplinary discussion

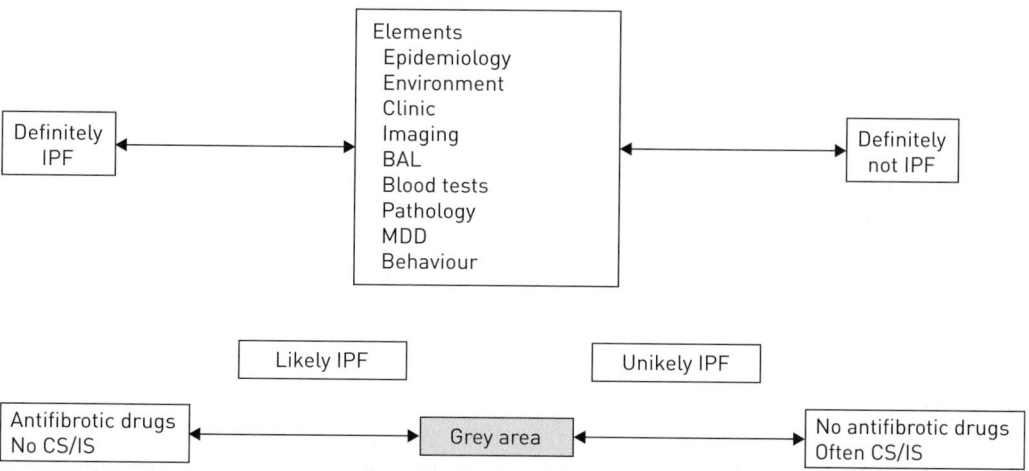

Figure 1. IPF diagnosis: the "grey area" and therapeutic consequences. The pro and con elements for IPF diagnosis are listed. MDD: multidisciplinary discussion; CS: corticosteroid; IS: immunosuppressants.

took place to determine whether the final diagnosis is or is not IPF. This approach was also very helpful in deciphering all steps leading to diagnosis and for unveiling the limitations of the guidelines.

Schematically, the limitations arise from cases for which some diagnostic elements are in a grey area: possible alternative diagnosis, particularly when occupational or environmental causes may be considered; difficult interpretation of CT, pathology or the conjunction of both; and cases for which CT or pathology do not precisely fit in boxes.

Differential diagnosis of UIP

A UIP pattern on either CT or pathology is not sufficient for diagnosing IPF [11]. The clinician has to exclude any UIP secondary to a known cause. That is easy when a cause is obvious or definitely absent according to the clinical history and clinical and paramedical investigations. However, many patients with IPF have been exposed, at a variable level, to different potentially harmful aerocontaminants or drugs. It is not always easy to accurately assess the level of exposure of an individual and compare it to a validated threshold, if there is one. Thus, differentiating true IPF from occupational or environmental diseases may be difficult. Moreover, the relationship between exposure to aerocontaminants and lung impact is not always very simple. Considering exposure to asbestos, three situations have been described and it is not always easy to determine the correct situation for individual patients: 1) typical asbestosis [12]; 2) true IPF in asbestos workers [13]; or 3) IPF impacted by exposure to aerocontaminants [14]. Sometimes exposure to asbestos is not known or appears minimal; however, an adequate search for asbestos bodies in lung specimens may lead to the clear diagnosis of asbestosis where an initial diagnosis of typical IPF had been made without dedicated mineralogical study [15]. Clinical signs may be helpful for some secondary UIP, for example, inspiratory squeaks or fever (favouring hypersensitivity pneumonitis), or systemic signs that may appear at a secondary level behind respiratory manifestations or may be delayed. CT may help consider alternative hypotheses: air trapping, centrilobular micronodules, upper predominance, or bridging which suggests hypersensitivity pneumonitis while pleural thickening or calcifications may favour asbestosis. Eventually, pathology may also indicate subtle signs that suggest either hypersensitivity pneumonitis [16], asbestosis (a lower level of inflammation although limited in IPF and a lower number of fibroblastic foci) [12], or connective tissue disease. Connective tissue disease-UIP may be indistinguishable from IPF when systemic manifestations are delayed. Secondary UIP may closely mimic IPF and very often, depending on the insufficient experience of some physicians in the ILD domain, a diagnosis of IPF may lead to the correct diagnosis being overlooked. In this chapter we will only mention the necessity of a systematic search for a familial fibrosis and a clinical or biological presentation compatible with a telomeropathy.

CT interpretation and interobserver agreement

CT has a long proven, high diagnostic specificity of 90–100% with a typical presentation [17]. Three levels of probability for IPF have been defined according to CT: UIP pattern, possible UIP pattern and inconsistent with UIP pattern. Four features are required to constitute a UIP pattern on CT: 1) subpleural and basal predominance; 2) reticular abnormality; 3) honeycombing with or without traction bronchiectasis; and 4) absence of features listed as inconsistent for UIP pattern [2, 18]. In possible UIP pattern, the evidence of typical honeycombing is lacking while in inconsistent with UIP pattern one of seven features inconsistent with UIP pattern and suggesting an alternative diagnosis is present. Evidence of typical honeycombing is a strong predictor of UIP [17], even though some disagreements concerning its imaging features remain [18]. Recently, some authors have customised a new CT probable UIP pattern category which might be highly predictive of UIP at pathology [19]. Differentiating honeycombing from traction bronchiectasis or emphysema may be particularly challenging even among radiologists and clinicians who are experts in the field of ILDs, as shown by the low level of interobserver agreement for the most difficult cases [20]. The sensitivity of CT for diagnosing IPF is significantly lower, estimated at ~50%. Finally, CT is not reliable for excluding UIP [21]. It is noteworthy that patients with an inconsistent UIP pattern may have UIP.

Pathology interpretation and interobserver agreement

KATZENSTEIN *et al.* [22] were the first to differentiate a UIP pattern from the NSIP pattern. In the 2011 ATS/ERS/JRS/ALAT guidelines [2], four levels of probability were considered at pathology: 1) UIP pattern; 2) probable UIP pattern; 3) possible UIP pattern; and 4) not UIP pattern. The UIP pattern was defined by the combination of evidence: 1) of fibrosis/architectural distortion±honeycombing in a predominantly subpleural/paraseptal distribution; 2) presence of patchy involvement of the lung parenchyma due to fibrosis; 3) presence of fibrotic foci; and 4) absence of features against a diagnosis of UIP and suggesting an alternative diagnosis. Although pathology has long been the gold standard for diagnosing IPF, evidence of a histopathological UIP pattern *per se* is not sufficient for diagnosing IPF. Pathological findings have to be interpreted by taking into account CT findings in a specific clinical setting. Moreover, the interobserver agreement level among pathologists is often low, as reported by some studies [23].

Multidisciplinary discussion

The benefits of multidisciplinary discussion involving a clinician, radiologist and pathologist have been reported previously [24–26]. Multidisciplinary discussion is now considered a standard for IPF diagnosis. The task of the multidisciplinary discussion team is ambitious and aims to: 1) estimate whether a diagnosis of IPF is reached or not before a surgical lung biopsy; 2) specify if a surgical lung biopsy is required for diagnosis and if it is feasible determine the best locations for biopsy specimens to be taken; 3) estimate if a diagnosis of IPF is met or excluded once the surgical biopsy has been performed; and 4) eventually plan the best treatment. Sometimes, the diagnostic input of an internist or rheumatologist involved in connective tissue disease, or a physician specialising in occupational or environmental diseases may also be helpful [24].

The place of BAL in diagnosing IPF

BAL may offer subtle information in some specific circumstances. For example, the extra value of BAL is very limited in typical UIP in patients for whom no alternative diagnosis of IPF is to be considered. However, BAL may be useful when alternative diagnoses are to be considered, such as hypersensitivity pneumonitis with a significant lymphocytosis [27], asbestosis for searching asbestos bodies [28] or even for considering fibrosing sarcoidosis in the case of a UIP pattern on CT [29]. Thus, BAL may be useful for differential diagnosis and helps, in some cases, to avoid unnecessary surgical biopsy.

Acute exacerbations of IPF

This chapter has only focused on initial diagnosis. Despite an acute exacerbation may rise *per se* diagnosis problems, it usually represents more an event during the course of a recognised IPF than a revealing manifestation of IPF [30, 31]. However, when an acute exacerbation occurs as the first manifestation of IPF the diagnosis can be supported by reviewing, when they are available, prior thoracic or abdominal CT when honeycombing can be seen *a posteriori*.

Delay in diagnosis

An early diagnosis of IPF greatly improves disease's prognosis. At present, the delay between initial symptoms and a final diagnosis of IPF is too long. All too frequently this delay reaches ⩾24 months. Several factors contribute to this delay: 1) the trivialisation of symptoms, such as persistent cough or dyspnoea, are too often attributed to smoking habits or age; and 2) when faced with symptoms of dyspnoea, general practitioners initially consider chronic heart failure or COPD and often overlook the hypothesis of IPF. General practitioners all too often do not consider IPF in the gamut of diagnoses in the presence of crackles. Doctors are often unaware of drugs that are efficient in slowing the course of IPF. In order to shorten the delay in diagnosis we must educate general practitioners and make general radiologists aware of the systematic research signs indicative of ILD on CT, whether CT is performed for cancer screening or other reasons (including CT for abdominal symptoms) as lung bases can often be analysed. Finally, familial history screening and searching for indices in favour of telomeropathies may make an earlier diagnosis possible in some patients.

Means and perspectives to improve diagnosis

Available tools

In 2010, FELL *et al.* [32] showed that combining age with CT might help specify the probability of a diagnosis of IPF in patients with compatible but not definite CT. This study suggested that for patients >70 years of age IPF was highly probable in this setting. Nevertheless, this very interesting study was conducted in a population for which biases could not be excluded and needs to be confirmed in further studies. Promoting screening for IPF as a "by-product" during HRCT for cancer screening strategies in smokers may help lead to diagnosis at a very early stage [33].

A significant or marginal decline of FVC has been shown to be more frequent at 6 months in IPF than in NSIP, indicating that the evidence of a confirmed short-term decline in some difficult contexts might be an extra element to take into account for diagnosis [34]. In patients who are difficult to classify, a classification based on observed disease behaviour may be very helpful [1]. Even though some validation is needed for this behavioural classification, it could help identify cases of IPF that are difficult to confirm, particularly for older people for whom surgical biopsy cannot reasonably be proposed. Transbronchial lung cryobiopsy is also a safe tool for obtaining pathological samples for IPF diagnosis when surgery appears excessively harmful in fragile patients or for those who prefer this option rather than surgery [35].

Tools for the future

For now, IPF is still mainly identified by morphological features (either radiological or pathological) in a specific clinical setting. The cause of IPF is still unknown and IPF could represent a common pathological reaction to various harmful agents. To date, only a few risk factors have been identified. It may be expected that new biological tools will help to accurately identify IPF, particularly from noninvasive sources such as blood specimens, evidencing a blood signature of the disease [10, 36]. Moreover, several elements converge to suggest that IPF presentation might be impacted by some predisposing factors, such as some polymorphisms leading to possible different behavioural responses to drugs, and that a more personalised medicine will be the rule in the near future for IPF.

Conclusion

Simplifications and clarifications of the 2011 guidelines have been an important step in improving IPF diagnosis. However, IPF diagnosis is still very challenging. The delay in diagnosis is excessively long and the diagnosis is still difficult for an important proportion of patients. Since an early and confident diagnosis is indispensable for improving the prognosis of this severe disease, there is an imperious necessity to improve the education of physicians from general practitioners, to radiologists and pulmonologists, as well as the population at large.

References

1. Travis WD, Costabel U, Hansell DM, *et al.* An official American Thoracic Society/European Respiratory Society statement: Update of the international multidisciplinary classification of the idiopathic interstitial pneumonias. *Am J Respir Crit Care Med* 2013; 188: 733–748.
2. Raghu G, Collard HR, Egan JJ, *et al.* An Official ATS/ERS/JRS/ALAT statement: idiopathic pulmonary fibrosis: evidence-based guidelines for diagnosis and management. *Am J Respir Crit Care Med* 2011; 183: 788–824.
3. Fidler L, Shapera S, Mittoo S, *et al.* Diagnostic disparity of previous and revised American Thoracic Society guidelines for idiopathic pulmonary fibrosis. *Can Respir J* 2015; 22: 86–90.
4. American Thoracic Society. Idiopathic pulmonary fibrosis: diagnosis and treatment. International consensus statement. American Thoracic Society (ATS), and the European Respiratory Society (ERS). *Am J Respir Crit Care Med* 2000; 161: 646–664.
5. Idiopathic Pulmonary Fibrosis Clinical Research Network, Raghu G, Anstrom KJ, *et al.* Prednisone, azathioprine, and N-acetylcysteine for pulmonary fibrosis. *N Engl J Med* 2012; 366: 1968–1977.
6. Noble PW, Albera C, Bradford WZ, *et al.* Pirfenidone in patients with idiopathic pulmonary fibrosis (CAPACITY): two randomised trials. *Lancet* 2011; 377: 1760–1769.
7. Richeldi L, Costabel U, Selman M, *et al.* Efficacy of a tyrosine kinase inhibitor in idiopathic pulmonary fibrosis. *N Engl J Med* 2011; 365: 1079–1087.
8. Richeldi L, du Bois RM, Raghu G, *et al.* Efficacy and safety of nintedanib in idiopathic pulmonary fibrosis. *N Engl J Med* 2014; 370: 2071–2082.
9. King TE Jr, Noble PW, Bradford WZ. Treatments for idiopathic pulmonary fibrosis. *N Engl J Med* 2014; 371: 783–784.
10. Spagnolo P, Tzouvelekis A, Maher TM. Personalized medicine in idiopathic pulmonary fibrosis: facts and promises. *Curr Opin Pulm Med* 2015; 21: 470–478.
11. Wuyts WA, Cavazza A, Rossi G, *et al.* Differential diagnosis of usual interstitial pneumonia: when is it truly idiopathic? *Eur Respir Rev* 2014; 23: 308–319.

12. Roggli VL, Gibbs AR, Attanoos R, *et al.* Pathology of asbestosis – an update of the diagnostic criteria: report of the asbestosis committee of the college of american pathologists and pulmonary pathology society. *Arch Pathol Lab Med* 2010; 134: 462–480.

13. Gaensler EA, Jederlinic PJ, Churg A. Idiopathic pulmonary fibrosis in asbestos-exposed workers. *Am Rev Respir Dis* 1991; 144: 689–696.

14. Lee SH, Kim DS, Kim YW, *et al.* Association between occupational dust exposure and prognosis of idiopathic pulmonary fibrosis: a Korean national survey. *Chest* 2015; 147: 465–474.

15. Monsó E, Tura JM, Pujadas J, *et al.* Lung dust content in idiopathic pulmonary fibrosis: a study with scanning electron microscopy and energy dispersive x ray analysis. *Br J Ind Med* 1991; 48: 327–331.

16. Morell F, Villar A, Montero MÁ, *et al.* Chronic hypersensitivity pneumonitis in patients diagnosed with idiopathic pulmonary fibrosis: a prospective case-cohort study. *Lancet Respir Med* 2013; 1: 685–694.

17. Hunninghake GW, Lynch DA, Galvin JR, *et al.* Radiologic findings are strongly associated with a pathologic diagnosis of usual interstitial pneumonia. *Chest* 2003; 124: 1215–1223.

18. Devaraj A. Imaging: how to recognise idiopathic pulmonary fibrosis. *Eur Respir Rev* 2014; 23: 215–219.

19. Chung JH, Chawla A, Peljto AL, *et al.* CT scan findings of probable usual interstitial pneumonitis have a high predictive value for histologic usual interstitial pneumonitis. *Chest* 2015; 147: 450–459.

20. Watadani T, Sakai F, Johkoh T, *et al.* Interobserver variability in the CT assessment of honeycombing in the lungs. *Radiology* 2013; 266: 936–944.

21. Sverzellati N, Wells AU, Tomassetti S, *et al.* Biopsy-proved idiopathic pulmonary fibrosis: spectrum of nondiagnostic thin-section CT diagnoses. *Radiology* 2010; 254: 957–964.

22. Katzenstein AL, Mukhopadhyay S, Myers JL. Diagnosis of usual interstitial pneumonia and distinction from other fibrosing interstitial lung diseases. *Hum Pathol* 2008; 39: 1275–1294.

23. Thomeer M, Demedts M, Behr J, *et al.* Multidisciplinary interobserver agreement in the diagnosis of idiopathic pulmonary fibrosis. *Eur Respir J* 2008; 31: 585–591.

24. Tomassetti S, Piciucchi S, Tantalocco P, *et al.* The multidisciplinary approach in the diagnosis of idiopathic pulmonary fibrosis: a patient case-based review. *Eur Respir Rev* 2015; 24: 69–77.

25. Flaherty KR, Andrei AC, King TE Jr, *et al.* Idiopathic interstitial pneumonia: do community and academic physicians agree on diagnosis? *Am J Respir Crit Care Med* 2007; 175: 1054–1060.

26. Flaherty KR, King TE Jr, Raghu G, *et al.* Idiopathic interstitial pneumonia: what is the effect of a multidisciplinary approach to diagnosis? *Am J Respir Crit Care Med* 2004; 170: 904–910.

27. Ohshimo S, Bonella F, Cui A, *et al.* Significance of bronchoalveolar lavage for the diagnosis of idiopathic pulmonary fibrosis. *Am J Respir Crit Care Med* 2009; 179: 1043–1047.

28. De Vuyst P, Karjalainen A, Dumortier P, *et al.* Guidelines for mineral fibre analyses in biological samples: report of the ERS Working Group, European Respiratory Society. *Eur Respir J* 1998; 11: 1416–1426.

29. Abehsera M, Valeyre D, Grenier P, *et al.* Sarcoidosis with pulmonary fibrosis: CT patterns and correlation with pulmonary function. *AJR Am J Roentgenol* 2000; 174: 1751–1757.

30. Collard HR, Moore BB, Flaherty KR, *et al.* Acute exacerbations of idiopathic pulmonary fibrosis. *Am J Respir Crit Care Med* 2007; 176: 636–643.

31. Ryerson CJ, Cottin V, Brown KK, *et al.* Acute exacerbation of idiopathic pulmonary fibrosis: shifting the paradigm. *Eur Respir J* 2015; 46: 512–520.

32. Fell CD, Martinez FJ, Liu LX, *et al.* Clinical predictors of a diagnosis of idiopathic pulmonary fibrosis. *Am J Respir Crit Care Med* 2010; 181: 832–837.

33. Cottin V, Richeldi L. Neglected evidence in idiopathic pulmonary fibrosis and the importance of early diagnosis and treatment. *Eur Respir Rev* 2014; 23: 106–110.

34. Zappala CJ, Latsi PI, Nicholson AG, *et al.* Marginal decline in forced vital capacity is associated with a poor outcome in idiopathic pulmonary fibrosis. *Eur Respir J* 2010; 35: 830–836.

35. Casoni GL, Tomassetti S, Cavazza A, *et al.* Transbronchial lung cryobiopsy in the diagnosis of fibrotic interstitial lung diseases. *PloS One* 2014; 9: e86716.

36. Meltzer EB, Barry WT, Yang IV, *et al.* Familial and sporadic idiopathic pulmonary fibrosis: making the diagnosis from peripheral blood. *BMC Genomics* 2014; 15: 902.

Disclosures: D. Valeyre reports personal fees for transport and accommodation at meetings from Roche, Intermune and Boehringer Ingelheim outside the submitted work. D. Valeyre is also the member of scientific boards for Roche, Intermune and Boehringer Ingelheim. O. Freynet is the co-investigator of clinical trials for Boehringer Ingelheim and Roche. H. Nunes is the investigator of clinical trials for Intermune, Roche, Boehringer Ingelheim, Sanfoi and Centocor.

Chapter 5

Histopathology and cryobiopsy

Venerino Poletti[1,2], Sara Tomassetti[2], Claudia Ravaglia[2],
Alessandra Dubini[3], Sara Piciucchi[4], Alberto Cavazza[5]
and Marco Chilosi[6]

The IIPs represent a subset of ILDs of unknown cause. Different histological patterns are linked to these entities. The UIP pattern is associated with IPF. Other histological patterns are: NSIP, respiratory bronchiolitis, desquamative interstitial pneumonia, organising pneumonia and diffuse alveolar damage. Lymphoid interstitial pneumonia is significantly rarer and the idiopathic form has been removed from the IIP category. New entities such as pleuroparenchymal fibroelastosis, acute fibrinous and organising pneumonia, and bronchiolocentric interstitial pneumonia have been recently considered. The "unclassifiable category" is nowadays also used in recognition of the difficulties that pathologists may meet. These patterns are usually identified on samples provided by surgical lung biopsy. Recently, new immunohistochemical analyses have better defined the boundaries of these patterns and a new endoscopic transbronchial approach using cryoprobes has been introduced in clinical practice. Using this approach, large samples are retrieved and identification of the UIP pattern or other complex patterns seems feasible on these samples. The complications are significantly less than those observed after a surgical lung biopsy and transbronchial cryobiopsy seems a promising diagnostic tool in patients with suspected IIP.

The morphological background of IPF was clearly defined only in the late 1990s [1, 2]. The histological hallmarks identifying the pattern observed in IPF subjects are: patchy fibrosis, fibroblastic foci and honeycombing. The combination of these hallmarks is termed the UIP pattern. Different patterns, previously included in the histopathological spectrum with which pulmonary fibrosis could manifest, were later recognised as independent entities and expression of disorders separate from IPF. More cogent criteria were used to define the NSIP pattern, the desquamative interstitial pneumonia (DIP) pattern and other patterns [1–3]. In addition, morphology was no longer considered the gold standard since disorders of known cause or appearing in specific contexts could have the same histological background and because the combination of information provided by different sources (clinical profile, laboratory tests, imaging features) could contribute more significantly to reach the diagnosis [4]. Recent progress includes the utilisation of new immunohistochemical markers to precisely define the histological patterns [5] and the use of transbronchial cryobiopsy (cryo-transbronchial biopsy (c-TBB)) in order to obtain sufficient lung tissue: c-TBB has been shown to be able to provide large samples, with limited and manageable complications [6].

[1]Dept of Respiratory Diseases and Allergology, University Hospital, Aarhus, Denmark. [2]Dept of Diseases of the Thorax, Ospedale GB Morgagni, Forlì, Italy. [3]Dept of Anatomic Pathology, Ospedale GB Morgagni, Forlì, Italy. [4]Dept of Radiology, Ospedale GB Morgagni, Forlì, Italy. [5]Pathology Unit, Arcispedale Santa Maria Nuova-IRCCS, Reggio Emilia, Italy. [6]Dept of Pathology, University of Verona, Verona, Italy.

Correspondence: Venerino Poletti, Ospedale GB Morgagni, Forlì, Via Carlo Forlanini 34, Forlì, Italy. E-mail: venerino.poletti@gmail.com

Copyright ©ERS 2016. Print ISBN: 978-1-84984-067-5. Online ISBN: 978-1-84984-068-2. Print ISSN: 2312-508X. Online ISSN: 2312-5098.

Histopathology

Usual interstitial pneumonia

The key morphological features identifying the UIP pattern are: patchy fibrosis, fibroblastic foci and honeycombing changes (table 1). The process has a "periacinar" distribution. The peripheral structures of the pulmonary acinus involved are therefore beneath the pleura, but also in the parenchyma around respiratory bronchioles (figure 1), within the centrilobular zone. Focal type II pneumocyte hyperplasia is commonly observed in affected areas, frequently associated with fibrosis and a mild chronic inflammatory infiltrate. This finding may represent the first pathogenic step in the complex pathogenesis of IPF, where frustrated pneumocyte renewal (due to cell senescence and/or stem cell exhaustion) is able to trigger abnormal signalling within the surrounding microenvironment [5].

In UIP, areas of advanced remodelling are common, where alveolar parenchyma is completely substituted by scarring rich in type III collagen and smooth muscle fibres. The significance of this smooth muscle hyperplasia has not yet been clearly defined, but it is likely secondary to an abnormal regeneration of bronchiolar walls. Accordingly, the accumulating smooth muscle cells are not myofibroblasts, but exhibit a marker profile consistent with bronchiolar wall derivation (α-smooth muscle actin-positive, caldesmon-positive) [7].

The boundaries between the fibrotic areas and the normal lung are sharp (this is the key element that confers the patchy aspect to the fibrotic lesion). Fibroblastic foci are dome-shaped structures (that appear pale bluish with haematoxylin–eosin staining and are clearly visualised by Alcian blue staining) since they are mainly formed by extracellular matrix rich in tenascin-C, do not contain vessels (as in Masson's bodies of organising pneumonia (OP)), and are mostly observed within interstitial spaces at the edges between the "acellular fibrotic" areas and normal lung, as well as in honeycomb lesions [8]. The α-smooth muscle actin-positive myofibroblasts with their long axis parallel to the long axis of the ellipsoid structure are embedded in the extracellular matrix. These foci are covered by cuboidal epithelial cells that express bronchiolar markers (presence of cytokeratin 5/6 and ΔN-p63 protein, and lack of pneumocyte

---

Table 1. Histological features of the UIP pattern

Hallmarks
"Patchy fibrosis"
Fibroblastic foci ("sandwich foci" using immunohistochemical investigations)
Honeycombing changes (bronchiolar dysplastic proliferation, accumulation of MUC5B-positive mucus in the cysts)
Periacinar distribution of the "patchy fibrosis"
Lack of significant inflammation/granulomas (acute lung injury features)

Ancillary findings
Bone metaplasia in remodelled areas
Pleural fat metaplasia
Centrilobular smoking-related lesions ("smoker's" macrophages, distorting fibrosis of the wall of terminal and respiratory bronchioles)

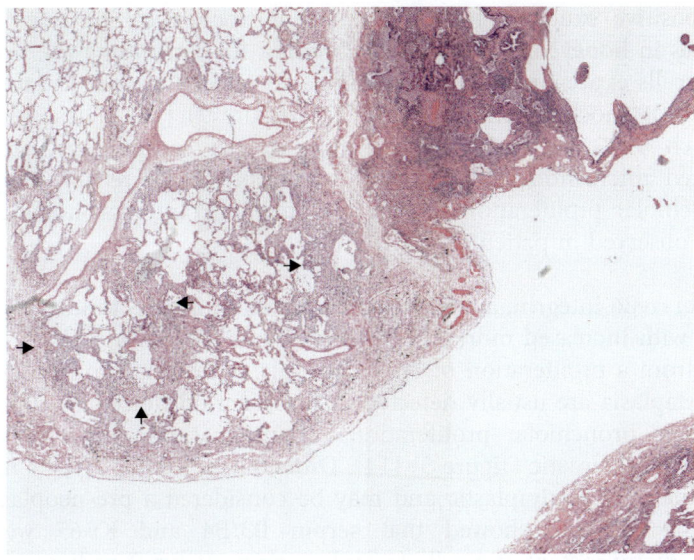

Figure 1. Bands of fibrotic tissue clearly define the boundaries (arrows) of acini contained in a secondary pulmonary lobule. Haematoxylin–eosin stain, low power.

markers) (figure 2) [9]. The epithelial cells may show squamoid or mucinous metaplasia and nuclear atypia may be focally prominent.

Honeycomb changes represent an important feature of the UIP pattern. Large cystic lesions (>1–2 mm in length) can be macroscopically recognised at necropsy or in large pulmonary excisions and can be demonstrated at HRCT analysis, representing a major diagnostic feature of the UIP pattern at imaging. Smaller "honeycomb" cysts (<1–2 mm) cannot be recognised at imaging, but can be easily demonstrated by histology (microscopic honeycombing). Honeycomb cysts are actually covered with epithelial bronchiolar cells that may abnormally express mucins (MUC5AC-negative, MUC5B-positive) and can contain a

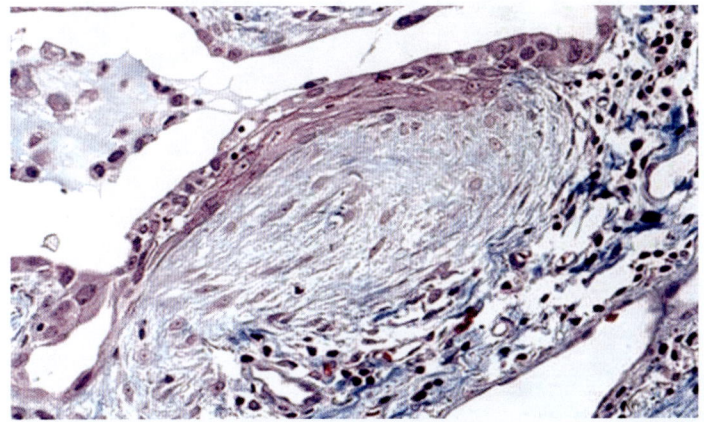

Figure 2. A typical fibroblastic focus. Elongated myofibroblasts are embedded in an extracellular matrix. The epithelial cells covering the dome-shaped structure are cuboidal and some appear ciliated. Mallory stain, high power.

thick MUC5B-positive exudate [10, 11]. Immunohistochemical analyses identify several abnormal features in honeycomb-associated fibroblast foci, including the presence of linear clusters of basal cells expressing migratory-associated molecules such as laminin-5 γ2 chain (LAM5γ2) and heat shock protein 27 (HSP-27) (figure 3) [12]. These lesions, which we named "sandwich foci" for their peculiar three-layered morphology, are fairly specific for IPF-associated micro-honeycombing and can represent a reliable diagnostic marker (figure 4). Bronchiolar proliferation is therefore an important morphologic component of the UIP pattern observed in patients with IPF [11].

The expression of αvβ6 integrin, an epithelial-restricted molecule, in lung biopsy was shown to be correlated with increased mortality in IPF patients [13]. Honeycomb cysts are at least in part derived from a proliferation of epithelial cells expressing bronchiolar markers. Foci of squamous metaplasia are usually detected in these remodelled areas. The morphological distinction between bronchiolar proliferation, squamous carcinoma and adenocarcinoma can sometimes be problematic (figure 5) [14]. Different molecular aspects indicate that this bronchiolar proliferation is dysplastic and may be considered a pre-neoplastic process [15, 16]. CALABRESE et al. [17] showed that serpin B3/B4 and Ki-67 were significantly overexpressed in many metaplastic cells (mainly squamous type) in lung samples obtained from IPF patients compared with control cases. Serpin B3/B4 expression was related to both TGF-β and Ki-67, and was higher in patients with high-grade dysplasia [17].

Inflammation is usually a minor component of the UIP pattern in patients with IPF. Ancillary findings are represented by areas of bone metaplasia in the fibrotic lung parenchyma, fat metaplasia in the pleural regions, and accumulation of "smoker's macrophages" and fibrosis in the wall of the terminal and respiratory bronchioles (table 1).

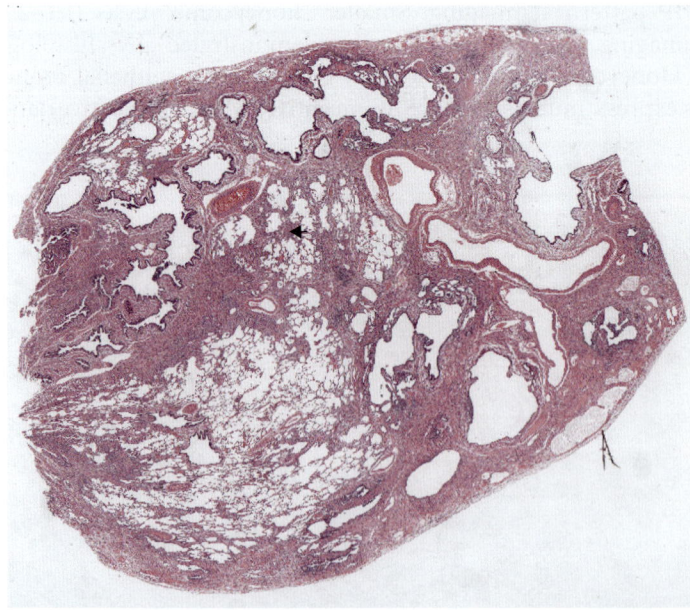

Figure 3. Honeycomb changes: cysts of irregular shape, covered by bronchiolar epithelium surrounded by fibrotic tissue. The periacinar distribution of the scarring tissue is still evident in adjacent areas (arrow). Haematoxylin–eosin stain, low power.

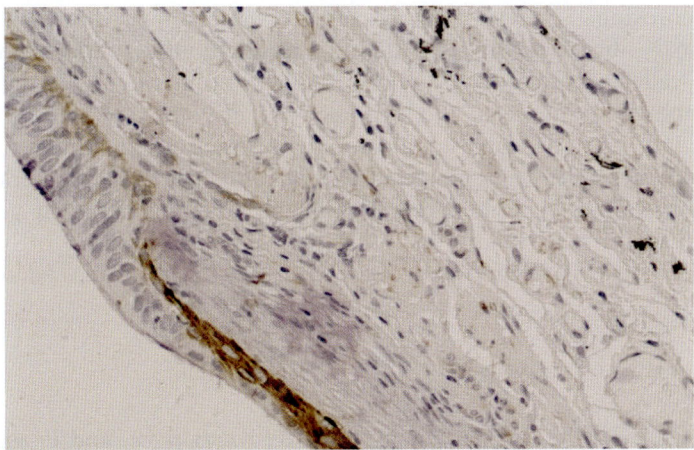

Figure 4. A "sandwich lesion". The basal epithelial cells covering an ellipsoid accumulation of extracellular matrix express the migratory-associated molecule heat shock protein 27. Immunohistochemical staining, high power.

The UIP pattern is recognised on surgical lung biopsy samples by pathologists with good interobserver agreement; evaluation of a second specimen does not increase recognition significantly [18]. When hyaline membranes, intra-alveolar and interstitial oedema, proliferation of dysplastic type II pneumocytes (diffuse alveolar damage (DAD) pattern), accumulation of granulation tissue in the alveolar spaces (OP pattern), or in the interalveolar septa or even capillaritis, are superimposed to the UIP pattern, a diagnosis of acute exacerbation of UIP should be strongly considered [19, 20]. Diagnostic challenges are represented by chronic hypersensitivity, collagen vascular diseases with lung involvement, end-stage fibrotic changes related to sarcoidosis, infectious disorders, Langerhan's cell

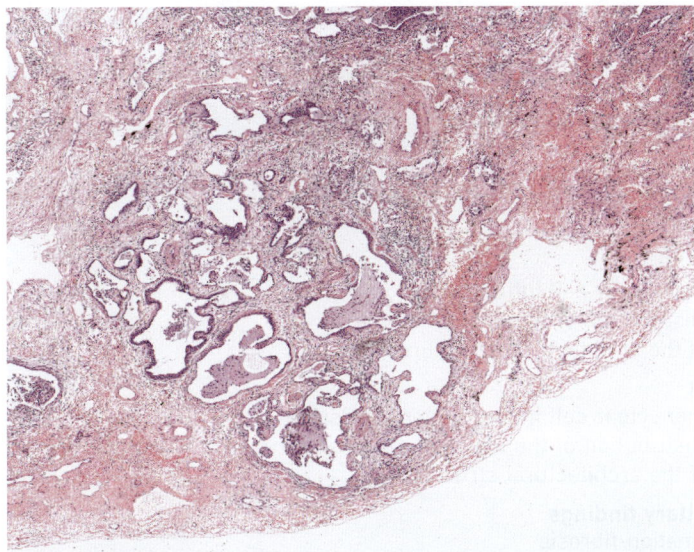

Figure 5. A prominent bronchiolar proliferation beneath the visceral pleura mimicking adenocarcinoma. Haematoxylin–eosin stain, low power.

histiocytosis, fibrosing NSIP, "airway-centred interstitial fibrosis lesions" and pleuroparenchymal fibroelastosis (PPFE) [20]. Bronchiolitis, peribronchiolar epithelial metaplasia (so-called "lambertosis"), centrilobular fibrosis, bridging fibrosis, OP, granulomas, scattered giant cells and lymphocytic alveolitis are clues in favour of a diagnosis of the UIP pattern related to chronic hypersensitivity pneumonitis [20]. Bridging fibrosis refers to fibrotic lesions connected to adjacent bronchioles, interlobular septa or pleural connective tissue [21]. The presence of lymphoid follicles with germinal centres, pleuritis and/or a significant inflammatory infiltrate consisting mainly of lymphocytes and plasma cells could suggest a diagnosis of secondary UIP in the context of collagen vascular disease [1].

Nonspecific interstitial pneumonia

In the seminal article on the histopathology of NSIP, KATZENTSEIN and FIORELLI [22] defined the NSIP pattern in 1994, introducing the concept of temporally and spatially homogenous interstitial fibrosis in contrast to the temporal and spatial heterogeneity evident in UIP for the presence of "patchy fibrosis". Two histological categories of NSIP were eventually identified: the cellular variant, characterised by interalveolar thickening due to the infiltration of inflammatory mononuclear cells (mainly lymphocytes), and the fibrotic variant, characterised by interalveolar thickening due to the presence of inflammation at different degrees of intensity and collagen [23]. This description is, however, too schematic. A deep analysis of the pathologic literature on idiopathic NSIP and clues provided by the analysis of lesions categorised as NSIP in patients with collagen vascular disease shows that at least three variants may be identified (table 2). 1) The mixed variant in which interstitial inflammation and acellular fibrosis are combined with the accumulation in granulation tissue in the alveolar spaces (OP pattern). The combination of the NSIP pattern and the OP pattern was reported by NAGAI et al. [24] to be prominent mainly in cellular NSIP. TRAVIS et al. [23] described a prominent OP pattern in samples classified as cellular NSIP in 29% of cases and the OP pattern was also identified as an ancillary finding in 32% of the fibrosing NSIP cases. This mixed pattern is also observed in cases of dermatomyositis/polymyositis or anti-synthetase syndrome (V. Poletti, unpublished data). 2) The cellular

---

Table 2. Histological features of the NSIP pattern

Mixed variant
  Interstitial inflammation (mainly mononuclear cells)
  Organising pneumonia

Cellular variant
  Interstitial mononuclear cell inflammation
  Homogenous distribution of the lesion
  Preservation of the architectural structure

Fibrosing variant
  Interstitial mononuclear cell inflammation/fibrosis
  Homogenous distribution of the lesion
  Preservation of the architectural structure

Histological ancillary findings
  Pleural inflammation/fibrosis
  Lymphoid follicles
  Intra-alveolar accumulation of fibrin (mainly in mixed and cellular variants)

---

variant with almost only interstitial inflammatory infiltration. 3) The fibrotic variant in which the interalveolar fibrosis is homogeneous and acellular. This last variant has as a prototype the histological pattern observed in patients with scleroderma [1].

The histological subsets of the NSIP pattern may be even more numerous if ancillary histological features are considered. KAMBOUCHNER *et al.* [25], reviewing 136 biopsy-proven NSIPs, identified essential NSIP and six overlap subgroups according to superimposed minor histological features: UIP overlap, chronic hypersensitivity overlap, OP overlap, organising DAD overlap, DIP overlap and lymphoid interstitial pneumonia (LIP) overlap.

Respiratory bronchiolitis/DIP and "smoking-related lung fibrosis"

Cigarette smokers commonly have a condition referred to as "respiratory bronchiolitis" where mild inflammation, fibrosis and pigmented airspace macrophages occur around distal bronchioles. A distinctive expansion of respiratory bronchiolitis foci, accentuated by a zone of macrophage accumulation in centrilobular alveolar spaces, is seen in symptomatic smokers with upper lung zone ground-glass opacities [1, 20]. Centriacinar emphysema is frequently present, but may be difficult to recognise in the biopsy sample.

First described by LIEBOW *et al.* [26] in 1965, and later expanded in detail by CARRINGTON *et al.* [27], DIP is a chronic interstitial pneumonia distinguished by the presence of abundant alveolar cells, thought initially to be sloughed epithelium (desquamation). The macrophage nature of the intra-alveolar cells was later confirmed by electron microscopy [1]. Therefore, DIP is a misnomer. However, the term was maintained in the recent classification with some reservations, recognising that the actual current incidence of DIP seems to be extremely low [28]. At scanning magnification, the lung architecture is preserved, with peribronchiolar and sometimes interstitial lymphoid aggregates visible. The alveolar walls are mildly thickened by uniform fibrosis, obscured by the presence of large numbers of macrophages filling the alveolar spaces. This extent of macrophage accumulation distinguishes DIP from respiratory bronchiolitis/ILD.

In smokers, the characteristic macrophage of DIP has abundant pale eosinophilic cytoplasm with finely granular tan-brown pigment (so-called smoker's macrophages). Iron stains are positive in these cells, but the pigment most often lacks the dense, golden, refractile pigment of the siderophages of pulmonary haemorrhage. In children with DIP, macrophages may lack such pigmentation. A few multinucleated giant cells are often admixed with the alveolar macrophages; eosinophils admixed with macrophages are usually present and occasionally they may be prominent, making the differential diagnosis with eosinophilic pneumonia difficult [29, 30]. Very rarely the intra-alveolar accumulation of neoplastic cells (primary lung cancers, metastatic tumours) may mimic the DIP pattern [31].

Respiratory bronchiolitis/ILD and DIP continue to be considered together as ends of a spectrum of ILD affecting cigarette smokers although this hypothesis does not seem to be strongly supported. It has only recently been acknowledged that the range of lung injury from cigarette smoke is wider than generally accepted; in particular, there is increasing recognition that fibrosis of alveolar walls occurs in smokers. Airspace enlargement with fibrosis and smoking-related interstitial fibrosis are almost synonymous terms that refer to smoking-related lung fibrosis [32, 33]. Histologically, it is characterised by alveolar enlargement ("alveolar cysts"), and by marked thickening of alveolar septa by fibrosis composed of thick collagen bundles that have a distinctive hyalinised quality and are often admixed with variable numbers of hyperplastic smooth muscle fibres. There is minimal accompanying inflammation. This fibrosis may, however, also be found in the centrilobular parenchyma. Respiratory bronchiolitis is usually an ancillary finding. Alveolar cysts without bronchiolisation and showing fibrotic walls are frequently identified in the upper lobes of the explants of patients affected by IPF [34].

Organising pneumonia

The characteristic histological features of OP are: patchy intra-alveolar accumulation of granulation tissue rich in extracellular myxoid matrix containing tenascin-C, in which myofibroblasts and neoformed capillaries are embedded; interalveolar and, less prominent, intra-alveolar inflammation consisting mainly of lymphocytes, scattered plasma cells, mast cells and eosinophils; and type II alveolar cell hyperplasia/dysplasia [1]. The intra-alveolar loose fibrotic buds have a serpiginous shape, and may extend to the respiratory and terminal bronchioles. A frequent ancillary finding is the presence of alveolar macrophages often having a vacuolated or foamy-appearing cytoplasm. Fibrin tends not to be a dominant feature in OP, but it can be present focally in the alveolar spaces. In patients with cryptogenic OP, intra-alveolar fibrin deposits were significantly associated with high C-reactive protein values in blood and predicted relapse of the disease within 6 months to 1 year [35, 36].

Diffuse alveolar damage

The histological findings of DAD vary depending on the time at which tissue sampling occurs [1, 37]. Three temporal phases of DAD are recognised: the exudative or acute phase, the proliferative or organising phase and the fibrotic stage.

The exudative phase takes place during the first week following the onset of the process, and is characterised by congestion of alveolar capillaries, interstitial and alveolar oedema, intra-alveolar haemorrhage, and hyaline membranes. The congestion of alveolar capillaries is less prominent compared with that observed in subjects with hydrostatic pulmonary oedema. Hyaline membranes are homogeneous eosinophilic material composed of cellular debris, plasma proteins and surfactant plastered against alveolar ducts and alveolar walls. Interstitial inflammation rich in neutrophils, but also containing mononuclear cells, is more prominent at the end of the first week of alveolar damage. Microvascular thrombi are frequently identified as well as the presence of megakaryocytes in the alveolar capillaries.

Alveolar capillaritis is a peculiar form of acute lung injury observed mainly in subjects with diffuse pulmonary haemorrhage syndromes. Capillaries are densely infiltrated by neutrophils: alveolar septa may be focally necrotic, and the alveolar spaces contain red cells, hemosiderin granules, focal deposits of fibrin and cellular debris. Nuclear dust or karyorrhectic debris may accompany the neutrophils.

The histological modification of the proliferative phase appears at the end of the first week. Extensive but more centrilobular-sited proliferation of type II pneumocytes and fibroblasts/ myofibroblasts is the hallmark of this phase. Epithelial cells may present dysplastic nuclei and show abundant eosinophilic, vacuolated cytoplasm. Squamous metaplasia appearing as hyaline Mallory's bodies or with the typical cytoplasmic modifications are detectable. The regenerating epithelial cells may also bridge the mouths of collapsed alveoli so that these airspaces never re-expand (atelectatic induration). The fibroblastic/myofibroblastic proliferation is evident in the interalveolar septa and in the alveolar spaces, and remnants of hyaline membranes may be identified embedded in the granulation tissue. Microvascular thrombi, small pulmonary infarcts and subsequently neoangiogenesis, and intimal and medial vascular remodelling are part of the morphological aspects of the proliferative phase of DAD.

The fibrotic phase of DAD is encountered in patients who survive 3–4 weeks after the acute alveolar injury. The reorganisation of the interstitium by fibroblast/myofibroblasts, proliferation of epithelium, and foci of epithelial squamous metaplasia could then result in multiple cysts resembling a honeycomb appearance. Deposition of collagen is more prominent around alveolar ducts and in the interalveolar septa [38].

It is important to note that the phases of DAD are not strictly sequential, that a great deal of overlap exists between these phases with many histological features occurring in tandem and that the timing of the appearance of the various histological findings is a rough approximation. The term "diffuse" in DAD is intended to convey the diffuse involvement of all constituents of the alveolar wall, *i.e.* the alveolar epithelium, basement membranes and capillary endothelium. DAD is the main histopathological feature superimposed to the UIP pattern in acute exacerbation of IPF [39].

Lymphoid interstitial pneumonia

The distinctive histological features of LIP are: a diffuse interstitial infiltration of mononuclear cells (lymphocytes, plasma cells, histiocytes); lymphoid follicles with germinal centres detectable along the bronchovascular bundles and beneath the visceral pleura, which may be prominent around bronchioles and partially occlude their lumen; scattered non-necrotising granulomas, giant cells containing cholesterol clefts and foci of OP [40]. The lymphoid infiltrate is mainly represented by CD4+ lymphocytes. B polyclonal lymphocytes are mainly identified in lymphoid nodules. In advanced cases, interstitial fibrosis with cysts bordered by hyperplastic epithelial cells may be prominent. As idiopathic LIP seems to be distinctively rare (it is mainly a morphological manifestation of immunologically driven diseases or of HIV infection) it has been removed from the category of IIPs [28]. However, idiopathic LIP cases are still reported in the literature [41] and we observed a few cases. The distinction between LIP and cellular NSIP may be arbitrary in the majority of cases, and rarely, hypersensitivity pneumonitis may present with a significant parenchymal lymphoid infiltrate mimicking LIP [42].

Pleuroparenchymal fibroelastosis

Pleural and subpleural obliterative fibrosis and a characteristic sharp interface with normal lung parenchyma are the histological hallmarks of PPFE at low power [43]. At higher power, the obliterative fibrosis appears characterised by prominent eosinophilic fragments of elastic lamellae (better visualised by elastic fibre stains). The areas of PPFE are present predominantly in a subpleural distribution, but in some cases they may also be paraseptal, centrilobular or more random (parenchymal) in distribution. Fibroblastic foci are usually present at the interface between fibroelastotic areas and normal lung parenchyma [44]. Scattered granulomas or foci of bronchiolitis may be ancillary findings.

Acute fibrinous and organising pneumonia

Acute fibrinous and OP was first reported in 17 patients with acute respiratory failure, and initially thought to represent a possible new IIP. The dominant histopathological pattern was intra-alveolar fibrin deposition ("fibrin balls") and associated OP in the absence of classical hyaline membranes of DAD or intra-alveolar eosinophils of acute eosinophilic pneumonia [45, 46]. Whether this pattern may be associated with an idiopathic diffuse lung disorder is still under investigation.

Bronchiolocentric interstitial pneumonia

In 2002, YOUSEM and DACIC [47] described 10 patients with a "distinctive idiopathic bronchiolocentric interstitial pneumonia". All 10 patients had airway-centred fibroinflammatory infiltrates with variable extension into surrounding lung. The authors noted histopathological similarities to hypersensitivity pneumonitis. CHURG et al. [48] presented 12 cases with "a distinctive pattern of airway-centered interstitial fibrosis centered on membranous and respiratory bronchioles" at scanning magnification. In both series, a distinction from the peripheral lobular distribution of fibrosis typical of UIP was emphasised. FUKUOKA et al. [49] reported a series consisting of 15 cases in which peribronchiolar metaplasia was the only major histological finding with a good prognosis compared with that reported in the two previous studies. The 2013 American Thoracic Society (ATS)/European Respiratory Society (ERS) consensus statement felt that these small series were insufficiently compelling from a clinical and radiological perspective to warrant inclusion as a formal IIP although the signal (an airway-centred remodelling fibrosis as histological background of a clinico-radiological IIP) needs to be considered [28].

Unclassifiable interstitial pneumonia

The ATS/ERS/Japanese Respiratory Society (JRS)/Latin-American Thoracic Association (ALAT) IPF guidelines introduced the concept that although lung samples may not have all the histological hallmarks of the UIP pattern, the histological features can still suggest a diagnosis of UIP [50]. The presence of patchy fibrosis and "fibroblastic foci" is considered diagnostic of the UIP pattern even in the absence of honeycomb changes; when one of these two aspects is not identified, with or without associated honeycomb changes, or when only honeycomb changes are detectable, the "probable" UIP pattern category is applied. Finally, the "possible" UIP pattern category is used when only fibrosis (not otherwise specifiable) is evident (table 3). However, the "probable" and "possible" categories actually define a "not classifiable" histological pattern [1]. The term "unclassifiable" should not be applied when the specimens are inadequate (as when insufficient alveolated tissue is present or in the presence of artefacts).

Cryobiopsy

Recently, cryoprobes were used to obtain lung tissue during a bronchoscopy. POLETTI et al. [51] provide a review on technical aspects of transbronchial lung biopsy using cryoprobes, and a review of the literature on its diagnostic yield and clinical value in patients with fibrosing

Table 3. Histological criteria for the UIP pattern

UIP pattern (all four criteria)	Probable UIP (any of the four criteria)	Possible UIP (all three criteria)	Not UIP pattern (any of the six criteria)
Evidence of marked fibrosis/architectural distortion with or without honeycombing in a predominantly subpleural/paraseptal distribution	Evidence of marked fibrosis/architectural distortion with or without honeycombing	Patchy or diffuse involvement of lung parenchyma by fibrosis, with or without interstitial inflammation	Hyaline membranes[¶,+] Organising pneumonia[¶,+]
Presence of patchy involvement of lung parenchyma by fibrosis	Absence of either patchy involvement or fibroblastic foci, but not both	Absence of other criteria for UIP (see UIP pattern)	Granulomas[+]
Presence of fibroblastic foci	Absence of features against a diagnosis of UIP suggesting an alternative diagnosis (see Not UIP pattern)	Absence of features against a diagnosis of UIP suggesting an alternative diagnosis (see Not UIP pattern)	Marked interstitial inflammatory cells infiltrate away from honeycombing
Absence of features against a diagnosis of UIP suggesting an alternative diagnosis (see Not UIP pattern)	Honeycomb changes only[#]		Predominant airway-centred changes
			Other features suggestive of an alternative diagnosis

[#]: this scenario usually represents end-stage fibrotic lung disease where honeycombed segments have been sampled, but where the UIP pattern might be present in other areas (such areas are usually represented by overt honeycombing on HRCT and can be avoided by pre-operative targeting of biopsy sites away from areas using HRCT); [¶]: can be associated with acute exacerbation of IPF; [+]: an isolated or occasional granuloma and/or a mild component of the organising pneumonia pattern may rarely coexist in lung biopsies with an otherwise UIP pattern. Reproduced and modified from [50] with permission from the publisher.

ILD and complications. The cryosurgical equipment operates by the Joule–Thomson effect, which dictates that a compressed gas released at high flow rapidly expands and creates a very low temperature. The cooling agent is applied under high pressure (45 bar) through the central canal of the probe (ERBOKRYO CA; ERBE, Tübingen, Germany). Carbon dioxide is the cooling agent most commonly used. The gas at the tip expands due to the sudden difference in pressure relative to the atmospheric pressure, resulting in a temperature drop at the tip of the probe.

c-TBB of lung tissue is carried out during flexible bronchoscopy in the majority of centres. Patients are deeply sedated with intravenous propofol with or without remifentanil and intubated with a spiral armoured endotracheal tube or a rigid tube. Oxygen is insufflated continuously through the tube. Spontaneous breathing is maintained during the whole procedure or, if patients are paralysed by the use of nondepolarising blocking agents, jet ventilation is used. Oxygen saturation, blood pressure, ECG and transcutaneous carbon dioxide partial pressure are monitored continuously. The bronchopulmonary segment for biopsy is determined prior to the procedure based on HRCT of the chest. A bronchial blocker (Fogarty balloon or other blocker) is positioned at the entrance of the pre-selected segmental bronchus. The cryoprobe is introduced into the selected area under fluoroscopic guidance *via* a flexible bronchoscope. A distance of ~10–20 mm from the thoracic wall and a perpendicular relation between the thoracic wall and the probe are considered optimal. Once brought into position, the probe is cooled for ~3–6 s. The frozen tissue attached to the probe tip is removed by pulling the cryoprobe together with the bronchoscope. This is because the biopsied tissue is larger than the working channel of the bronchoscope and the frozen distal end of the cryoprobe might damage the working channel of the scope during retraction of the biopsy. The frozen specimen is thawed in saline and fixed in formalin. The number of biopsies taken is usually between three and six. c-TBB is carried out in a few centres using a flexible bronchoscope without intubation [52].

Studies on the clinical role of c-TBB in fibrosing ILDs are increasing and the results are promising. In the "nonintubated group", the mean sample size reported so far varies 9–17 mm^2 [53, 54]. In the "intubated group", the mean size of samples varies 9.5–64.2 mm^2 [55–61].

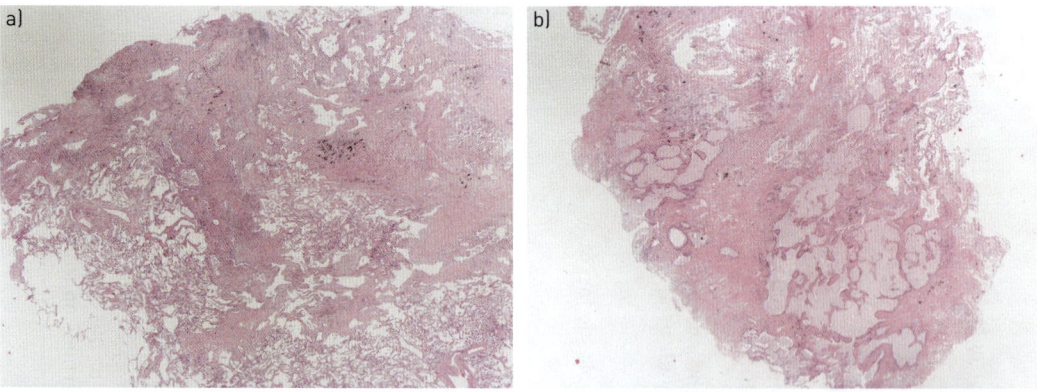

Figure 6. Transbronchial cryobiopsy samples from the same patient. a) Bands of fibrotic tissue with a periacinar distribution. The boundaries between fibrotic lung tissue and normal lung parenchyma are sharp ("patchy fibrosis"). Numerous dome-shaped foci of "pale" fibrosis (fibroblastic foci) are evident at the edges between the scarring areas and the normal lung parenchyma. b) Cystic spaces containing mucus in a fibrotic context are clearly evident (honeycomb changes). Haematoxylin–eosin stain, low power.

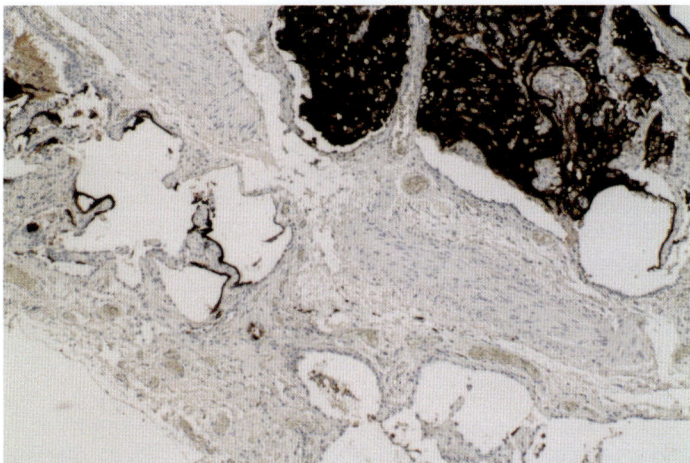

Figure 7. Transbronchial cryobiopsy sample. Honeycomb cysts containing MUC5B-positive mucus. Immunohistochemical staining, high power.

Samples do not present crash artefacts and frequently contain peripheral structures of the secondary pulmonary lobules. The diagnostic yield of c-TBB in patients with diffuse parenchymal lung disease varies 68–100%. The UIP pattern may be identified with high confidence because in the majority of cases fibroblastic foci, patchy fibrosis and even honeycomb changes are easily identified in samples obtained in a patient (figure 6). Agreement between pathologists in the detection of UIP has been reported to be very good with a κ coefficient of 0.83 (95% CI 0.69–0.97); in the same study, the diagnosis of UIP pattern was made by the pathologists involved with high confidence in 77% of the cases [59].

Immunohistochemical analysis may be performed easily in samples obtained by cryobiopsy. In the near future, new markers such as LAM5γ2, fascin, HSP-27, β-catenin and MUC5B (figure 7), identified on the basis of new pathogenetic hypotheses, will be useful to clearly

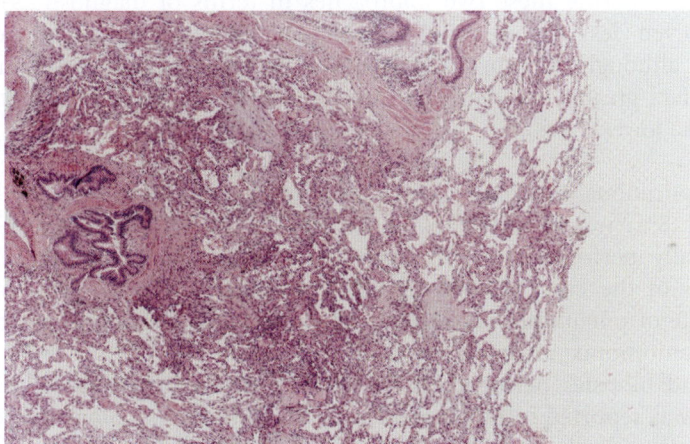

Figure 8. Transbronchial cryobiopsy: a mixed organising pneumonia/NSIP pattern is evident. Scattered serpiginous alveolar buds of loose fibrotic tissue and a homogenous interstitial chronic inflammation are identifiable. Haematoxylin–eosin stain, low power.

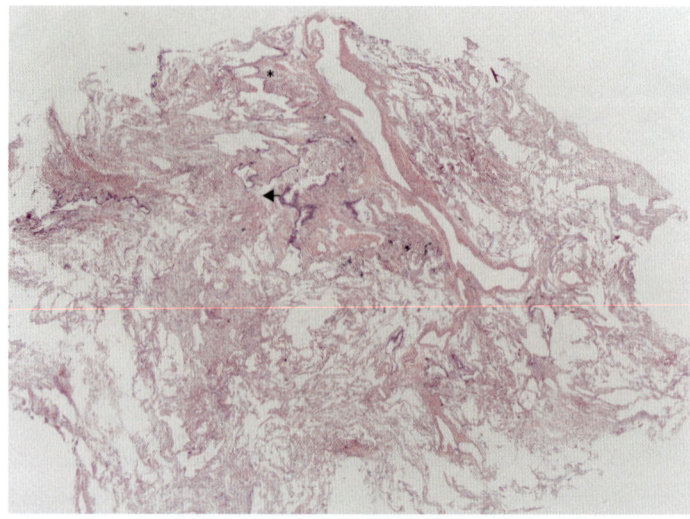

Figure 9. Transbronchial cryobiopsy from the right upper lobe. The typical pleuroparenchymal fibroelastosis features are present: dense collagenous fibrotic bands also containing eosinophilic fragments of elastic lamellae extending from the subpleural region deep into the alveolated tissue (arrow). The interface with uninvolved parenchyma is abrupt. The visceral pleura is easily identifiable (*). Haematoxylin–eosin stain, low power.

and objectively recognise the morphological background of IPF. Less high-quality evidence studies are available for NSIP and DIP. However, the combination of morphological information provided by c-TBB and BAL profiles (a lymphocytosis in subjects with NSIP or an increase of smoker's macrophages and eosinophils in patients with the DIP pattern) might be considered diagnostic and avoid a surgical lung biopsy (figure 8).

The strategies used to collect samples are not yet standardised [52]. The majority of authors reported retrieving lung tissue from one segment and only a minority collected lung samples from different segments of the same lobe. No perspective studies have yet been published comparing these two approaches in terms of diagnostic yield and rate of complications. Even less information is available on biopsies performed in different ipsilateral lobes, although this approach seems to be reasonable in cases in which the CT scan pattern differs greatly in different lobes (*i.e.* PPFE in the upper lobes (figure 9) and reticulation in the lower lobes).

The main complications reported are pneumothorax and bleeding. The highest rate of pneumothorax (28%) was reported by CASONI *et al.* [59]. However, the biopsies in their study were usually performed ⩽1 cm from the visceral pleura and a UIP pattern was detected in 75% of the cases. Pneumothorax was significantly lower in other series and nowadays the rate of pneumothorax seems to be ∼10% when all series are considered. Risk factors for pneumothorax after the procedure seem to be: UIP pattern, a HRCT scan fibrotic score and biopsies performed close to the pleura (unpublished data, V. Poletti). Severe bleeding was reported to be frequent only when bronchial blockers were not inserted in advance [61]. One death due to acute exacerbation of IPF has been reported so far [59]. The clinical role of c-TBB in diffuse parenchymal lung disease is still under investigation. Only a few studies suggest that the information provided by c-TBB has a value similar to that provided by surgical lung biopsy in the context of a multidisciplinary discussion [60–62].

However, c-TBB appears promising as recognition of the UIP pattern is possible in the lung samples retrieved.

References

1. Colby TV, Carrington CB. Interstitial lung disease. *In*: Thurlbeck WM, Churg AM, eds. Pathology of the Lung. 2nd Edn. New York, Thieme, 1995; pp. 589–737.

2. Katzenstein AL, Mukhopadhyay S, Myers JL. Diagnosis of usual interstitial pneumonia and distinction from other fibrosing interstitial lung diseases. *Human Pathol* 2008; 39: 1275–1294.

3. Nicholson AG, Colby TV, du Bois RM, *et al*. The prognostic significance of the histologic pattern of interstitial pneumonia in patients presenting with the clinical entity of cryptogenic fibrosing alveolitis. *Am J Respir Crit Care Med* 2000; 162: 2213–2217.

4. Wells AU. Histopathologic diagnosis in diffuse lung disease: an ailing gold standard. *Am J Respir Crit care Med* 2004; 170: 828–829.

5. Chilosi M, Carloni A, Rossi A, *et al*. Premature lung aging and cellular senescence in the pathogenesis of idiopathic pulmonary fibrosis and COPD/emphysema. *Transl Res* 2013; 162: 156–173.

6. Poletti V, Benzaquen S. Transbronchial cryo-biopsy in diffuse parenchymal lung disease. A new star in the horizon. *Sarcoidosis Vasc Diffuse Lung Dis* 2014; 20: 178–180.

7. Chilosi M, Poletti V, Murer B, *et al*. Bronchiolar epithelium in idiopathic fibrosis/usual interstitial fibrosis. *In*: Lynch JPIII, ed. Idiopathic Pulmonary Fibrosis. New York, Marcel Dekker, 2004; pp. 631–664.

8. Estany S, Vicenz-Zygmut V, Llatjós R, *et al*. Lung fibrotic tenascin-C upregulation is associated with other extracellular matrix proteins and induced by TGFβ1. *BMC Pulm Med* 2014; 14: 120–129.

9. Chilosi M, Poletti V, Murer B, *et al*. Abnormal re-epithelialization and lung remodeling in idiopathic pulmonary fibrosis: the role of deltaN-p63. *Lab Invest* 2002; 82: 1335–1345.

10. Seibold MA, Smith RW, Urbanek C, *et al*. The idiopathic pulmonary fibrosis honeycomb cyst contains a mucociliary pseudostratified epithelium. *PLoS One* 2013; 8: e58658.

11. Plantier L, Crestani B, Wert SE, *et al*. Ectopic respiratory epithelial cell differentiation in broncholised distal airspaces in idiopathic pulmonary fibrosis. *Thorax* 2011; 66: 651–657.

12. Chilosi M, Zamò A, Doglioni C, *et al*. Migratory marker expression in fibroblast foci of idiopathic pulmonary fibrosis. *Respir Res* 2006; 7: 95.

13. Saini G, Porte J, Weinreb PH, *et al*. αvβ6 integrin may be a potential prognostic biomarker in interstitial lung disease. *Eur Respir J* 2015; 46: 486–494.

14. Haddad R, Massaro D. Idiopathic diffuse interstitial pulmonary fibrosis (fibrosing alveolitis). Atypical epithelial proliferation and lung cancer. *Am J Med* 1968; 45: 211–219.

15. Hironaka M, Fukayama M. Pulmonary fibrosis and lung carcinoma: a comparative study of metaplastic epithelia in honeycombed areas of usual interstitial pneumonia with or without lung carcinoma. *Pathol Int* 1999; 49: 1060–1066.

16. Calabrese F, Lunardi F, Giacometti C, *et al*. Overexpression of squamous cell carcinoma antigen in idiopathic pulmonary fibrosis: clinicopathological correlations. *Thorax* 2008; 63: 795–802.

17. Calabrese F, Lunardi F, Balestro E, *et al*. Serpin B4 isoform overexpression is associated with aberrant epithelial proliferation and lung cancer in idiopathic pulmonary fibrosis. *Pathology* 2012; 44: 192–198.

18. Nicholson AG, Addis BJ, Bharucha H, *et al*. Inter-observer variation between pathologists in diffuse parenchymal lung disease. *Thorax* 2004; 59: 500–505.

19. Ryu HJ, Moua T, Daniels CE, *et al*. Idiopathic pulmonary fibrosis: evolving concepts. *Mayo Clin Proc* 2014; 89: 1130–1142.

20. Tabaj GC, Fernandez CF, Sabbagh E, *et al*. Histopathology of the idiopathic interstitial pneumonias (IIP): a review. *Respirology* 2015; 20: 873–883.

21. Akashi T, Takemura T, Ando N, *et al*. Histopathologic analysis of sixteen autopsy cases of chronic hypersensitivity pneumonitis. and comparison with idiopathic pulmonary fibrosis/usual interstitial pneumonia. *Am J Clin Pathol* 2009; 131: 405–415.

22. Katzenstein AL, Fiorelli RF. Nonspecific interstitial pneumonia/fibrosis. Histologic features and clinical significance. *Am J Surg Pathol* 1994; 18: 136–147.

23. Travis WD, Matsui K, Moss J, *et al*. Idiopathic nonspecific interstitial pneumonia: prognostic significance of cellular and fibrosing patterns: survival comparison with usual interstitial pneumonia and desquamative interstitial pneumonia. *Am J Surg Pathol* 2000; 24: 19–33.

24. Nagai S, Kitaichi M, Itoh H, *et al*. Idiopathic nonspecific interstitial pneumonia/fibrosis: comparison with idiopathic pulmonary fibrosis and BOOP. *Eur Respir J* 1998; 12: 1010–1019.

25. Kambouchner M, Levy P, Nicholson AG, *et al*. Prognostic relevance of histological variants in nonspecific interstitial pneumonia. *Histopathology* 2014; 65: 549–560.

26. Liebow A, Steer A, Billingsley J. Desquamative interstitial pneumonia. *Am J Med Sci* 1965; 39: 369–404.

27. Carrington CB, Gaensler EA, Coutu RE, *et al.* Natural history and treated course of usual and desquamative interstitial pneumonia. *N Engl J Med* 1978; 298: 801–809.

28. Travis WD, Costabel U, Hansell DM, *et al.* An official American Thoracic Society/European Respiratory Society statement: update of the international multidisciplinary classification of the idiopathic interstitial pneumonias. *Am J Respir Crit Care Med* 2013; 188: 733–748.

29. Kawabata Y, Takemura T, Hebisawa A, *et al.* Eosinophilia in bronchoalveolar lavage fluid and architectural destruction are features of desquamative interstitial pneumonia. *Histopathology* 2008; 52: 194–202.

30. Tazelaar H, Wright J, Churg A. Desquamative interstitial pneumonia. *Histopathology* 2011; 58: 509–516.

31. Raparia K, Ketterer J, Dalurzo ML, *et al.* Lung tumors masquerading as desquamative interstitial pneumonia (DIP): report of 7 cases and review of the literature. *Am J Surg Pathol* 2014; 38: 921–924.

32. Franks TJ, Galvin JR. Smoking-related "interstitial" lung disease. *Arch Pathol Lab Med* 2015; 139: 974–977.

33. Katzenstein A-LA, Mukhopadhyay S, Zanardi C, *et al.* Clinically occult interstitial fibrosis in smokers: classification and significance of a surprisingly common finding in lobectomy specimens. *Hum Pathol* 2010; 41: 316–325.

34. Rabeyrin M, Thivolet F, Ferretti GR, *et al.* Usual interstitial pneumonia end-stage features from explants with radiologic and pathologic correlations. *Ann Diagn Pathol* 2015; 19: 269–276.

35. Nagata N, Wakamatsu K, Kumazoe H, *et al.* Clinical significance of intra-alveolar fibrin deposition in transbronchial lung biopsy in patients with organizing pneumonia. *Lung* 2015; 193: 203–208.

36. Nishino M, Mathai SK, Schoengeld D, *et al.* Clinicopathologic features associated with relapse in cryptogenic organizing pneumonia. *Hum Pathol* 2014; 45: 342–351.

37. Poletti V, Casoni GL, Cancellieri A, *et al.* Diffuse alveolar damage. *Pathologica* 2010; 102: 453–463.

38. Fukuda Y, Ishizaki M, Masuda Y, *et al.* The role of intraalveolar fibrosis in the process of pulmonary structural remodeling in patients with diffuse alveolar damage. *Am J Pathol* 1987; 126: 171–182.

39. Ryerson CJ, Cottin V, Brown KK, *et al.* Acute exacerbation of idiopathic pulmonary fibrosis: shifting the paradigm. *Eur Respir J* 2015; 46: 512–520.

40. Tian X, Yi ES, Ryu JH. Lymphocytic interstitial pneumonia and other benign lymphoid disorders. *Semin Respir Crit Care Med* 2012; 33: 450–461.

41. Abdarbashi P, Abrudescu A. Rare case of idiopathic lymphocytic interstitial pneumonia exhibits good response to mycophenolate mofetil. *Respir Med Case Rep* 2013; 9: 27–29.

42. Grunes D, Beasley MB. Hypersensitivity pneumonitis: a review and update of histologic findings. *J Clin Pathol* 2013; 66: 888–895.

43. Piciucchi S, Tomassetti S, Casoni G, *et al.* High resolution CT and histological findings in idiopathic pleuroparenchymal fibroelastosis: features and differential diagnosis. *Respir Res* 2011; 12: 111.

44. Rosenbaum JN, Butt YM, Johns KA, *et al.* Pleuroparenchymal fibroelastosis: a pattern of chronic lung injury. *Hum Pathol* 2015; 46: 137–146.

45. Beasley MB, Franks TJ, Galvin JR, *et al.* Acute fibrinous and organising pneumonia: a histological pattern of lung injury and possible variant of diffuse alveolar damage. *Arch Pathol Lab Med* 2002; 126: 1064–1070.

46. Piciucchi S, Dubini A, Tomassetti S, *et al.* A case of amiodarone-induced acute fibrinous and organizing pneumonia mimicking mesothelioma. *Am J Respir Crit Care Med* 2015; 191: 104–106.

47. Yousem SA, Dacic S. Idiopathic bronchiolocentric interstitial pneumonia. *Mod Pathol* 2002; 15: 1148–1153.

48. Churg A, Myers J, Suarez T, *et al.* Airway-centred interstitial fibrosis: a distinct form of aggressive diffuse lung disease. *Am J Surg Pathol* 2004; 28: 62–68.

49. Fukuoka J, Franks TJ, Colby TV, *et al.* Peribronchiolar metaplasia: a common histologic lesion in diffuse lung disease and a rare cause of interstitial lung disease: clinicopathologic features of 15 cases. *Am J Surg Pathol* 2005; 29: 948–954.

50. Raghu G, Collard HR, Egan JJ, *et al.* An Official ATS/ERS/JRS/ALAT statement: idiopathic pulmonary fibrosis: evidence-based guidelines for diagnosis and management. *Am J Respir Crit Care Med* 2011; 183: 788–824.

51. Poletti V, Casoni GL, Gurioli C, *et al.* Lung cryobiopsies: a paradigm shift in diagnostic bronchoscopy? *Respirology* 2014; 19: 645–654.

52. Poletti V, Hetzel J. Transbronchial cryobiopsy in diffuse parenchymal lung disease: need for procedural standardization. *Respiration* 2015; 90: 275–278.

53. Fruchter O, Fridel L, El Raouf BA, *et al.* Histological diagnosis of interstitial lung diseases by cryo-transbronchial biopsy. *Respirology* 2014; 19: 683–688.

54. Fruchter O, Fridel L, Rosengarten D, *et al.* Transbronchial cryo-biopsy in immunocompromised patients with pulmonary infiltrates: a pilot study. *Lung* 2013; 191: 619–624.

55. Babiak A, Hetzel J, Krishna G, *et al.* Transbronchial cryobiopsy: a new tool for lung biopsies. *Respiration* 2009; 78: 203–208.

56. Pajares V, Torrego A, Puzo C, *et al.* Utilizacion de criosondas para la realizacion de la biopsia pulmonar transbronquial. [Transbronchial lung biopsy using cryoprobes]. *Arch Bronconeumol* 2010; 46: 111–115.

57. Griff S, Ammenwerth W, Schönfeld N, *et al.* Morphometrical analysis of transbronchial cryobiopsies. *Diagn Pathol* 2011; 6: 53.

58. Kropski JA, Pritchett JM, Mason WR, *et al.* Bronchoscopic cryobiopsy for the diagnosis of diffuse parenchymal lung disease. *PLoS One* 2013; 12: e78674.

59. Casoni GL, Tomassetti S, Cavazza A, *et al.* Transbronchial lung cryobiopsy in the diagnosis of fibrotic interstitial lung diseases. *PLoS One* 2014; 9: e86716.

60. Pajares V, Puzo C, Castillo D, *et al.* Diagnostic yield of transbronchial cryobiopsy in interstitial lung disease: a randomized trial. *Respirology* 2014; 19: 900–906.

61. Hagmeyer L, Theegarten D, Wohlschläger J, *et al.* The role of transbronchial cryobiopsy and surgical lung biopsy in the diagnostic algorithm of interstitial lung disease. *Clin Respir J* 2015 [in press DOI: 10.1111/crj.12261].

62. Tomassetti S, Wells AU, Costabel U, *et al.* Bronchoscopic lung cryobiopsy increases confidence in the multidisciplinary diagnosis of idiopathic pulmonary fibrosis. *Am J Respir Crit Care Med* 2015 [in press; DOI: 10.1164/rccm.201504-0711OC].

Disclosures: None declared.

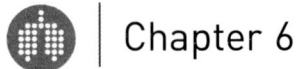

Chapter 6

Bronchoalveolar lavage

Tiago M. Alfaro and Carlos Robalo Cordeiro

In this chapter we will discuss the role of BAL in IPF from clinical and research perspectives, presenting a review of the most recent advances in both areas. Although guidelines on the diagnosis and management of IPF do not recommend the use of BAL, its use is argued in excluding differential diagnosis and in patients without a confident diagnosis on HRCT, which is driven by the centre's experience and expertise. As a research tool, BAL has been useful in the study of the pathogenesis of pulmonary fibrosis, as well as in the identification of disease subtypes and response to therapy. After discussing the safety of the technique and less invasive alternatives, we will highlight some areas where further research is needed.

The study of both cellular and acellular components of the lower respiratory tract is performed using BAL, a minimally invasive bronchoscopic procedure. The technique was first reported in the USA in 1974 by REYNOLDS and NEWBALL [1] and provided a new way for assessing the pathophysiology of diffuse parenchymal lung diseases without the need for surgical biopsy. Being a safe and informative procedure, there was rapid widespread adoption of the technique for two reasons: 1) the analysis of the different cell populations is used for differential diagnosis between different ILDs, while at the same time excluding infections and malignancy with high confidence; and 2) the collection of both live cells and supernatant allows the development of both cell-based fundamental research and quantification of mediators. These studies have been the source of most of our current knowledge about the pulmonary immune mechanisms during both physiological and pathological conditions.

The number of PubMed papers using BAL for diagnosis and research has been steadily increasing, despite the 40 years that have passed since the first published report. The development of news ways and techniques that could compete with BAL for sample analysis of the lower respiratory tract environment is also increasing.

At present, the clinical and research application of BAL presents some significant challenges. When evaluating the acellular components of the collected fluid, variable dilution of the alveolar lining fluid is to be expected. Concerning the cell population analysis, the initial promises of a straightforward BAL-derived diagnosis for most ILDs did not turn out to be an easy task [2]. Most ILDs are rare or infrequent, complicating the development of adequate clinical trials. A significant number of small studies have shown

Centre of Pneumology, Coimbra University Hospital, Coimbra, Portugal.

Correspondence: Carlos Robalo Cordeiro, Centre of Pneumology, Coimbra University Hospital, Rua Mota Pinta, 3000 Coimbra, Portugal. E-mail: carlos.crobalo@gmail.com

ERS Monogr 2016; 71: 74–81. DOI: 10.1183/2312508X.10005115

that most diseases do not have a specific cell pattern. This is common in all tests for the diagnosis of ILD. Accordingly, the gold standard for the diagnosis of ILD is a multidisciplinary discussion, where the clinical findings are combined with the results from multiple tests, such as BAL, imaging and biopsies, by a team of physicians that includes a pulmonologist, radiologist and pathologist [3, 4]. It should be noted, however, that in some cases the BAL findings may be very specific and so can directly confirm a particular diagnosis and, thus, can then replace lung biopsy. This is the case for rare ILDs such as pulmonary alveolar proteinosis, Langerhans' cell histiocytosis, diffuse alveolar haemorrhage and ILDs due to mineral dust exposure [5].

Concerning IPF, whereas the role of BAL as a research tool is generally accepted, its place in the clinical management of patients with suspected or confirmed disease is still a matter of discussion. In this chapter we present a review of the most recent advances in both areas, as well as a small discussion on the safety of this technique in this unique population. We will conclude by proposing some areas where further research is required.

Clinical management

The creation of an adequate definition and classification for ILDs has proved to be a large and difficult task, especially for the IIPs. Accordingly, the term IPF has suffered significant changes in its meaning, particularly prior to and after 2000 [6]. These changes render the current interpretation of many previous studies on BAL quite difficult or even impossible. Another issue is the improvement in diagnostic accuracy of alternative tests, especially HRCT [7]. This means that in older studies the diagnostic importance of BAL could be higher, because the imaging findings were not as clear. In this chapter we will focus on the current role of BAL in IPF within the typical circumstances of a specialist ILD centre.

Diagnosis

The recent and widely accepted American Thoracic Society/European Respiratory Society/ Japanese Respiratory Society/Latin American Thoracic Association guidelines on the diagnosis and management of IPF do not recommend the usage of BAL for diagnosis. The committee placed a high value on the additional risk and cost of BAL in patients with IPF and a low value on possible improved specificity of diagnosis [8]. Similarly, the 2012 American Thoracic Society guidelines on clinical utility of BAL in ILD recommend that BAL is not needed when there is a diagnostic HRCT scan, as might be the case in IPF patients with a definite UIP HRCT pattern [5].

The typical BAL cell profile in a patient with IPF shows a predominance of macrophages, with a moderate increase in neutrophils and eosinophils, and normal lymphocyte numbers. This profile is not specific, as other diseases might show the exact same findings, *e.g.* fibrotic NSIP, desquamative interstitial pneumonia or collagen vascular disease-related ILD (table 1) [5]. The main clinical scenario where BAL could be of diagnostic importance is when hypersensitivity pneumonitis is a concern. A seminal study by OHSHIMO *et al.* [9] analysed the BAL profile of 74 patients fulfilling the criteria for diagnosis of IPF according to the 2002 guidelines. Six (8%) of these patients had an increase in lymphocytes of >30%. Upon further clinical investigation, all patients were shown to have an alternative diagnosis (hypersensitivity pneumonitis: n=3; NSIP: n=3). The authors argue that a 30% lymphocyte threshold can be used for the exclusion of IPF, thus underlining the importance of BAL

Table 1. BAL changes in IPF and some differential diagnoses

Disease	Macrophages	Neutrophils	Eosinophils	Lymphocytes	Other findings
IPF	Increased	Increased	Increased	Normal	
NSIP	Increased	Normal/increased	Normal	Increased	
HP	Normal	Normal/increased	Normal	Very high	Increased total cell count, foamy macrophages, mast cells, plasma cells
DIP/RBILD	Increased	Normal/increased	Normal/increased	Normal	Pigmented AM
Sarcoidosis	Normal	Normal/increased	Normal	Increased	Elevated CD4/CD8 ratio
CVD	Normal/increased	Elevated	Normal/elevated	Elevated	

HP: hypersensitivity pneumonitis; DIP: desquamative interstitial pneumonia; RBILD: respiratory bronchiolitis with ILD; CVD: collagen vascular disease; AM: alveolar macrophage.

even in patients with an otherwise clear IPF diagnosis [9]. It is recognised that chronic hypersensitivity pneumonitis and IPF may show identical clinical, imaging and even pathological findings [10]. Some authors have subsequently argued that BAL should only be considered when there is a high local prevalence of hypersensitivity pneumonitis [11]. This is still an active area of discussion. Nevertheless, most authors agree that local experience and expertise will influence the decision on whether or not to perform BAL in patients with suspected IPF [8]. A recent German clinical practice IPF cohort study reported the use of BAL in 310 out of 502 patients, confirming frequent use of BAL in European IPF patients [12]. Some authors have argued that the guidelines on the diagnosis of IPF should make different recommendations for the cases when the clinical and HRCT findings are typical of IPF (definite IPF) *versus* the cases where clinical and imaging findings do not allow a confident diagnosis [13]. In patients with an unclear history and/or imaging findings for IPF, the performance of BAL is more accepted. A cultural difference on the use of BAL between Europe and USA is also acknowledged [13]. For discussion and guidelines on the performance and interpretation of BAL, readers are referred to the updated and comprehensive guidelines on this subject published in 2012 by the American Thoracic Society [5].

Prognosis

Recent studies have not found a consistent benefit of BAL for the evaluation of the prognosis of an individual patient. One study found a correlation between BAL lymphocytosis and survival in patients with fibrotic IIPs [14], while another found increased mortality in patients with increased neutrophils [15]. A third study found no significant associations [16]. There have been no studies on prediction of response to the currently available anti-fibrotic therapies. One interesting finding is the association between chronic aspiration and IPF [17]. Several studies have evaluated the utility of BAL pepsin for identification of chronic aspiration [18]. It is currently unknown whether the quantification of pepsin in the BAL of IPF patients could predict the response to anti-acid therapy.

In conclusion, most authors currently agree that there is no role for BAL in the assessment of prognosis in IPF patients [5].

Exacerbations

Patients with IPF are at risk of episodes of clinical deterioration called acute exacerbations following the exclusion of a number of other causes besides the disease itself. The generally accepted diagnostic criteria for acute exacerbations of IPF require the use of BAL for the exclusion of infection [19]. Some authors have argued that this could lead to unnecessary risks and proposed an algorithm where BAL is only performed in a subset of these patients [20]. The cellular BAL analysis from patients with acute exacerbations of IPF usually shows increased neutrophils [21, 22]. It is important to remember that BAL can be valuable in other causes of deterioration in a patient with IPF, such as drug toxicity and possibly gastric aspiration [20]. In conclusion, BAL should be considered for IPF patients with disease worsening, although a proportion will not need it or tolerate it.

Research tool

The main advantages for using BAL as a research tool are its safety, broad availability and capacity to reflect the global pathophysiology of normal or diseased lung. Although BAL was classically used in the study of parenchymal disorders, its application in airway diseases such as asthma and COPD has been increasing, further strengthening the importance of this procedure [23]. Since BAL recovers both live cells and fluid with soluble mediators, these aspects can be mutually studied in each subject. The broad usage of BAL for clinical reasons means that part of the recovered fluid and cells can be preserved for research, without causing further risk or discomfort to the patient. A final advantage is that BAL can be performed serially, reflecting change with time, although this is not normally performed in clinical practice [23].

Researchers are also faced with some problems when using BAL. Safety should always be a concern as the procedure is not completely free of risk. Secondly, there are significant variations between centres regarding the technique, despite published recommendations for homogenisation [5]. Finally, when studying soluble components, a dilution of the epithelial lining fluid is expected. For the precise quantification of any mediator, this dilution factor should be known. However, different methods have been used [24] and an accurate estimation of the dilution has never been accepted. Published international guidelines have recommended the use of non-corrected quantifications [25]. This limitation has probably prevented the use of BAL quantification methods in clinical practice.

Some of the areas where BAL has been instrumental in IPF research include the study of disease pathophysiology, disease subtypes and response to therapy. Concerning pathophysiology, studies in BAL cells and mediators were helpful in showing IPF to be a fibroblast driven, noninflammatory fibrotic process [26]. Many of the recent discoveries on the importance of microorganisms in the pathogenesis of IPF are also based on BAL [27]. Concerning disease subtypes, SELMAN et al. [28] studied rapid IPF progressors and showed increased BAL concentrations of the A2B adenosine receptor and activated matrix metalloproteinase-9. Finally, the preclinical and clinical development of both pirfenidone and nintedanib benefited from studies using BAL [29, 30].

Safety

BAL is a minimally invasive technique with a favourable risk/benefit ratio. The contraindications and risk factors for complications from BAL are the same as for bronchoscopy. The rate of complications varies from 0% to 2.3%. Post-procedure fever is expected to occur in 3–30% of patients. Its frequency is correlated to total volume used and the mechanism is local release of inflammatory mediators. A transient loss of lung function (possibly leading to hypoxaemia and intubation in severe patients) [31], and radiological infiltrates can also be seen (figure 1). Patients with airway hyperreactivity can develop wheezing, and recommendations for the use of BAL in asthmatic patients are available [32].

However, the main concern when considering BAL in IPF patients is BAL-induced acute exacerbation. A recent Japanese cohort study evaluated the risk of acute exacerbations of IPF following BAL and found significantly increased risk in the 30 days post-procedure. Importantly, none of the four reported events occurred after a first (diagnostic) BAL. The authors also reviewed all the previous reports of BAL-induced acute exacerbations of IPF [33]. A total of 12 cases were described. Most patients had functional impairment and peripheral inflammation before BAL [33].

In conclusion, BAL is a generally safe procedure in IPF patients. The small number of BAL-induced exacerbations that have been described should not deter clinicians from performing this important procedure when indicated.

Alternatives

Although BAL is considered a safe and minimally invasive procedure, several research groups have tried to develop techniques that offer similar information in a less invasive or safer way. Some of these technologies are induced sputum, exhaled breath condensate and bronchoscopic microprobe collection of pulmonary epithelial lining fluid.

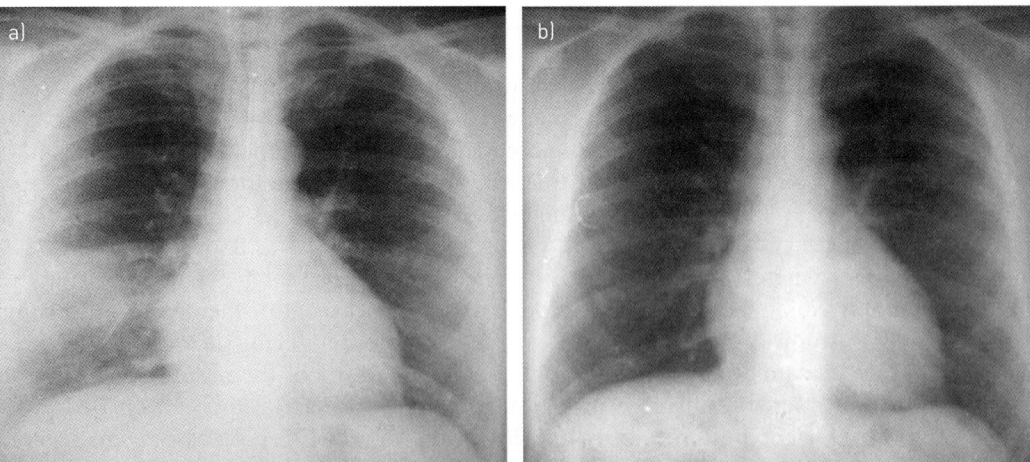

Figure 1. Chest radiograph showing a transient segmental infiltrate in the right middle lobe a) directly following BAL and b) 24 h after BAL.

Induced sputum has been widely used for the study of airways disorders. The technique involves the nebulisation of saline in isotonic or hypertonic concentrations, leading to increased production of sputum that can then be collected and analysed. Similar to BAL, both the cellular and acellular components of induced sputum can be studied. The advantages are a reduced invasiveness with increased possibility for developing serial studies, as well as less need for technology and expertise. The main disadvantage is that induced sputum studies a different component from BAL, since the sputum mostly reflects airway changes. It is generally accepted that induced sputum will not replace BAL in the clinical management and research of IPF, although some authors argue that both methods might be complementary. All in all, the data on induced sputum in IPF is still scarce and uncertain [34, 35].

Exhaled breath condensate is a completely noninvasive method for evaluating the exhaled non-volatile components of the epithelial lining fluid. The technique is quite simple and consists of directing the subject's exhaled breath over a cooled condenser system. Within a few minutes of calm breathing, a small quantity of condensate can be collected for analysis. The procedure can be safely used in children, the elderly and patients of any severity. This method allows for only non-cellular studies. The main use for exhaled breath condensate in IPF is the development of noninvasive biomarkers. The main disadvantage of the method is the extensive dilution of the solutes. This requires extremely sensitive quantification techniques and presently unavailable robust and accepted dilution markers. There is also a problem with significant methodological heterogeneity between different centres and studies [36].

Bronchoscopic microprobe sampling uses a small probe with an absorptive tip, which is introduced through the working channel of a bronchoscope to collect undiluted epithelial lining fluid from the tracheobronchial tree. The technique has been applied in studies on COPD, lung cancer, acute respiratory distress syndrome and epithelial lining fluid drug penetration. Some of the advantages of bronchoscopic microprobe over BAL are the lack of dilution, precise location of sampling and less contamination with serum proteins. The high concentration of proteins on bronchoscopic microprobe samples makes this technique particularly promising for proteomic studies. A non-bronchoscopic method has also been applied in rabbits [37].

Further research

Worldwide, many centres have been using BAL for the study of patients with suspected IPF for decades. It is therefore surprising that there is still significant discussion around the simple recommendation for its use in the diagnosis of IPF. This reflects the major need for large-scale, well-conducted studies on the benefits of BAL for the clinical management of suspected IPF patients. An example of the successful application of such studies can be found with transbronchial cryobiopsy, a new technique that can be useful in the diagnosis of IPF [38]. An equally important consideration is the interest of novel recommendations that clearly distinguish between those cases with typical features from the nondiagnostic clinical and imaging characteristics [13].

Another future clinical application of BAL in IPF is the development of biomarkers for diagnosis, evolution and response to therapy. However, biomarkers should be noninvasive and cheap, so the peripheral blood would be a better source for clinical application. We argue that BAL studies could facilitate the development phase, followed later by studies of blood [39].

The use of omics technologies, comprehensively studying a related set of biological molecules in an unbiased fashion, has been a valuable source of information on the causes, pathophysiology and treatment for human disease. Concerning BAL in IPF, the use of protein studies (proteomics) is particularly promising. In a recent study, FOSTER *et al.* [40] identified and validated pro-fibrotic cytokines in BALF of IPF patients. Marker profiling and targeted quantitation of soluble markers through proteomic approach can give insight into IPF pathology and response to therapy.

Finally, we propose greater use of BAL as a source of live cells for basic research on new therapeutic targets. The currently available animal models of IPF have significant limitations, including major differences in pathogenesis and inter-species differences in pharmacological targets when compared to human IPF [41]. BAL cells collected from IPF patients under normal clinical management can be used as a source of identification for modulators of fibrogenesis [40] and eventually for identifying new targets for therapy.

References

1. Reynolds HY, Newball HH. Analysis of proteins and respiratory cells obtained from human lungs by bronchial lavage. *J Lab Clin Med* 1974; 84: 559–573.
2. Meyer KC, Raghu G. Bronchoalveolar lavage for the evaluation of interstitial lung disease: is it clinically useful? *Eur Respir J* 2011; 38: 761–769.
3. Maher TM. A clinical approach to diffuse parenchymal lung disease. *Immunol Allergy Clin North Am* 2012; 32: 453–472.
4. Tomassetti S, Piciucchi S, Tantalocco P, *et al.* The multidisciplinary approach in the diagnosis of idiopathic pulmonary fibrosis: a patient case-based review. *Eur Respir Rev* 2015; 24: 69–77.
5. Meyer KC, Raghu G, Baughman RP, *et al.* An official American Thoracic Society clinical practice guideline: the clinical utility of bronchoalveolar lavage cellular analysis in interstitial lung disease. *Am J Respir Crit Care Med* 2012; 185: 1004–1014.
6. Travis WD, Costabel U, Hansell DM, *et al.* An official American Thoracic Society/European Respiratory Society statement: Update of the international multidisciplinary classification of the idiopathic interstitial pneumonias. *Am J Respir Crit Care Med* 2013; 188: 733–748.
7. Walsh SL, Hansell DM. High-resolution CT of interstitial lung disease: a continuous evolution. *Semin Respir Crit Care Med* 2014; 35: 129–144.
8. Raghu G, Collard HR, Egan JJ, *et al.* An official ATS/ERS/JRS/ALAT statement: idiopathic pulmonary fibrosis: evidence-based guidelines for diagnosis and management. *Am J Respir Crit Care Med* 2011; 183: 788–824.
9. Ohshimo S, Bonella F, Cui A, *et al.* Significance of bronchoalveolar lavage for the diagnosis of idiopathic pulmonary fibrosis. *Am J Respir Crit Care Med* 2009; 179: 1043–1047.
10. Cordeiro CR, Alfaro TM, Freitas S. Clinical case: differential diagnosis of idiopathic pulmonary fibrosis. *BMC Res Notes* 2013; 6: Suppl. 1, S1.
11. Kinder BW, Wells AU. The art and science of diagnosing interstitial lung diseases. *Am J Respir Crit Care Med* 2009; 179: 974–975.
12. Behr J, Kreuter M, Hoeper MM, *et al.* Management of patients with idiopathic pulmonary fibrosis in clinical practice: the INSIGHTS-IPF registry. *Eur Respir J* 2015; 46: 186–196.
13. Wells AU. Managing diagnostic procedures in idiopathic pulmonary fibrosis. *Eur Respir Rev* 2013; 22: 158–162.
14. Ryu YJ, Chung MP, Han J, *et al.* Bronchoalveolar lavage in fibrotic idiopathic interstitial pneumonias. *Respir Med* 2007; 101: 655–660.
15. Kinder BW, Brown KK, Schwarz MI, *et al.* Baseline BAL neutrophilia predicts early mortality in idiopathic pulmonary fibrosis. *Chest* 2008; 133: 226–232.
16. Veeraraghavan S, Latsi PI, Wells AU, *et al.* BAL findings in idiopathic nonspecific interstitial pneumonia and usual interstitial pneumonia. *Eur Respir J* 2003; 22: 239–244.
17. Raghu G, Meyer KC. Silent gastro-oesophageal reflux and microaspiration in IPF: mounting evidence for anti-reflux therapy? *Eur Respir J* 2012; 39: 242–245.
18. Meyer KC. Gastroesophageal reflux and lung disease. *Expert Rev Respir Med* 2015; 9: 383–385.
19. Collard HR, Moore BB, Flaherty KR Jr, *et al.* Acute exacerbations of idiopathic pulmonary fibrosis. *Am J Respir Crit Care Med* 2007; 176: 636–643.

20. Petrosyan F, Culver DA, Reddy AJ. Role of bronchoalveolar lavage in the diagnosis of acute exacerbations of idiopathic pulmonary fibrosis: a retrospective study. *BMC Pulm Med* 2015; 15: 70.

21. Ambrosini V, Cancellieri A, Chilosi M, *et al.* Acute exacerbation of idiopathic pulmonary fibrosis: report of a series. *Eur Respir J* 2003; 22: 821–826.

22. Parambil JG, Myers JL, Ryu JH. Histopathologic features and outcome of patients with acute exacerbation of idiopathic pulmonary fibrosis undergoing surgical lung biopsy. *Chest* 2005; 128: 3310–3315.

23. Rose AS, Knox KS. Bronchoalveolar lavage as a research tool. *Semin Respir Crit Care Med* 2007; 28: 561–573.

24. Haslam PL, Baughman RP. Report of ERS Task Force: guidelines for measurement of acellular components and standardization of BAL. *Eur Respir J* 1999; 14: 245–248.

25. Baughman RP. Technical aspects of bronchoalveolar lavage: recommendations for a standard procedure. *Semin Respir Crit Care Med* 2007; 28: 475–485.

26. Buckley S, Shi W, Xu W, *et al.* Increased alveolar soluble annexin V promotes lung inflammation and fibrosis. *Eur Respir J* 2015; 46: 1417–1429.

27. Molyneaux PL, Cox MJ, Willis-Owen SA, *et al.* The role of bacteria in the pathogenesis and progression of idiopathic pulmonary fibrosis. *Am J Respir Crit Care Med* 2014; 190: 906–913.

28. Selman M, Carrillo G, Estrada A, *et al.* Accelerated variant of idiopathic pulmonary fibrosis: clinical behavior and gene expression pattern. *PLoS One* 2007; 2: e482.

29. Iyer SN, Gurujeyalakshmi G, Giri SN. Effects of pirfenidone on transforming growth factor-β gene expression at the transcriptional level in bleomycin hamster model of lung fibrosis. *J Pharmacol Exp Ther* 1999; 291: 367–373.

30. Wollin L, Maillet I, Quesniaux V, *et al.* Antifibrotic and anti-inflammatory activity of the tyrosine kinase inhibitor nintedanib in experimental models of lung fibrosis. *J Pharmacol Exp Ther* 2014; 349: 209–220.

31. Bonella F, Ohshimo S, Bauer P, *et al.* Bronchoalveolar lavage. *In*: Strausz J Bolliger CT, eds. Interventional Pulmonology (ERS Monograph). Sheffield, European Respiratory Society, 2010; 48: pp. 59–72.

32. Summary and recommendations of a workshop on the investigative use of fiberoptic bronchoscopy and bronchoalveolar lavage in asthmatics. *Am Rev Respir Dis* 1985; 132: 180–182.

33. Sakamoto K, Taniguchi H, Kondoh Y, *et al.* Acute exacerbation of IPF following diagnostic bronchoalveolar lavage procedures. *Respir Med* 2012; 106: 436–442.

34. Araujo L, Beltrao M, Palmares C, *et al.* Induced sputum in interstitial lung diseases – a pilot study. *Rev Port Pneumol* 2013; 19: 53–58.

35. Economidou F, Samara KD, Antoniou KM, *et al.* Induced sputum in interstitial lung diseases: novel insights in the diagnosis, evaluation and research. *Respiration* 2009; 77: 351–358.

36. Dompeling E, Rosias PPR, Jobsis Q. Exhaled breath condensate sample collection: standards and open issues. *In*: Horvath I de Jongste JC, eds. Exhaled Biomarkers (ERS Monograph). Sheffield, European Respiratory Society, 2010; 49: pp. 152–161.

37. Franciosi L, Govorukhina N, Fusetti F, *et al.* Proteomic analysis of human epithelial lining fluid by microfluidics-based nanoLC-MS/MS: a feasibility study. *Electrophoresis* 2013; 34: 2683–2694.

38. Tomassetti S, Wells AU, Costabel U, *et al.* Bronchoscopic lung cryobiopsy increases diagnostic confidence in the multidisciplinary diagnosis of idiopathic pulmonary fibrosis. *Am J Respir Crit Care Med* 2015; [In press; DOI: 10.1164/rccm.201504-0711OC].

39. O'Riordan TG, Smith V, Raghu G. Development of novel agents for idiopathic pulmonary fibrosis: progress in target selection and clinical trial design. *Chest* 2015; 148: 1083–1092.

40. Foster MW, Morrison LD, Todd JL, *et al.* Quantitative proteomics of bronchoalveolar lavage fluid in idiopathic pulmonary fibrosis. *J Proteome Res* 2015; 14: 1238–1249.

41. Degryse AL, Lawson WE. Progress toward improving animal models for idiopathic pulmonary fibrosis. *Am J Med Sci* 2011; 341: 444–449.

Disclosures: None declared.

| Chapter 7

Imaging

Simon L.F. Walsh

HRCT is central to the evaluation of patients with suspected IPF. Based on the most up-to-date diagnostic guidelines, which were published as a collaborative effort by American Thoracic Society (ATS), European Respiratory Society (ERS), Japanese Respiratory Society (JRS) and the Latin American Thoracic Association (ALAT) in 2011, in the correct clinical setting a pattern of UIP on HRCT allows a diagnosis of IPF to be made without the need for surgical lung biopsy. An important difficulty applying these guidelines is that a significant proportion of patients with IPF, do not present with typical HRCT appearances and, at the same time, are unable to undergo surgical lung biopsy. Recognising this limitation, there have been several recent attempts to expand the range of HRCT appearances, which are considered sufficiently accurate for IPF to preclude the need to proceed to biopsy. Detection and diagnosis of early IPF also represents an important challenge for the radiologist particularly given the recent licensing of new therapeutic agents for IPF. Finally, there is a growing perception that the initial HRCT appearances of patients with suspected IPF are best considered the starting point of a diagnostic process which is dynamic, rather than representing an immutable diagnosis in the absence of biopsy material.

IPF is a progressive fibrotic lung disease of unknown aetiology with a median survival from time of diagnosis of 2–3 years [1–5]. Accurate diagnosis of IPF is crucial to ensure prompt initiation of appropriate treatment and enrolment of patients in clinical trials. HRCT plays a key role in the initial evaluation of patients with suspected IPF and, based on the most recent diagnostic guidelines published in 2011 by the American Thoracic Society (ATS), European Respiratory Society (ERS), Japanese Respiratory Society (JRS) and the Latin American Thoracic Association (ALAT), a typical pattern of UIP on HRCT obviates the need for surgical lung biopsy [6]. When HRCT features are not those of UIP, surgical lung biopsy is mandated. Since the publication of the 2011 statement, this paradigm has faced several challenges. First, a significant minority of patients with IPF does not present with typical HRCT features of UIP and are also unable to undergo surgical lung biopsy due to advanced age or preclusive comorbidities, thus debarring them from a secure diagnosis based on these criteria [7]. Second, there is a growing perception that selected patients whose HRCT appearances do not meet criteria for UIP, have histopathological UIP [8–11]. Third, evidence from two recent IPF trials suggests that, if therapeutic benefit is to be optimised, early initiation of treatment is highly desirable, yet paradoxically, a HRCT-based diagnosis of IPF requires the presence of honeycombing, which is a relatively late HRCT sign [12–14]. Fourth, there is emerging evidence that interobserver agreement for the current 2011 HRCT criteria for a UIP pattern is

King's College Hospital Foundation Trust, London, UK.

Correspondence: Simon L.F. Walsh, King's College Hospital Foundation Trust, Denmark Hill, London SE5 9RS. E-mail: slfwalsh@gmail.com suboptimal [15]. Notwithstanding these limitations, HRCT and the 2011 ATS/ERS/JRS/ALAT recommendations remain central to the initial evaluation of patients with suspected IPF. These issues, as they relate to the imaging of IPF, will form the focus of discussion in the first part of this manuscript. A discussion on the prognostic role HRCT plays in IPF will follow.

Diagnosis

Current guidelines: defining a UIP pattern

The most recent evidence based guidelines for the diagnosis and management of IPF represent the collaborative effort of the ATS, ERS, JRS and ALAT and were published in 2011 [6]. These guidelines, which are based upon evidence published until 2011 and expert opinion when evidence was lacking, state that in correct clinical context, a typical pattern of UIP on HRCT may be sufficient to diagnosis IPF without the need to perform surgical lung biopsy [16, 17]. Therefore, HRCT has a primary role in the diagnosis of patients with suspected IPF and, once performed, greatly influences subsequent management decisions.

HRCT evaluation of patients with suspected IPF is based upon three separate HRCT diagnosis categories clearly defined in the 2011 ATS/ERS/JRS/ALAT statement: "UIP", "possible UIP" and "inconsistent with UIP" (table 1). HRCT criteria for a diagnosis of UIP include the presence of honeycombing in a basal and subpleural distribution without features considered incompatible with a diagnosis of IPF (figure 1a). The HRCT features of honeycombing are clustered cystic airspaces usually of consistent diameter (3–10 mm, but occasionally larger), with characteristically thick, well-defined walls. Traction bronchiectasis

Table 1. ATS/ERS/JRS/ALAT HRCT criteria for a UIP pattern

UIP pattern (all four features)	Possible UIP pattern (all three features)	Inconsistent with UIP pattern (any of the seven features)
Subpleural, basal predominance	Subpleural, basal predominance	Upper or mid-lung predominance
Reticular abnormality	Reticular abnormality	Peribronchovascular predominance
Honeycombing with or without traction bronchiectasis	Absence of features listed as inconsistent with UIP pattern (see third column)	Extensive ground-glass abnormality (extent reticular abnormality)
Absence of features listed as inconsistent with UIP pattern (see third column)		Profuse micronodules (bilateral, predominantly upper lobes)
		Discrete cysts (multiple, bilateral, away from areas of honeycombing)
		Diffuse mosaic attenuation/ air-trapping (bilateral, in three or more lobes)
		Consolidation in bronchopulmonary segment(s)/lobe(s)

ATS: American Thoracic Society; ERS: European Respiratory Society; JRS: Japanese Respiratory Society; ALAT: Latin American Thoracic Association. Reproduced and modified from [6] with permission from the publisher.

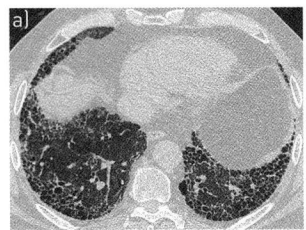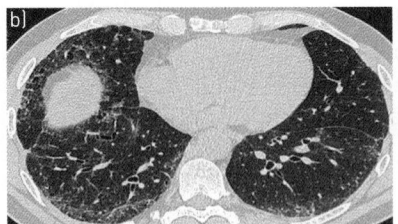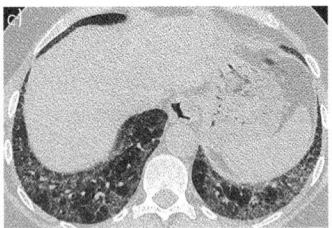

Figure 1. Axial HRCT images demonstrating: a) UIP, characterised by subpleural basal predominant honeycombing without atypical features (table 1); b) possible UIP pattern, showing basal subpleural reticular abnormalities containing traction bronchiectasis without evidence of honeycombing; and c) inconsistent with UIP pattern showing areas of ground-glass opacification and reticulation containing traction bronchiectasis.

is invariably present. When the HRCT lacks honeycombing but otherwise demonstrates basal reticular abnormalities typical of UIP, the HRCT meets criteria for a diagnosis of "possible UIP" (figure 1b). For HRCT appearances to be considered "inconsistent with a UIP pattern", one or more specific features must be present (figure 1c). If the HRCT appearances are not those of UIP, the diagnosis of IPF cannot be made on imaging alone and surgical lung biopsy is recommended.

Numerous retrospective and prospective studies have demonstrated that the positive predictive value of a radiological diagnosis of UIP on HRCT for a pathologic diagnosis of UIP is between 90–100%, although all of these studies included only patients with a biopsy-proven diagnosis, therefore introducing a selection bias [16–23]. Regardless, current recommendations recognise a UIP pattern on HRCT to be highly accurate for the presence of UIP on lung biopsy. Despite this, a substantial minority of patients with histopathological UIP (30–50%) do not fulfil the current HRCT criteria for a UIP pattern [16, 17, 21, 22]. This point is highlighted in a recent IPF drug trial in which "definite UIP" (as described by the study protocol and corresponding to the current ATS/ERS/JRS/ALAT HRCT criteria for UIP) was found in only 32.6% of enrolled patients [24]. The range of HRCT appearances of pathological UIP, not presenting with typical imaging features on HRCT, has been investigated by SVERZELLATI et al. [25]. In that study, 55 biopsy proven cases of IPF were stratified based on their HRCT appearances being typical or atypical for a radiological diagnosis of IPF. A total of 34 (62%) of the cases were considered to have atypical imaging features; the most common radiological diagnosis was NSIP (18 out of 34) followed by chronic hypersensitivity pneumonitis (four out of 34), sarcoidosis (three out of 34), organising pneumonia (one out of 34) and, in eight cases, no consensus diagnosis could be reached. Finally, it is noteworthy that although a UIP pattern on HRCT is accurate for pathological UIP in more than 90% of cases, fibrotic NSIP, chronic hypersensitivity pneumonitis and very rarely sarcoidosis may present with HRCT features compatible with UIP [26, 27].

Diagnostic challenges for the radiologist

Clarification of possible UIP on HRCT

A prevalent diagnostic problem encountered is the IPF patient whose HRCT lacks honeycombing but otherwise has basal subpleural reticular abnormalities typical of UIP. These patients often meet imaging criteria for a "possible UIP pattern" and in this setting, the 2011 ATS/ERS/JRS/ALAT statement mandates that biopsy evidence of UIP is needed to secure a diagnosis of IPF. This is appropriate as there is significant overlap between the imaging features of possible UIP, fibrotic NSIP and chronic hypersensitivity pneumonitis (CHP).

In one study, within a cohort of 66 patients with CHP, IPF or NSIP, although a correct first-choice HRCT diagnosis was made in 92 (81%) of 113 readings, confident distinction between these disease entities could be made in only approximately 50% of patients [28]. A common difficulty applying this recommendation is that a significant minority of these patients is unable to undergo lung biopsy because of comorbidities, severity of disease or age and this ultimately prevents them access to treatments only licensed for use in patients with a secure diagnosis of IPF.

Given this limitation, being able to secure an accurate diagnosis of IPF in patients whose imaging meets possible UIP criteria without proceeding to surgical lung biopsy would be desirable. This has been the goal of several recent radiological studies. In a cohort of 44 patients with biopsy-proven UIP, GRUDEN et al. [10] defined four patterns of fibrosis: classic UIP, fibrosis with no honeycombing, minimal fibrosis and a ground-glass present pattern. The authors reported that both classic UIP and fibrosis with no honeycombing patterns consistently demonstrated a heterogeneous pattern of fibrosis and concluded that heterogeneity of fibrosis may be diagnostic of pathological UIP in the appropriate clinical setting. More recently, CHUNG et al. [9] addressed this problem directly by dividing the current "possible UIP" category into "probable UIP" and "indeterminate". Probable UIP was defined as peripheral and basilar predominant pulmonary fibrosis with reticulation, little or no honeycombing, and absence of features to suggest another specific diagnosis [9]. From a cohort of 201 patients with pulmonary fibrosis, those meeting "probable UIP" imaging criteria were reported as more likely to have histopathological UIP/definite UIP than those with indeterminate UIP (82.4% versus 54.2%).

Lastly, the age of the patient, which is available to radiologist at the time of reporting, appears to be highly predictive of IPF when HRCT features are not typical. In a study of 135 patients with biopsy-proven IIP (97 of whom had IPF), FELL et al. [8] demonstrated that increasing age was associated with an increasing likelihood of a diagnosis of IPF, with a positive predictive value of 100% when the patient is more than 75 years old. It is worth noting that these findings support the evolving concept of IPF as a degenerative disease of the lung [29, 30]. Furthermore, it has been suggested by some that confirmation of these findings in a larger cohort is of particular importance, as it would allow the current criteria for a definite diagnosis of IPF to be expanded [7].

Identification of early IPF on HRCT

Based upon the 2011 ATS/ERS/JRS/ALAT statement, an HRCT-based diagnosis of IPF requires the presence of honeycombing; arguably implicit in this definition is that established fibrosis must be present. In contrast, with the recent licensing of two new drugs for treatment of IPF in mild-to-moderate disease, early and accurate diagnosis of IPF is crucial for improvement of clinical outcome [13, 14]. This requires radiologists to be vigilant to early signs of fibrosis on HRCT. For example, although a very limited subpleural reticular abnormality on HRCT without honeycombing may not meet criteria for a UIP pattern, in a patient over the age of 75 years without an identifiable cause, these findings point to an IPF diagnosis, and present an opportunity for early intervention [8]. It should be highlighted, that the spectrum of HRCT patterns seen in early IPF has not been investigated. Although there is some evidence that reticulation on HRCT may progress to honeycombing [31], this author recognises that cases of IPF presenting with very limited subpleural honeycomb change do occur. Several studies suggest that limited fibrotic lung disease on HRCT is important. Using low-dose CT imaging from a lung cancer screening trial, JIN et al. [32] documented the presence of interstitial lung abnormalities (ILA) in a cohort of 884 smokers. A total of 86 (9.7%) demonstrated some form of ILA, of which 19 were designated as fibrotic (ground glass with reticulation, reticulation, or honeycombing present). All of these patients demonstrated progression of disease at 2 year follow up, in contrast to the non-fibrotic ILAs, which improved or resolved. Furthermore, early fibrotic lung disease may be apparent on HRCT before physiological impairment can be detected. KONDOH et al. [33] evaluated the HRCT imaging of 16 patients with biopsy confirmed IPF but no evidence of physiological impairment on lung function testing. After a median time of 19.9±12.3 months, 11 out of 16 showed at least 10% decline in FVC or at least 15% decline in DLCO. The existence and extent of honeycombing at baseline was reported as predictive of this decline.

Observer agreement issues

Reasonable levels of observer agreement are a requisite for 2011 ATS/ERS/JRS/ALAT HRCT criteria for a UIP pattern to be useful in clinical practice. This issue can be discussed at two levels. First, because a diagnosis of definite UIP on HRCT requires the presence of honeycombing, the degree to which radiologists agree on the presence of this pattern is clinically important. The key difficulties in this regard are the distinction between honeycombing and traction bronchiectasis and the distinction between honeycombing and emphysema. Second, among radiologists who evaluate cases of suspected IPF, how well do they agree on the assignment of the three HRCT diagnosis categories specified in the 2011 recommendations?

The definition of honeycombing has undergone multiple revisions since its first description more than 60 years ago [34–38]. Several studies have reported on the observer agreement for honeycombing with conflicting results [39–41]. Perhaps the best illustration of this comes from a study by LYNCH et al. [39] in which interobserver agreement for the presence of honeycombing among expert thoracic radiologists, as assessed by a weighted kappa coefficient, was reported as no greater than 0.31, a result that would hardly be considered an acceptable level of agreement in clinical practice. Similar results have been described in several other studies [40, 41]. Most recently, a study by WATADANI et al. [36] reported interobserver agreement for honeycombing as moderate (weighted $\kappa=0.40–0.58$) among 43 observers from various subspecialties and geographic locations scoring 80 HRCT images. Disagreement on the presence of honeycombing occurred in 29% of cases and was, in most cases, due to the presence of subpleural pathology mimicking honeycombing such as traction bronchiolectasis, paraseptal emphysema and subpleural cysts (figure 2a–d). One possible limitation of this study was that observers were asked to score honeycombing on single slice CT images rather than full volumetric CT datasets.

Although in the hands of experienced observers, the accuracy of a radiological diagnosis for a specific ILD is approximately 80–90% [20, 42], less experienced observers, who also routinely report HRCT studies in patients with ILD, may be much less accurate. In a recent survey performed at a Europe-wide IPF meeting, a majority of clinicians stated that they found an HRCT diagnosis of IPF to be reliable in less than one-third of radiologists [7]. This finding supports the results of FLAHERTY et al. [43], who reported high levels of disagreement between community and academic radiologists/physicians for diagnosis in a review of 39 patients with diffuse parenchymal lung disease. Despite the clinical importance of the 2011 ATS/ERS/JRS/ALAT HRCT diagnosis categories for UIP, the interobserver agreement for these criteria is not known. Several studies, which predate the 2011 ATS/ERS/JRS/ALAT statement, have reported on the observer agreement for a confident diagnosis of UIP with conflicting results [39, 44, 45]. A limitation of these studies

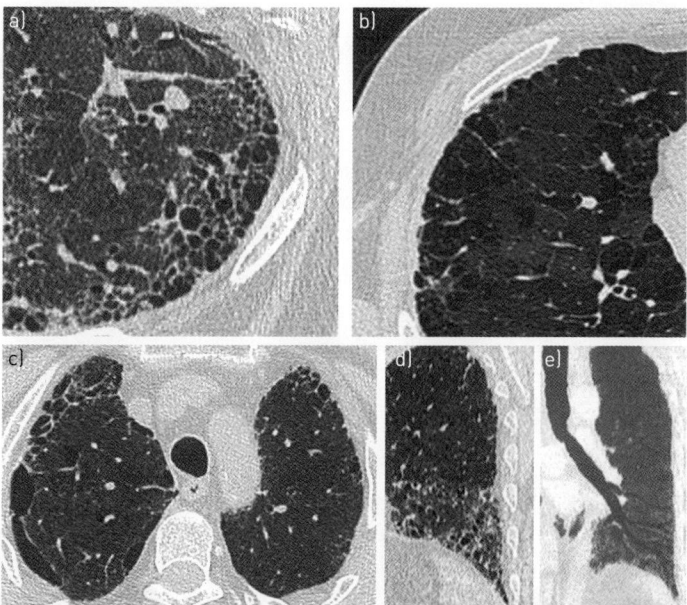

Figure 2. Honeycombing and its mimickers. a) Typical honeycombing showing multi-layered subpleural cystic spaces with thick walls in a patient with UIP. b) Paraseptal emphysema showing subpleural regions of low attenuation separated by fine intact interlobular septa. c) Honeycombing modified by co-existent paraseptal emphysema demonstrated in the subpleural lung of the right upper lobe. d) Subpleural traction bronchiectasis and bronchiolectasis in the left lower lobe. e) The minimum intensity projection image that accompanies clearly demonstrates the non-tapering airways extending into the subpleural lung responsible for this "honeycombing-like" appearance.

is that all employed small numbers of academic radiologists from tertiary referral centres with specific expertise in the evaluation of patients with IPF [39, 45].

More recently, observer agreement for the 2011 ATS/ERS/JRS/ALAT HRCT diagnosis categories for a UIP pattern has been evaluated directly in 112 thoracic radiologists from five international thoracic imaging societies, across five continents [15]. Observers were invited to evaluate 150 cases of fibrotic lung disease and provide a diagnosis score (UIP, possible UIP, inconsistent with UIP). Critically, observer agreement for the diagnosis categories was moderate (weighted $\kappa=0.47\pm0.05–0.51\pm0.11$) with thoracic radiologists of greater than 25 years of experience (n=22, 0.48±0.14) demonstrating levels of agreement no better than thoracic imaging fellows (n=5, 0.47±0.05). In this study, coexistent emphysema and fibrosis impacting observer interpretation of the presence and predominant distribution of honeycombing may have been an important source of disagreement (figure 3).

Prognosis and staging

The role of HRCT in predicting prognosis: basic patterns

The prognostic role of HRCT in the setting of IPF has been extensively reported on. At the simplest level, the radiological presentation may be prognostic significance. In the setting of biopsy-proven IPF, FLAHERTY *et al.* [46] demonstrated that a typical UIP pattern on HRCT, indicating radiological–histopathological concordance, was associated with increased

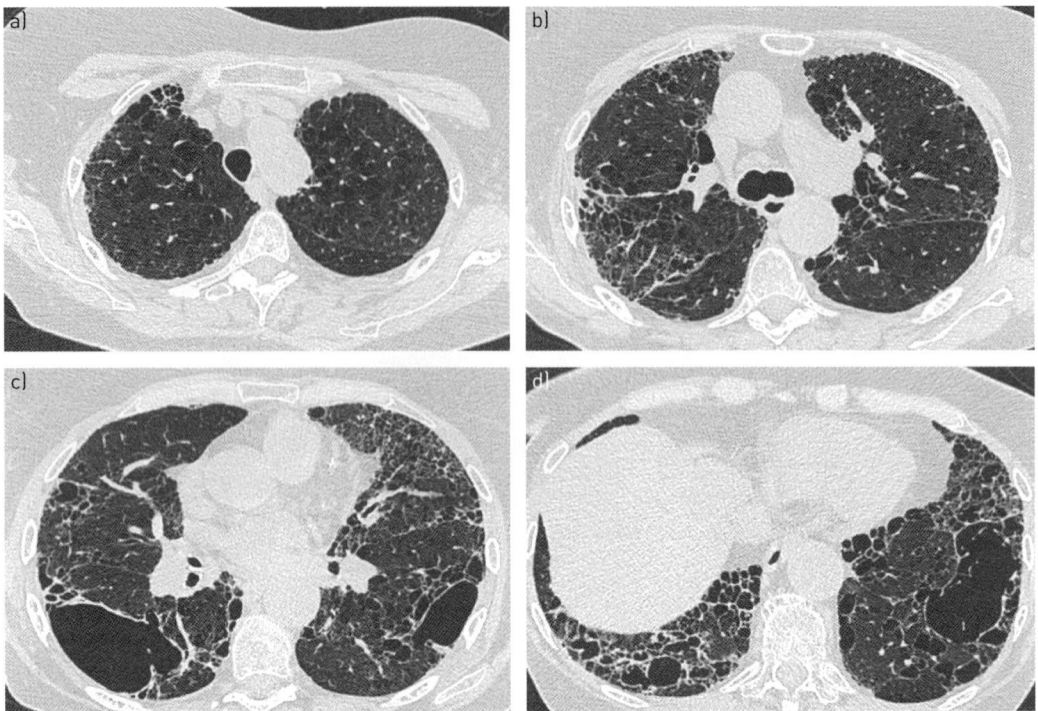

Figure 3. Axial HRCT images from a patient with a multidisciplinary team diagnosis of IPF scored by 112 thoracic radiologists on the presence/absence of emphysema and honeycombing and the diagnosis based on the American Thoracic Society (ATS)/European Respiratory Society (ERS)/Japanese Respiratory Society (JRS)/Latin American Thoracic Association (ALAT) HRCT criteria for a UIP pattern. 78% emphysema present, 82% honeycombing present. UIP 35.7%; possible UIP 36.5%; inconsistent with UIP 27.0%.

mortality when compared with those patients with an atypical UIP or fibrotic NSIP pattern on HRCT.

Honeycombing is a diagnostic HRCT pattern in patients with IPF and has consistently been reported as predicting survival in many studies over the past 15 years [40, 41, 47–49]. As discussed previously however, accurately identifying honeycombing on HRCT may not always be straightforward. Given this potential limitation, other predictive HRCT patterns, which may be more easily identified, are perhaps more useful in routine practice. Traction bronchiectasis is defined as "irregular bronchial and bronchiolar dilatation caused by surrounding retractile pulmonary fibrosis" [38] and might be considered to be as definitive an indicator of fibrotic lung disease as honeycombing. Despite this, a review of the last 20 years of HRCT outcome studies in the setting of fibrotic lung disease suggests that traction bronchiectasis has been largely been ignored; although recently this has changed. Traction bronchiectasis has emerged in several studies recently to be an important predictor of mortality in a variety of different fibrotic lung diseases, including IPF [50–54]. These findings might be explained by a recent study which has demonstrated that the severity of traction bronchiectasis on HRCT is a marker of fibroblastic foci profusion in patients with IPF [55].

Overall extent of fibrosis on HRCT may also be predictive of mortality in IPF. To quantify fibrosis, several studies have combined the extent of reticular abnormalities and honeycombing to form a CT-fibrosis score, which has been reported as predictive of mortality [51, 56, 57]. In the largest study to date, 315 well-characterised IPF patients enrolled in a clinical trial of interferon-γ1b, LYNCH et al. [39] reported that overall extent of fibrosis, also defined as extent of reticular and honeycombing patterns combined, was the strongest predictor of mortality. It is noteworthy that, in this study, HRCT was a better predictor of mortality than pulmonary function in IPF.

A specific clinical situation in which HRCT has shown interesting results, particularly when compared to pulmonary function, is acute exacerbation of IPF. AKIRA et al. [58], in a study of 34 patients with acute exacerbation of IPF, identified total disease extent on HRCT and the distribution of disease (multifocal and diffuse patterns of disease being associated with higher mortality than a predominantly peripheral distribution of disease) as being the strongest predictors of survival. Importantly, pulmonary function offered no further prognostic information once HRCT findings were accounted for. In another study by FUJIMOTO et al. [49], an HRCT score based upon extent of disease calculated from CT attenuation values was used to predict prognosis in 60 patients with acute exacerbation of IPF. From these results, a prognostic threshold value for the HRCT score was generated for stratifying clinical risk. Again, this threshold proved to be stronger predictor of mortality than pulmonary function.

The data on the impact of serial HRCT change on prognosis in IPF is relatively limited. Although honeycombing progresses over time most patients with IPF [31, 59–61] few studies have evaluated the prognostic impact of these changes over a specific follow-up period. In a study by FLAHERTY et al. [62] who evaluated the prognostic impact of changes in physiological and HRCT data over a 6-month follow-up period in 109 patients with idiopathic fibrotic lung disease, semiquantitative HRCT scoring failed to demonstrate prognostic short-term changes in HRCT fibrosis scores. In contrast, HWANG et al. [63] using a median 12-month follow-up period, reported that baseline extent of honeycombing and progression of honeycombing in a cohort of 72 patients fibrotic lung disease (42 idiopathic, 30 connective tissue related) were the only predictors of mortality. Interestingly, in this study, neither baseline nor serial change in pulmonary function predicted survival.

Automated prognostic evaluation of HRCT in IPF

In several studies, physiological surrogates of disease progression in IPF, such as changes in FVC or DLCO over 6–12 months have proven to be superior predictors of mortality than their baseline counterparts [62, 64–66]. In contrast, although baseline HRCT patterns have prognostic value in patients with IPF, studies evaluating longitudinal changes in disease extent or qualitative pattern changes on HRCT have been less impressive [62]. The likely explanation for this is that HRCT evaluation by human observers is subjective and, as previously discussed, coexistent pulmonary pathology, experience or even viewing conditions may adversely impact observer agreement [36]. These limitations have prompted evaluation of various objective, computer-based image analysis tools for assessing disease extent and disease progression on HRCT.

The CT attenuation histogram, which reflects lung density, may be used to characterise and quantify diffuse lung disease. Several studies have evaluated histogram-based measurements such as mean lung attenuation, skew and kurtosis from HRCT images in patients with IPF and have demonstrated a correlation with physiological markers of disease severity [67–69]. In one study, which included a subgroup of 95 IPF patients with both baseline and follow-up HRCT and lung function data, only a visually estimated fibrosis score, skewness and kurtosis (derived from the CT histogram) predicted mortality [68]. A limitation of histogram analysis is that it uses only one feature to evaluate diffuse lung disease: lung density. In the setting of mixed disease, such as emphysema with fibrosis a discriminatory assessment is not possible using these techniques. Textural analysis involves identification of different CT patterns (such as honeycombing, reticulation or ground-glass opacification) using multiple texture features computed from CT data. UPPALURI et al. [70], using this technique, reported high levels of accuracy (when evaluated against human observers) for the identification of six different CT patterns (honeycombing, ground glass, bronchovascular, nodular, emphysema-like, and normal lung). More recently, IWASAWA et al. [71] demonstrated that an automated analysis of fibrosis extent using a multi-feature CT frequency histogram based system, may be used to predict prognosis in patients with IPF.

The most recent and perhaps the most promising imaging analysis technique to be evaluated in patients with IPF is the CALIPER (Computer-Aided Lung Informatics for Pathology Evaluation and Ratings) developed by the Biomedical Imaging Resource Laboratory at the Mayo Clinic [72]. This system is based upon histogram signature mapping techniques and is trained using pathologically confirmed imaging data evaluated by expert radiologist consensus. In a study by MALDONADO et al. [72] the HRCTs of 55 patients with IPF were evaluated at baseline and follow up (mean 289 days) by expert thoracic radiologists and by CALIPER. Although the interpretation of global disease progression by both the radiologists and CALIPER predicted mortality, the CALIPER quantification of progression of reticular changes was also predictive of mortality [72]. These findings, might suggest that automated evaluation of lung patterns by CALIPER may allow the identification of subtle qualitative changes that are imperceptible to human observers (figure 4).

HRCT and staging of IPF

Numerous studies have evaluated predictors of mortality in patients with IPF, and clearly from the previous discussion, HRCT has a part to play. In addition to imaging data, other prognostic variables include patient-reported symptoms, baseline lung function [73–76] and changes in lung function over time [62, 64, 74, 76, 77], composite measures of physiological impairment, 6MWT data [78, 79], serum/BAL biomarkers [80–91] and histopathological features, in particular, fibroblastic foci profusion [1, 92–94]. Despite this extensive effort, use of individual parameters to guide management decisions in clinical practice has been limited, possibly because no one variable appears to accurately predict prognosis is isolation. Furthermore, in patients with IPF, management strategies are often dichotomous: does the patient have progressive but potentially modifiable disease warranting treatment, or do they have stable disease, or disease that is inexorably progressive which is unlikely to respond to treatment. A limitation of the data discussed up to now, by virtue of them being continuous, is that they are not easily applied to these dichotomous management strategies in individual patients. One approach, which addresses both of these issues, is to generate staging algorithms by combining prognostic variables, which stratify patients into clear groups based on prognosis. As an example, this approach has been successfully applied to patients with systemic sclerosis-related ILD, for which a sharp dichotomous separation of patients with good and poor prognosis based on the extent of disease extent on HRCT (using a threshold of 20%) and the FVC (using a threshold of 70%) has been reported [95]. A similar approach to staging ILD, which incorporates HRCT, has recently been reported in pulmonary sarcoidosis [96].

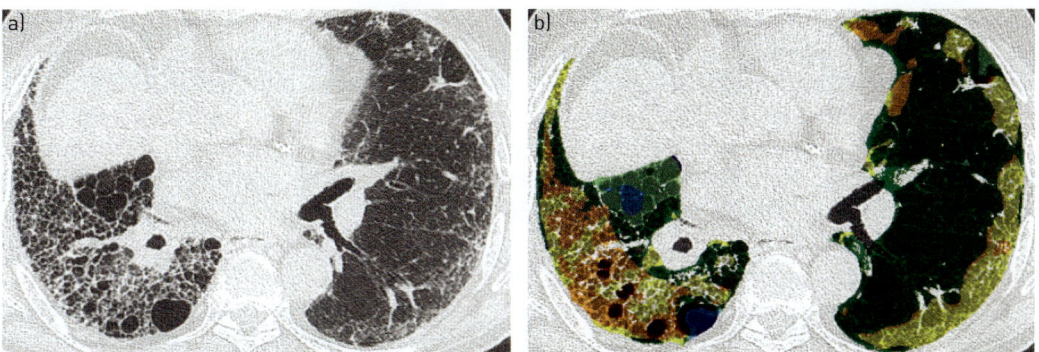

Figure 4. Representative images from the quantitative analysis of CALIPER (Computer-Aided Lung Informatics for Pathology Evaluation and Ratings). a) The individual regions of lung are classified using histogram signature mapping techniques and b) colour-coded into one of the classes of parenchymal abnormality. Courtesy of J. Jacob, Royal Brompton Hospital, London, UK and B. Bartholmai, Mayo Clinic, Rochester, MN, USA.

In the past, patients with IPF have been classified as having "mild", "moderate" or "severe" disease based on lung function tests however these stages do not represent distinct clinical phenotypes and their ability to predict therapeutic response or mortality is limited. Therefore, there is a pressing need to develop a reliable means to stage patients with IPF, which usefully informs management decisions [97]. Recently, LEY et al. [98] reported the GAP model: a multidimensional risk prediction model for IPF based upon patient age, sex, FVC and DLCO which separates patients into one of three prognostically distinct groups. This model has subsequently been validated in a separate Asian population of patients with IPF [99], successfully applied to a large all-comers ILD group made up of patients with idiopathic fibrotic lung disease, connective tissue disease related ILD, chronic hypersensitivity pneumonitis and unclassifiable ILD [100] and most recently expanded to include longitudinal physiological data [101]. What is interesting about this staging model from an imaging perspective is that a modified GAP model has been proposed using HRCT-pattern extent scores [102]. In a retrospective study, the HRCT scans from 348 patients with IPF were evaluated for extent of fibrosis and extent of emphysema using a visual scoring method. A CT–GAP score was calculated by replacing the DLCO from the original GAP model with a CT fibrosis score. This CT–GAP score was reported as providing an equally robust prognostic separation of patients with IPF, as the original GAP model. In patients who cannot perform lung function tests, this CT–GAP score provides a useful alternative. In the future, incorporation of predictive biomarkers and longitudinal imaging/physiological data may help to refine these staging models further. In this regard, two important issues warrant consideration: first, while it may be desirable to only include the strongest prognostic data in any staging model, it is also important that this data can be obtained from tests that are readily available in clinical practice; and second, a staging model should be easy to apply and allow swift and robust management decisions to be made, even by less experienced observers.

HRCT and clinical trials in IPF

The role of HRCT in IPF clinical trials can be discussed in terms of HRCT-defined trial entry criteria and HRCT-defined endpoints. Although the 2011 ATS/ERS/JRS/ALAT statement clearly defines the requirements for a HRCT-based diagnosis of IPF (essentially basal predominant subpleural honeycombing [6]), emerging evidence, which has previously been discussed, suggests that selected participants who meet criteria for a possible UIP pattern usually have histopathological UIP [8–11]. This was reflected in the inclusion criteria of a recent IPF trial evaluating the efficacy and safety of nintedanib, in which patients with basal predominant reticular abnormalities but without honeycombing or atypical features (essentially meeting "possible UIP" criteria), qualified for inclusion without the need for histopathological proof of UIP [13]. By performing a central review of imaging by radiologists with specialist expertise in diagnosing IPF, inclusion of homogenous patient populations in clinical trials is made more likely [13, 14].

Optimum design and implementation of clinical trials in IPF requires the selection of appropriate endpoints, but the question of which outcome measures represent the best end points has been the source of debate [103–105]. Although mortality has commonly been regarded as the "gold-standard" endpoint in IPF, its practical use may be limited to large cohorts enriched by patients with advanced or rapidly progressive disease. Smaller, shorter duration and less costly trials require surrogate endpoints, which indirectly measure clinically meaningful endpoints. Several on-going clinical trials have incorporated HRCT-defined endpoints in their protocols [106]. A potential limitation of HRCT-defined endpoints, when compared to objective measures of disease severity such as lung function tests are the variable levels of observer agreement reported for important HRCT patterns such as honeycombing [36, 39, 41]. Furthermore, the apparent lack of sensitivity of HRCT in depicting marginal disease progression over short follow up periods may also be perceived as a weakness [62]. Both of these concerns might be addressed by the use of objective, automated imaging analysis tools discussed earlier [72]. An advantage HRCT has over pulmonary function is that when pulmonary fibrosis and emphysema coexist (a common occurrence in IPF patients), HRCT allows quantification of morphologic disease severity due to pulmonary fibrosis in isolation, while pulmonary function often shows spurious preservation of lung volumes with severe depression of the D_{LCO} [107]. In addition, as HRCT patterns of fibrosis are predictive of mortality in IPF, HRCT may also have a role in identifying patients with advanced disease with a view to cohort enrichment [14].

Conclusion

In patients with suspected IPF, HRCT broadly has two roles. First, if current diagnostic guidelines are followed rigidly, the need for surgical lung biopsy to secure a diagnosis of IPF hinges on the HRCT appearances at presentation. As discussed, this approach presents problems in patients unable or unwilling to undergo lung biopsy. Current challenges for the radiologist which relate to these guidelines are: 1) identifying patients with IPF whose HRCT appearances do not meet current criteria for UIP; 2) identifying early IPF with a view to early intervention; and 3) identifying and resolving sources of interobserver disagreement when applying diagnostic criteria. In the future, the best use of HRCT may be as the starting point of a diagnostic process which is dynamic, includes disease behaviour and prognostic biomarkers, and which focuses less stringently on specific HRCT patterns. Second, HRCT may have a prognostic role in patients with IPF. Although early studies focused on the prognostic value of individual HRCT patterns, the optimum use of HRCT in this setting appears to be in combination with other prognostic variables to form staging algorithms. As automated image analysis techniques become more sophisticated, subtle quantitative or qualitative changes in disease patterns over time, which are imperceptible to human observers, may help to sharpen our existing prognostic tools.

References

1.   King TE Jr, Schwarz MI, Brown K, *et al.* Idiopathic pulmonary fibrosis: relationship between histopathologic features and mortality. *Am J Respir Crit Care Med* 2001; 164: 1025–1032.

2.   Raghu G, Weycker D, Edelsberg J, *et al.* Incidence and prevalence of idiopathic pulmonary fibrosis. *Am J Respir Crit Care Med* 2006; 174: 810–816.

3.   Rudd RM, Prescott RJ, Chalmers JC, *et al.* Fibrosing Alveolitis Subcommittee of the Research Committee of the British Thoracic S. British Thoracic Society Study on cryptogenic fibrosing alveolitis: Response to treatment and survival. *Thorax* 2007; 62: 62–66.

4.   Bjoraker JA, Ryu JH, Edwin MK, *et al.* Prognostic significance of histopathologic subsets in idiopathic pulmonary fibrosis. *Am J Respir Crit Care Med* 1998; 157: 199–203.

5.   Flaherty KR, Toews GB, Travis WD, *et al.* Clinical significance of histological classification of idiopathic interstitial pneumonia. *Eur Respir J* 2002; 19: 275–283.

6.   Raghu G, Collard HR, Egan JJ, *et al.* An official ATS/ERS/JRS/ALAT statement: idiopathic pulmonary fibrosis: evidence-based guidelines for diagnosis and management. *Am J Respir Crit Care Med* 2011; 183: 788–824.

7.   Wells AU. The revised ATS/ERS/JRS/ALAT diagnostic criteria for idiopathic pulmonary fibrosis (IPF)--practical implications. *Respir Res* 2013; 14: Suppl 1, S2.

8.   Fell CD, Martinez FJ, Liu LX, *et al.* Clinical predictors of a diagnosis of idiopathic pulmonary fibrosis. *Am J Respir Crit Care Med* 2010; 181: 832–837.

9.   Chung JH, Chawla A, Peljto AL, *et al.* CT scan findings of probable usual interstitial pneumonitis have a high predictive value for histologic usual interstitial pneumonitis. *Chest* 2015; 147: 450–459.

10. Gruden JF, Panse PM, Leslie KO, *et al.* UIP diagnosed at surgical lung biopsy, 2000–2009: HRCT patterns and proposed classification system. *AJR Am J Roentgenol* 2013; 200: W458–W467.

11. Raghu G, Lynch D, Godwin JD, *et al.* Diagnosis of idiopathic pulmonary fibrosis with high-resolution CT in patients with little or no radiological evidence of honeycombing: secondary analysis of a randomised, controlled trial. *Lancet Respir Med* 2014; 2: 277–284.

12. Cottin V, Richeldi L. Neglected evidence in idiopathic pulmonary fibrosis and the importance of early diagnosis and treatment. *Eur Respir Rev* 2014; 23: 106–110.

13. Richeldi L, du Bois RM, Raghu G, *et al.* Efficacy and safety of nintedanib in idiopathic pulmonary fibrosis. *N Engl J Med* 2014; 370: 2071–2082.

14. King TEJr, Bradford WZ, Castro-Bernardini S, *et al.* A phase 3 trial of pirfenidone in patients with idiopathic pulmonary fibrosis. *N Engl J Med* 2014; 370: 2083–2092.

15. Walsh SL, Calandriello L, Sverzellati N, *et al.* Interobserver agreement for the ATS/ERS/JRS/ALAT criteria for a UIP pattern on CT. *Thorax* 2016; 71: 45–51.

16. Hunninghake GW, Zimmerman MB, Schwartz DA, *et al.* Utility of a lung biopsy for the diagnosis of idiopathic pulmonary fibrosis. *Am J Respir Crit Care Med* 2001; 164: 193–196.

17. Raghu G, Mageto YN, Lockhart D, *et al.* The accuracy of the clinical diagnosis of new-onset idiopathic pulmonary fibrosis and other interstitial lung disease: A prospective study. *Chest* 1999; 116: 1168–1174.

18. Johkoh T, Muller NL, Cartier Y, *et al.* Idiopathic interstitial pneumonias: diagnostic accuracy of thin-section CT in 129 patients. *Radiology* 1999; 211: 555–560.

19. Nishimura K, Izumi T, Kitaichi M, *et al.* The diagnostic accuracy of high-resolution computed tomography in diffuse infiltrative lung diseases. *Chest* 1993; 104: 1149–1155.

20. Tung KT, Wells AU, Rubens MB, *et al.* Accuracy of the typical computed tomographic appearances of fibrosing alveolitis. *Thorax* 1993; 48: 334–338.

21. Swensen SJ, Aughenbaugh GL, Myers JL. Diffuse lung disease: diagnostic accuracy of CT in patients undergoing surgical biopsy of the lung. *Radiology* 1997; 205: 229–234.

22. Mathieson JR, Mayo JR, Staples CA, *et al.* Chronic diffuse infiltrative lung disease: comparison of diagnostic accuracy of CT and chest radiography. *Radiology* 1989; 171: 111–116.

23. Lee KS, Primack SL, Staples CA, *et al.* Chronic infiltrative lung disease: comparison of diagnostic accuracies of radiography and low- and conventional-dose thin-section CT. *Radiology* 1994; 191: 669–673.

24. Richeldi L, Costabel U, Selman M, *et al.* Efficacy of a tyrosine kinase inhibitor in idiopathic pulmonary fibrosis. *N Engl J Med* 2011; 365: 1079–1087.

25. Sverzellati N, Wells AU, Tomassetti S, *et al.* Biopsy-proved idiopathic pulmonary fibrosis: spectrum of nondiagnostic thin-section CT diagnoses. *Radiology* 2010; 254: 957–964.

26. Padley SP, Padhani AR, Nicholson A, *et al.* Pulmonary sarcoidosis mimicking cryptogenic fibrosing alveolitis on CT. *Clin Radiol* 1996; 51: 807–810.

27. Vourlekis JS, Schwarz MI, Cherniack RM, *et al.* The effect of pulmonary fibrosis on survival in patients with hypersensitivity pneumonitis. *Am J Med* 2004; 116: 662–668.

28. Silva CI, Muller NL, Lynch DA, *et al.* Chronic hypersensitivity pneumonitis: differentiation from idiopathic pulmonary fibrosis and nonspecific interstitial pneumonia by using thin-section CT. *Radiology* 2008; 246: 288–297.

29. Selman M, Pardo A. Revealing the pathogenic and aging-related mechanisms of the enigmatic idiopathic pulmonary fibrosis. an integral model. *Am J Respir Crit Care Med* 2014; 189: 1161–1172.

30. Thannickal VJ, Loyd JE. Idiopathic pulmonary fibrosis: a disorder of lung regeneration? *Am J Respir Crit Care Med* 2008; 178: 663–665.

31. Lee HY, Lee KS, Jeong YJ, *et al.* High-resolution CT findings in fibrotic idiopathic interstitial pneumonias with little honeycombing: serial changes and prognostic implications. *AJR Am J Roentgenol* 2012; 199: 982–989.

32. Jin GY, Lynch D, Chawla A, *et al.* Interstitial lung abnormalities in a CT lung cancer screening population: prevalence and progression rate. *Radiology* 2013; 268: 563–571.

33. Kondoh Y, Taniguchi H, Ogura T, *et al.* Disease progression in idiopathic pulmonary fibrosis without pulmonary function impairment. *Respirology* 2013; 18: 820–826.

34. Oswald N, Parkinson T. Honeycomb lungs. *Q J Med* 1949; 18: 1–20.

35. Johnson TH, Jr. Radiology and honeycomb lung disease. *Am J Roentgenol Radium Ther Nucl Med* 1968; 104: 810–821.

36. Watadani T, Sakai F, Johkoh T, *et al.* Interobserver Variability in the CT Assessment of Honeycombing in the Lungs. *Radiology* 2012.

37. Heppleston AG. The pathology of honeycomb lung. *Thorax* 1956; 11: 77–93.

38. Hansell DM, Bankier AA, MacMahon H, *et al.* Fleischner Society: glossary of terms for thoracic imaging. *Radiology* 2008; 246: 697–722.

39. Lynch DA, Godwin JD, Safrin S, *et al.* High-resolution computed tomography in idiopathic pulmonary fibrosis: diagnosis and prognosis. *Am J Respir Crit Care Med* 2005; 172: 488–493.

40. Sundaram B, Gross BH, Martinez FJ, *et al.* Accuracy of high-resolution CT in the diagnosis of diffuse lung disease: effect of predominance and distribution of findings. *AJR Am J Roentgenol* 2008; 191: 1032–1039.

41. Goldin J, Elashoff R, Kim HJ, *et al.* Treatment of scleroderma-interstitial lung disease with cyclophosphamide is associated with less progressive fibrosis on serial thoracic high-resolution CT scan than placebo: findings from the scleroderma lung study. *Chest* 2009; 136: 1333–1340.

42. Grenier P, Valeyre D, Cluzel P, *et al.* Chronic diffuse interstitial lung disease: diagnostic value of chest radiography and high-resolution CT. *Radiology* 1991; 179: 123–132.

43. Flaherty KR, Andrei AC, King TE, Jr, *et al.* Idiopathic interstitial pneumonia: do community and academic physicians agree on diagnosis? *Am J Respir Crit Care Med* 2007; 175: 1054–1060.

44. Aziz ZA, Wells AU, Hansell DM, *et al.* HRCT diagnosis of diffuse parenchymal lung disease: inter-observer variation. *Thorax* 2004; 59: 506–511.

45. Thomeer M, Demedts M, Behr J, *et al.* Multidisciplinary interobserver agreement in the diagnosis of idiopathic pulmonary fibrosis. *Eur Respir J* 2008; 31: 585–591.

46. Flaherty KR, Thwaite EL, Kazerooni EA, *et al.* Radiological versus histological diagnosis in UIP and NSIP: survival implications. *Thorax* 2003; 58: 143–148.

47. Wells AU, Hansell DM, Rubens MB, *et al.* The predictive value of appearances on thin-section computed tomography in fibrosing alveolitis. *Am Rev Respir Dis* 1993; 148: 1076–1082.

48. Akira M, Inoue Y, Arai T, *et al.* Long-term follow-up high-resolution CT findings in non-specific interstitial pneumonia. *Thorax* 2011; 66: 61–65.

49. Fujimoto K, Taniguchi H, Johkoh T, *et al.* Acute exacerbation of idiopathic pulmonary fibrosis: high-resolution CT scores predict mortality. *Eur Radiol* 2012; 22: 83–92.

50. Edey AJ, Devaraj AA, Barker RP, *et al.* Fibrotic idiopathic interstitial pneumonias: HRCT findings that predict mortality. *Eur Radiol* 2011; 21: 1586–1593.

51. Sumikawa H, Johkoh T, Colby TV, *et al.* Computed tomography findings in pathological usual interstitial pneumonia: relationship to survival. *Am J Respir Crit Care Med* 2008; 177: 433–439.

52. Walsh SL, Sverzellati N, Devaraj A, *et al.* Chronic hypersensitivity pneumonitis: high resolution computed tomography patterns and pulmonary function indices as prognostic determinants. *Eur Radiol* 2012; 22: 1672–1679.

53. Kim EJ, Elicker BM, Maldonado F, *et al.* Usual interstitial pneumonia in rheumatoid arthritis-associated interstitial lung disease. *Eur Respir J* 2010; 35: 1322–1328.

54. Walsh SL, Sverzellati N, Devaraj A, *et al.* Connective tissue disease related fibrotic lung disease: high resolution computed tomographic and pulmonary function indices as prognostic determinants. *Thorax* 2014; 69: 216–222.

55. Walsh SLF, Wells AU, Sverzellati N, *et al.* Relationship between fibroblastic focus profusion and high resolution CT morphology in fibrotic lung disease. *BMC Med* 2015. (in press).

56. Gay SE, Kazerooni EA, Toews GB, *et al.* Idiopathic pulmonary fibrosis: predicting response to therapy and survival. *Am J Respir Crit Care Med* 1998; 157: 1063–1072.

57. Mogulkoc N, Brutsche MH, Bishop PW, *et al.* Pulmonary function in idiopathic pulmonary fibrosis and referral for lung transplantation. *Am J Respir Crit Care Med* 2001; 164: 103–108.

58. Akira M, Kozuka T, Yamamoto S, *et al.* Computed tomography findings in acute exacerbation of idiopathic pulmonary fibrosis. *Am J Respir Crit Care Med* 2008; 178: 372–378.

59. Akira M, Sakatani M, Ueda E. Idiopathic pulmonary fibrosis: progression of honeycombing at thin-section CT. *Radiology* 1993; 189: 687–691.

60. Lee JS, Gong G, Song KS, *et al.* Usual interstitial pneumonia: relationship between disease activity and the progression of honeycombing at thin-section computed tomography. *J Thorac Imaging* 1998; 13: 199–203.

61. Xaubet A, Agusti C, Luburich P, *et al.* Pulmonary function tests and CT scan in the management of idiopathic pulmonary fibrosis. *Am J Respir Crit Care Med* 1998; 158: 431–436.

62. Flaherty KR, Mumford JA, Murray S, *et al.* Prognostic implications of physiologic and radiographic changes in idiopathic interstitial pneumonia. *Am J Respir Crit Care Med* 2003; 168: 543–548.

63. Hwang JH, Misumi S, Curran-Everett D, *et al.* Longitudinal follow-up of fibrosing interstitial pneumonia: relationship between physiologic testing, computed tomography changes, and survival rate. *J Thorac Imaging* 2011; 26: 209–217.

64. Collard HR, King TEJr, Bartelson BB, *et al.* Changes in clinical and physiologic variables predict survival in idiopathic pulmonary fibrosis. *Am J Respir Crit Care Med* 2003; 168: 538–542.

65. Zappala CJ, Latsi PI, Nicholson AG, *et al.* Marginal decline in forced vital capacity is associated with a poor outcome in idiopathic pulmonary fibrosis. *Eur Respir J* 2010; 35: 830–836.

66. Flaherty KR, Andrei AC, Murray S, *et al.* Idiopathic pulmonary fibrosis: prognostic value of changes in physiology and six-minute-walk test. *Am J Respir Crit Care Med* 2006; 174: 803–809.

67. Best AC, Lynch AM, Bozic CM, *et al.* Quantitative CT indexes in idiopathic pulmonary fibrosis: relationship with physiologic impairment. *Radiology* 2003; 228: 407–414.

68. Best AC, Meng J, Lynch AM, *et al.* Idiopathic pulmonary fibrosis: physiologic tests, quantitative CT indexes, and CT visual scores as predictors of mortality. *Radiology* 2008; 246: 935–940.

69. Sverzellati N, Calabro E, Chetta A, *et al.* Visual score and quantitative CT indices in pulmonary fibrosis: Relationship with physiologic impairment. *Radiol Med* 2007; 112: 1160–1172.

70. Uppaluri R, Hoffman EA, Sonka M, *et al.* Computer recognition of regional lung disease patterns. *Am J Respir Crit Care Med* 1999; 160: 648–654.

71. Iwasawa T, Asakura A, Sakai F, *et al.* Assessment of prognosis of patients with idiopathic pulmonary fibrosis by computer-aided analysis of CT images. *J Thorac Imaging* 2009; 24: 216–222.

72. Maldonado F, Moua T, Rajagopalan S, *et al.* Automated quantification of radiological patterns predicts survival in idiopathic pulmonary fibrosis. *Eur Respir J* 2014; 43: 204–212.

73. Collard HR, King TEJr, Bartelson BB, *et al.* Changes in clinical and physiologic variables predict survival in idiopathic pulmonary fibrosis. *Am J Respir Crit Care Med* 2003; 168: 538–542.

74. King TE Jr, Safrin S, Starko KM, *et al.* Analyses of efficacy end points in a controlled trial of interferon-gamma1b for idiopathic pulmonary fibrosis. *Chest* 2005; 127: 171–177.

75. Egan JJ, Martinez FJ, Wells AU, *et al.* Lung function estimates in idiopathic pulmonary fibrosis: the potential for a simple classification. *Thorax* 2005; 60: 270–273.

76. Latsi PI, du Bois RM, Nicholson AG, *et al.* Fibrotic idiopathic interstitial pneumonia: the prognostic value of longitudinal functional trends. *Am J Respir Crit Care Med* 2003; 168: 531–537.

77. Jegal Y, Kim DS, Shim TS, *et al.* Physiology is a stronger predictor of survival than pathology in fibrotic interstitial pneumonia. *Am J Respir Crit Care Med* 2005; 171: 639–644.

78. Hallstrand TS, Boitano LJ, Johnson WC, *et al.* The timed walk test as a measure of severity and survival in idiopathic pulmonary fibrosis. *Eur Respir J* 2005; 25: 96–103.

79. Lama VN, Flaherty KR, Toews GB, *et al.* Prognostic value of desaturation during a 6-minute walk test in idiopathic interstitial pneumonia. *Am J Respir Crit Care Med* 2003; 168: 1084–1090.

80. Kohno N, Kyoizumi S, Awaya Y, *et al.* New serum indicator of interstitial pneumonitis activity. Sialylated carbohydrate antigen KL-6. *Chest* 1989; 96: 68–73.

81. Yokoyama A, Kondo K, Nakajima M, *et al.* Prognostic value of circulating KL-6 in idiopathic pulmonary fibrosis. *Respirology* 2006; 11: 164–168.

82. Greene KE, King TE Jr, Kuroki Y, *et al.* Serum surfactant proteins-A and -D as biomarkers in idiopathic pulmonary fibrosis. *Eur Respir J* 2002; 19: 439–446.

83. Kinder BW, Brown KK, McCormack FX, *et al.* Serum surfactant protein-A is a strong predictor of early mortality in idiopathic pulmonary fibrosis. *Chest* 2009; 135: 1557–1563.

84. Takahashi H, Fujishima T, Koba H, *et al.* Serum surfactant proteins A and D as prognostic factors in idiopathic pulmonary fibrosis and their relationship to disease extent. *Am J Respir Crit Care Med* 2000; 162: 1109–1114.

85. Prasse A, Probst C, Bargagli E, *et al.* Serum CC-chemokine ligand 18 concentration predicts outcome in idiopathic pulmonary fibrosis. *Am J Respir Crit Care Med* 2009; 179: 717–723.

86. Leuchte HH, Baumgartner RA, Nounou ME, *et al.* Brain natriuretic peptide is a prognostic parameter in chronic lung disease. *Am J Respir Crit Care Med* 2006; 173: 744–750.

87. Song JW, Song JK, Kim DS. Echocardiography and brain natriuretic peptide as prognostic indicators in idiopathic pulmonary fibrosis. *Respir Med* 2009; 103: 180–186.

88. Shinoda H, Tasaka S, Fujishima S, *et al.* Elevated CC chemokine level in bronchoalveolar lavage fluid is predictive of a poor outcome of idiopathic pulmonary fibrosis. *Respiration* 2009; 78: 285–292.

89. Rosas IO, Richards TJ, Konishi K, *et al.* MMP1 and MMP7 as potential peripheral blood biomarkers in idiopathic pulmonary fibrosis. *PLoS Med* 2008; 5: e93.

90. Phelps DS, Umstead TM, Rose RM, *et al.* Surfactant protein-A levels increase during Pneumocystis carinii pneumonia in the rat. *Eur Respir J* 1996; 9: 565–570.

91. McCormack FX, King TEJr, Bucher BL, *et al.* Surfactant protein A predicts survival in idiopathic pulmonary fibrosis. *Am J Respir Crit Care Med* 1995; 152: 751–759.

92. Enomoto N, Suda T, Kato M, *et al.* Quantitative analysis of fibroblastic foci in usual interstitial pneumonia. *Chest* 2006; 130: 22–29.

93. Nicholson AG, Fulford LG, Colby TV, *et al.* The relationship between individual histologic features and disease progression in idiopathic pulmonary fibrosis. *Am J Respir Crit Care Med* 2002; 166: 173–177.

94. Flaherty KR, Colby TV, Travis WD, *et al.* Fibroblastic foci in usual interstitial pneumonia: idiopathic versus collagen vascular disease. *Am J Respir Crit Care Med* 2003; 167: 1410–1415.

95. Goh NS, Desai SR, Veeraraghavan S, *et al.* Interstitial lung disease in systemic sclerosis: a simple staging system. *Am J Respir Crit Care Med* 2008; 177: 1248–1254.

96. Walsh SL, Wells AU, Sverzellati N, *et al.* An integrated clinicoradiological staging system for pulmonary sarcoidosis: a case-cohort study. *Lancet Respir Med* 2014; 2: 123–130.

97. Wells AU, Antoniou KM. The prognostic value of the GAP model in chronic interstitial lung disease: the quest for a staging system. *Chest* 2014; 145: 672–674.

98. Ley B, Ryerson CJ, Vittinghoff E, *et al.* A multidimensional index and staging system for idiopathic pulmonary fibrosis. *Ann Intern Med* 2012; 156: 684–691.

99. Kim ES, Choi SM, Lee J, *et al.* Validation of the GAP score in Korean patients with idiopathic pulmonary fibrosis. *Chest* 2015; 147: 430–437.

100. Ryerson CJ, Vittinghoff E, Ley B, *et al.* Predicting survival across chronic interstitial lung disease: the ILD-GAP model. *Chest* 2014; 145: 723–728.

101. Ley B, Bradford WZ, Weycker D, *et al.* Unified baseline and longitudinal mortality prediction in idiopathic pulmonary fibrosis. *Eur Respir J* 2015; 45: 1374–1381.

102. Ley B, Elicker BM, Hartman TE, *et al.* Idiopathic pulmonary fibrosis: CT and risk of death. *Radiology* 2014; 273: 570–579.

103. Raghu G, Collard HR, Anstrom KJ, r, *et al.* Idiopathic pulmonary fibrosis: clinically meaningful primary endpoints in phase 3 clinical trials. *Am J Respir Crit Care Med* 2012; 185: 1044–1048.

104. Nathan SD, Meyer KC. IPF clinical trial design and endpoints. *Curr Opin Pulm Med* 2014; 20: 463–471.

105. Wells AU. Forced vital capacity as a primary end point in idiopathic pulmonary fibrosis treatment trials: making a silk purse from a sow's ear. *Thorax* 2013; 68: 309–310.

106. Hansell DM, Goldin JG, King TE Jr, *et al.* CT staging and monitoring of fibrotic interstitial lung diseases in clinical practice and treatment trials: a position paper from the Fleischner Society. *Lancet Respir Med* 2015; 3: 483–496.

107. Wells AU, Desai SR, Rubens MB, *et al.* Idiopathic pulmonary fibrosis: a composite physiologic index derived from disease extent observed by computed tomography. *Am J Respir Crit Care Med* 2003; 167: 962–969.

Disclosures: None declared.

Chapter 8

The evaluation of disease severity/staging for prognosis

Oisin J. O'Connell and Jim J. Egan

The natural history of IPF is poorly defined and has a variable clinical course. There has been debate in the international literature as to the appropriate clinically meaningful end-points for clinical trials. Recent US Food and Drug Administration approval for pirfenidone and nintedanib was granted primarily based on showing efficacy in stabilising or reducing the decline in FVC. However, there is some controversy over the use of nonvalidated end-points that have not definitively been proven to be clinically meaningful, such as the use of FVC, 6MWD or D_{LCO} for clinical trials in IPF. Some IPF experts have suggested that all-cause mortality and hospitalisation rates are the most appropriate clinically meaningful end-points for clinical trials in IPF. Single clinical end-point measurements have their own limitations, including effect measure modification, the concept that a therapy may only influence a single part of a process but have less of an effect at a different stage of the same process. To date, the international guidelines have not implemented a standardised staging system in IPF. This chapter reviews the evidence and background for a number of staging systems described for patients with IPF.

Guidelines from the American Thoracic Society, European Respiratory Society, Japanese Respiratory Society and Latin American Thoracic Association have yet to implement a formal staging system for IPF [1]. This lack of a recognised staging system poses problems in a number of clinical aspects of the care of patients with IPF [2]. Studies on pulmonary fibrosis from the 1990s used poorly defined criteria for the diagnosis of IPF, meaning other interstitial pneumonitides with variable natural histories were mixed in with the true IPF patients. This resulted in difficulty in the accurate prognosis of survival for patients with IPF in these studies. Furthermore, the estimation of patient survival is influenced by the time of diagnosis [3]. IPF is often only diagnosed after patients have been evaluated for dyspnoea, rather than from incidental radiological pick-up, which can result in variability in the time of diagnosis. Thus, mean reported survival rates have been quite variable, ranging from 2 to 4 years from the time of diagnosis [4, 5].

The standardisation of the diagnostic criteria for IPF has resulted in a number of more recent studies addressing staging and disease severity assessment for patients with IPF [6]. This accurate assessment of disease severity has implications for both clinical and research studies, as well as for the timing of lung transplantation in patients with IPF. Patients with

Dept of Lung Transplantation and Interventional Pulmonology, Mater Misericordiae University Hospital, Dublin, Ireland.

Correspondence: Jim J. Egan, Dept of Lung Transplantation and Interventional Pulmonology, Mater Misericordiae University Hospital, Eccles St, Dublin 7, Ireland. E-mail: jegan@mater.ie

IPF have been shown to have the highest mortality among lung transplant waiting lists [7], probably as a result of the heterogeneity in clinical course, making optimal timing of lung transplantation difficult.

There has been no consensus on the optimal "clinically meaningful end-point" for clinical trials in IPF. Clinically meaningful end-points refer to end-points that directly measure how a patient feels, functions or survives [8]. There have been numerous clinical end-points studied in clinical trials for IPF, ranging from hospitalisation rate, acute exacerbation rate, patient-reported outcomes, surrogate end-points such as FVC or 6MWD decline, and composite end-points, to lung transplantation or death. Each of these isolated end-points has its respective limitation. HANSELL et al. [9] highlighted the fact that the use of a severity threshold, such as an FVC of 70% predicted, may represent a reduction in FVC of between 10% and 50% from baseline, depending on premorbid values. Therefore, indeterminate values that lie close to the threshold values are intrinsically unreliable. One solution they suggested is to use the most accurate prognostic test to stage the disease when the test value is distant from the threshold (i.e. clearly mild or severe disease), and to use a second test when the index test is indeterminate. GOH et al. [10] previously proposed this contingent staging approach when assessing prognosis for patients with scleroderma lung. They categorised patients as "restricted disease" when the abnormality on CT was estimated visually as <10% and as "extensive disease" when >30%. For patients with an estimated CT disease extent between 10% and 30%, stratification was based on whether FVC was ⩾70% pred [10].

Another suggested approach is to use a composite scoring system, incorporating clinical, radiological and physiological assessments to develop an integrated prediction model, which is likely to be more accurate than any single test. When developing a staging model, one must remain cognisant of "statistical interaction" or "effect measure modification", a situation in which the magnitude of the effect of an exposure of interest differs depending on another variable (a classic example being the development of Reye's syndrome upon exposure to aspirin in childhood, which is much more common than the same exceedingly rare phenomenon in adulthood) [11]. This lack of an isolated single clinically meaningful end-point for IPF staging has resulted in significant debate on appropriate clinical trial end-points [12].

The clinical trials for pirfenidone and nintedanib both used FVC as a surrogate end-point, while the interferon gamma-1b trial used mortality as a primary end-point [13–16]. RAGHU et al. [17] argued that there were no validated surrogate end-points in IPF at that time. They highlighted that a surrogate end-point is an indirect measure intended to substitute for a clinically meaningful end-point, such that clinical trials can be designed with smaller sample sizes, shortened durations and lower costs. Validation of a surrogate end-point requires substantial evidence that the effect of the intervention on the clinically meaningful end-point is reliably predicted by the effect of the intervention on the surrogate end-point, and this process generally requires an understanding of the causal pathway. RAGHU et al. [17] acknowledged that, while a decline of 10% in an individual's FVC has been correlated with survival time in multiple cohorts of patients with IPF [18–20], there is a lack of evidence establishing that treatment-induced changes in this end-point reliably predict a clinically meaningful outcome. They have suggested that all-cause mortality and all-cause non-elective hospitalisation rates should be used as clinical trial end-points for IPF in the absence of other validated surrogate end-points [17].

However, another expert international panel of IPF experts (n=52) strongly opposed this suggestion of all-cause mortality as the primary clinical end-point required for clinical trials, highlighting that this end-point is impractical and sets a standard not required for drug registration in other respiratory diseases, including lung cancer, cystic fibrosis and COPD [21]. KING et al. [22] performed an analysis of the mortality data from the INSPIRE and CAPACITY trials in IPF (which studied use of interferon gamma-1b and pirfenidone, respectively) to help establish the sample size necessary for a clinical trial using all-cause mortality as the primary clinical end-point. They calculated that the estimated number of subjects necessary to enrol over 3 years in order to perform a clinical trial to detect a 25% reduction in mortality, with 90% power and 5 years of follow-up, was 2582 patients. This is an impractical and unfeasible number of patients required for clinical trials for IPF.

The US Food and Drug Administration (FDA) recently issued their perspective of the issue of FVC as a clinically meaningful end-point [23]. They highlighted that five of the six trials involving pirfenidone and nintedanib found a slower rate of decline in FVC in the intervention arm compared with the placebo arm. While these studies were not powered to detect a decline in mortality, in the five studies that revealed a significant difference in FVC decline, there was a numerical trend towards improvement in mortality [23]. The FDA authors suggested that these trial results strengthen the ability to rely on FVC as a clinically relevant efficacy measure in IPF, and highlighted the increasing amount of data on a relationship between FVC and mortality.

The second clinically meaningful end-point suggested by RAGHU et al. [17] was hospitalisation rate, which could be further categorised into all-cause hospitalisation, respiratory hospitalisation and IPF-related hospitalisation. Certainly hospitalisation rate is easy to measure and is a well-defined outcome, although its limitations would include non-disease-related hospitalisation rates and national/international variability in access to healthcare. DURHEIM et al. [24] performed an analysis of 517 patients with IPF from three randomised controlled trials, using Cox proportional hazard ratios to compare two outcomes (incidence of non-elective hospital admission and $\geqslant$10% reduction in FVC) across strata in IPF patients with mild to moderate physiological impairment. 7% (38 out of 510) of patients required hospitalisation during the study period, while 11% (58 out of 510) had $\geqslant$10% decrease in FVC. The majority of patients requiring hospitalisation did not have $\geqslant$10% decline in FVC (30 versus eight), suggesting these surrogate markers may be independent markers for composite end-points in clinical trials of IPF (hazard ratio (HR) for admission 4.05, 95% CI 1.36–12.11; HR for $\geqslant$10% decline in FVC 4.68, 95% CI 1.83–11.99).

A significant factor influencing the opposing views on appropriate clinical trial end-points is the lack of an international standardised staging system in clinical trial enrolment [2, 12]. In clinical trials for IPF, the response to therapy is influenced by the disease burden at presentation and on entry to the clinical trial [12]. Therefore, a single clinical end-point in a clinical trial for IPF will be insufficient if applied to all patients with IPF. An ideal system for severity staging should use readily available tests that are routine at the time of patient presentation and assessment [9]. We will review some of the recent literature addressing staging and survival analyses as it applies to the current definition of IPF patients (table 1).

Staging models in IPF

Manchester model

MOGULKOC et al. [7] performed a study on 115 patients with IPF aged 45–65 years. They found that 12 variables correlated with mortality on univariate analysis; however, only two

Table 1 Recent studies addressing staging and survival analyses for IPF patients

First author [ref.]	Patients n	Model	Variables	Outcomes
Mogulkoc [7]	115	Manchester model	D_{LCO}; HRCT score	Increased mortality for "advanced disease" when D_{LCO} ≤39% pred, compared with "limited disease"
Wells [25]	212	CPI	Extent of disease on CT=91.0−[0.65×D_{LCO} % pred]−[0.53×FVC % pred]+[0.34×FEV1 % pred]	Mortality predicted more accurately by the CPI than by PFTs alone
du Bois [18]	830	Mortality risk scoring system	Age; respiratory hospitalisation; FVC % pred; 24-week change in FVC	1-year risk of death dependent on score from four variables
Ley [26]	558	GAP	Gender; age; physiology (FVC % pred and D_{LCO} % pred)	1-, 2- and 3-year mortality rates, respectively: GAP I 6%, 11%, 16% GAP II 16%, 30%, 42% GAP III 39%, 62%, 77%
Mura [3]	138	ROSE	MRCDS; 6MWD; CPI	MRCDS >3, 6MWD ≤72% pred and CPI >41 predicted 3-year survival with 100% specificity and 39% sensitivity
Ley [27]	348	CT-GAP	CT fibrosis score; gender; age; physiology (FVC % pred)	1-, 2- and 3-year mortality rates, respectively: CT-GAP I 5%, 10%, 17% CT-GAP II 19%, 34%, 49% CT-GAP III 43%, 67%, 84%

CPI: composite physiological index; ROSE: Risk stratificatiOn ScorE; MRCDS: Medical Research Council dyspnoea score.

variables retained significance following multivariate stepwise regression analysis. They identified D_{LCO} % pred and HRCT fibrosis score as the two independent predictors of 2-year survival. Receiver operating characteristic analysis of D_{LCO} % pred gave an area under the curve (AUC) of 0.8 (95% CI 0.7–0.9) and HRCT fibrosis score gave an AUC of 0.86 (95% CI 0.77–0.95). A D_{LCO} of 39% pred combined with a HRCT fibrosis score of 2.25 gave an 82% sensitivity and 84% specificity for predicting the risk of death within 2 years. This prompted a staging system of IPF disease severity into those with "limited disease" defined by D_{LCO} >39% and those with "advanced disease" defined by D_{LCO} ⩽39% pred. LATSI et al. [20] also demonstrated that a median D_{LCO} of 39% pred was associated with an increased risk of 2-year mortality, and for idiopathic fibrotic interstitial pneumonia, D_{LCO} >35% had a 2-year survival >75%, while D_{LCO} <35% had only a 50% chance of survival. EGAN et al. [28] suggested that in those with "limited IPF disease", serial lung function monitoring is more likely to have prognostic value, while in those with "advanced IPF disease" other outcome variables, such as all-cause mortality, are likely to be beneficial in clinical trials.

Clinical, radiographic and physiological scoring system

In 1986, WATTERS et al. [29] developed the clinical, radiographic and physiological (CRP) scoring system to help assess the clinical status of patients with IPF. This scoring system was based on seven variables: dyspnoea, chest radiography, spirometry, lung volume, diffusion capacity, resting alveolar–arterial oxygen tension difference and exercise arterial oxygen saturation. This CRP score correlated with the extent of pathology seen on open lung biopsy. The study has been criticised for failing to perform stepwise regression analysis to adjust for collinearity between lung function indices and not taking into account the effect of emphysema. This original CRP scoring system was not found to predict survival consistently in patients with IPF [30].

More recently, KING et al. [5] published a new CRP scoring system and correlated this scoring system with survival in a larger cohort of patients with UIP (n=238). This model included a simplified physiological component, derived from TLC and arterial oxygen levels on maximal exertion. This model also adjusted for collinearity between lung function indices. The factors found to predict survival in this model (with maximal potential score for each category in parentheses) were: increasing age (25.6 points), smoking status (13.6 points), presence of digital clubbing (10.7 points), extent of profusion of interstitial opacities (18.3 points), the presence of PH on chest radiography (10.3 points), TLC % pred (11.0 points) and arterial oxygen tension (P_{aO_2}) at the end of maximal exercise (10.5 points). Patients can get scores up to 100 points in the complete model, and a second abbreviated model was developed with the exclusion of P_{aO_2} during maximal exercise, which had a maximal potential score of 89.5 points. This study illustrated the predicted survival curves for patients with a given CRP score at 10-point intervals, up to ~115 months. The calculated 5-year survival from CRP scores of 20, 40, 60 and 80 were 89%, 53%, 4% and <1%, respectively. Both the new CRP score and the abbreviated new CRP models were shown to have significant prognostic information for patients with IPF, and incorporated a measurement that aided adjustment for the presence of emphysema.

Composite physiological index

WELLS et al. [25] developed the composite physiological index (CPI) score based on the extent of disease on HRCT. While several studies have confirmed the finding that D_{LCO} has the strongest correlation with morphological extent of disease both by histology and CT, the interpretation of PFTs in IPF patients with emphysema can result in preservation of lung volumes and depression of gas transfer [31]. The CPI is a scoring system marked out of 15 points and is based on the proportion of ground-glass attenuation, and both the proportion and the coarseness of reticular abnormalities at five pre-specified levels on a HRCT scan of the thorax in patients with IPF. It had been found that >20% of patients with IPF had concomitant emphysema, which confounds the interpretation of PFTs in IPF [32]. Three variables (D_{LCO}, FVC % pred and FEV1 % pred) were found to be predictive of disease severity in the CPI. The multivariate regression model for CPI found that the extent of disease on CT=91.0–(0.65×D_{LCO} % pred)–(0.53×FVC % pred)+(0.34×FEV1 % pred) [25]. The median survival in the IPF study population was 22 months, with a 23% 5-year survival in the entire cohort. WELLS *et al.* [25] found that the CPI was the most powerful independent prognostic indicator, compared with other univariate candidates examined, with a regression coefficient of 0.092 (95% CI 0.043–0.141) and p<0.0005. They concluded that the CPI correlates more strongly with mortality than any individual pulmonary function index, and attributed this prognostic value to the ability of the CPI to account for coexisting emphysema, although the authors did find in patients without emphysema on CT that the CPI reflected the extent of fibrosis no better than D_{LCO} levels alone.

GAP index

LEY *et al.* [26] published the GAP index in 2012. This index is a clinical prediction rule based on modelling for mortality over 3 years in a cohort of 558 patients with IPF derived from retrospective cohorts in two US centres and one Italian centre. The univariate candidate variables used to develop this model included age, gender, body mass index, smoking status, supplemental oxygen use, FVC, FEV1, TLC and D_{LCO}. Four variables from the univariate analysis were significant predictors of the primary end-point of time to death or lung transplantation in the multivariate analysis using Fine–Gray competing risk modelling. The four variables found to be significant predictors on multivariate modelling (with respective scores in parentheses) were: gender (male=1, female=0), age (≤60 years=0, 61–65 years=1, ≥65 years=2), FVC % pred (>75%=0, 50–75%=1, <50%=2), D_{LCO} % pred (>55%=0, 36–55%=1, ≤35%=2, cannot perform=3). The staging system was divided into three stages: stage I was a low-risk group with a score of 0–3, stage II was an intermediate-risk group with a score of 4–5 and stage III was a high-risk group with a score of 6–8. The mortality rates for GAP stage I are 6%, 11% and 16% at years 1, 2 and 3, respectively; this increased to 16%, 30% and 42% for GAP stage II and to 39%, 62% and 77% for GAP stage III at years 1–3. The c-index for the GAP index was 69.3 and 68.7 in the derivation and validation cohorts, respectively. Strengths of this study included the large study population (228 patients in the derivation cohort and 325 patients in the validation cohort), although the retrospective nature of the study could bias against patients who died rapidly. Furthermore, no exercise testing component was used as part of the model development [33]. Interestingly, RYERSON *et al.* [34] demonstrated the outcomes using a modified ILD-GAP score and found similar accuracy for mortality prediction in other interstitial pneumonitides including chronic hypersensitivity pneumonitis and NSIP, when compared with IPF (c-index 74.6 in the combined cohort).

Risk stratificatiOn ScorE

MURA *et al.* [3] studied demographic, functional and radiographic factors to develop a scoring system (the Risk stratificatiOn ScorE (ROSE)) to determine 3-year survival based on clinical indicators collected at the time of diagnosis and re-evaluated at 6 months.

70 patients were used in the derivation cohort and 68 in the confirmatory arm. 24 (34%) patients had concomitant emphysema on CT. The authors performed a univariate and subsequent multivariate model to predict survival. Three variables present at diagnosis were found to be predictive of 3-year mortality in the multivariate analysis: modified Medical Research Council dyspnoea score (MRCDS) >3, 6MWD ⩽72% pred and CPI >41. These three variables were divided into three groups to give low-risk, intermediate-risk and high-risk groups. The low-risk group had MRCDS ⩽3, 6MWD >72% pred and CPI ⩽41; the 3-year mortality rate was 19%. The intermediate group had one of: MRCDS >3, 6MWD ⩽72% pred or CPI >41; the 3-year mortality was 42% in this group. The high-risk group had all three of: MRCDS >3, 6MWD ⩽72% pred and CPI >41; in this group the 3-year mortality was 100%. The ROSE predicted 3-year survival with 39% sensitivity and 100% specificity. Furthermore, an increase in category grouping from the initial ROSE group at the 6-month re-evaluation was a sensitive predictor of 3-year mortality (94% sensitivity and 40% specificity). The authors also recorded the incidence of acute exacerbations of IPF, with 13 (18.6%) out of 70 patients experiencing acute exacerbations, three of which were fatal and six of which were associated with death within a 3-month window. The only independent predictors for acute IPF exacerbations at the time of diagnosis were the D_{LCO} and the presence of concomitant emphysema. Limitations of this study were its small sample size, the lack of assessment for PH and a lack of specificity in the definition of an adverse effect.

CT-GAP model

LEY *et al.* [27] recently developed the CT-GAP score, where D_{LCO} was substituted with a CT fibrosis extent score. Analysing the data of 348 patients with IPF, the authors assessed the prognostic value of both the original GAP score plus the addition of a CT scoring system, and the replacement of variables in the GAP score with the CT scoring system. Given an increasing availability of reliable CT automation, the fact that all patients with IPF will require a CT, and the difficulty in measuring D_{LCO} in some patients with IPF, the authors reasoned that CT may be a useful additional prognostic factor for patients with IPF. The authors found that their prediction model had comparable accuracy with the original GAP model, and that it may be clinically useful due to the known inter-facility and intra-patient variability of D_{LCO} [35, 36]. The predicted mortality using the CT-GAP model for stage I disease was 5.3%, 10.3% and 16.6% for years 1, 2 and 3, respectively; for stage II predicted mortality was 18.7%, 33.6% and 49.0% for years 1, 2 and 3, respectively; and for stage III predicted mortality was 42.8%, 67.2% and 84.3% for years 1, 2 and 3, respectively. Limitations of this study were the lack of data on other clinical variables, such as 6MWD, desaturation levels, comorbidities, dynamic changes in FVC and D_{LCO} over time and the levels of serum or BAL biomarkers. That said, the CT-GAP model, if validated, may be useful for some cohorts over time.

Conclusion

IPF is a complex disease characterised by acute exacerbations and periods of stability, with intercurrent stepwise periods of rapid decline. Functional tests alone have proven to be insufficient in staging patients with IPF. This has led to the development of multidimensional staging systems, which have increased discrimination and predictive power. The ideal multidimensional index or staging system will need to be simple to calculate, include parameters that are easy to measure, be safe, inexpensive and validated, and should ideally be calibrated if it is to influence clinical decision making. The optimal multidimensional staging system has yet to be defined and yet to be incorporated into the consensus guidelines for IPF. Future research will need to incorporate both baseline information and longitudinal parameters, and probably will need to integrate the use of serum biomarkers and biological data [37, 38]. In the interim, we have a number of multidimensional staging systems that have been shown to be better at predicting mortality than isolated functional tests alone.

References

1. Raghu G, Collard HR, Egan JJ, *et al.* An official ATS/ERS/JRS/ALAT statement: idiopathic pulmonary fibrosis: evidence-based guidelines for diagnosis and management. *Am J Respir Crit Care Med* 2011; 183: 788–824.
2. O'Connell OJ, Riddell P, Egan JJ. Importance of idiopathic pulmonary fibrosis staging for clinical trial endpoints. *Am J Respir Crit Care Med* 2013; 187: 1271.
3. Mura M, Porretta MA, Bargagli E, *et al.* Predicting survival in newly diagnosed idiopathic pulmonary fibrosis: a 3-year prospective study. *Eur Respir J* 2012; 40: 101–109.
4. Selman M, Carrillo G, Estrada A, *et al.* Accelerated variant of idiopathic pulmonary fibrosis: clinical behavior and gene expression pattern. *PLoS One* 2007; 2: e482.
5. King TE Jr, Tooze JA, Schwarz MI, *et al.* Predicting survival in idiopathic pulmonary fibrosis: scoring system and survival model. *Am J Respir Crit Care Med* 2001; 164: 1171–1181.
6. Idiopathic pulmonary fibrosis: diagnosis and treatment. International consensus statement. American Thoracic Society (ATS), and the European Respiratory Society (ERS). *Am J Respir Crit Care Med* 2000; 161: 646–664.
7. Mogulkoc N, Brutsche MH, Bishop PW, *et al.* Pulmonary function in idiopathic pulmonary fibrosis and referral for lung transplantation. *Am J Respir Crit Care Med* 2001; 164: 103–108.
8. Biomarkers Definitions Working Group. Biomarkers and surrogate endpoints: preferred definitions and conceptual framework. *Clin Pharmacol Ther* 2001; 69: 89–95.
9. Hansell DM, Goldin JG, King TE Jr, *et al.* CT staging and monitoring of fibrotic interstitial lung diseases in clinical practice and treatment trials: a position paper from the Fleischner Society. *Lancet Respir Med* 2015; 3: 483–496.
10. Goh NS, Desai SR, Veeraraghavan S, *et al.* Interstitial lung disease in systemic sclerosis: a simple staging system. *Am J Respir Crit Care Med* 2008; 177: 1248–1254.
11. Brumback BA, Bouldin ED, Zheng HW, *et al.* Testing and estimating model-adjusted effect-measure modification using marginal structural models and complex survey data. *Am J Epidemiol* 2010; 172: 1085–1091.
12. O'Connell OJ, Egan JJ. The burden of disease and the need for a simple staging system in idiopathic pulmonary fibrosis. *Am J Respir Crit Care Med* 2014; 189: 765–767.
13. Raghu G, Rochwerg B, Zhang Y, *et al.* An official ATS/ERS/JRS/ALAT clinical practice guideline: treatment of idiopathic pulmonary fibrosis. An update of the 2011 clinical practice guideline. *Am J Respir Crit Care Med* 2015; 192: e3–e19.
14. King TE Jr, Albera C, Bradford WZ, *et al.* Effect of interferon gamma-1b on survival in patients with idiopathic pulmonary fibrosis (INSPIRE): a multicentre, randomised, placebo-controlled trial. *Lancet* 2009; 374: 222–228.
15. Richeldi L, du Bois RM, Raghu G, *et al.* Efficacy and safety of nintedanib in idiopathic pulmonary fibrosis. *N Engl J Med* 2014; 370: 2071–2082.
16. King TE Jr, Bradford WZ, Castro-Bernardini S, *et al.* A phase 3 trial of pirfenidone in patients with idiopathic pulmonary fibrosis. *N Engl J Med* 2014; 370: 2083–2092.
17. Raghu G, Collard HR, Anstrom KJ, *et al.* Idiopathic pulmonary fibrosis: clinically meaningful primary endpoints in phase 3 clinical trials. *Am J Respir Crit Care Med* 2012; 185: 1044–1048.
18. du Bois RM, Weycker D, Albera C, *et al.* Forced vital capacity in patients with idiopathic pulmonary fibrosis: test properties and minimal clinically important difference. *Am J Respir Crit Care Med* 2011; 184: 1382–1389.
19. Collard HR, King TE Jr, Bartelson BB, *et al.* Changes in clinical and physiologic variables predict survival in idiopathic pulmonary fibrosis. *Am J Respir Crit Care Med* 2003; 168: 538–542.
20. Latsi PI, du Bois RM, Nicholson AG, *et al.* Fibrotic idiopathic interstitial pneumonia: the prognostic value of longitudinal functional trends. *Am J Respir Crit Care Med* 2003; 168: 531–537.
21. Wells AU, Behr J, Costabel U, *et al.* Hot of the breath: mortality as a primary end-point in IPF treatment trials: the best is the enemy of the good. *Thorax* 2012; 67: 938–940.
22. King TE Jr, Albera C, Bradford WZ, *et al.* All-cause mortality rate in patients with idiopathic pulmonary fibrosis. Implications for the design and execution of clinical trials. *Am J Respir Crit Care Med* 2014; 189: 825–831.
23. Karimi-Shah BA, Chowdhury BA. Forced vital capacity in idiopathic pulmonary fibrosis – FDA review of pirfenidone and nintetanib. *N Engl J Med* 2015; 372: 1189–1191.

24. Durheim MT, Collard HR, Roberts RS, *et al.* Association of hospital admission and forced vital capacity endpoints with survival in patients with idiopathic pulmonary fibrosis: analysis of a pooled cohort from three clinical trials. *Lancet Respir Med* 2015; 3: 388–396.

25. Wells AU, Desai SR, Rubens MB, *et al.* Idiopathic pulmonary fibrosis: a composite physiologic index derived from disease extent observed by computed tomography. *Am J Respir Crit Care Med* 2003; 167: 962–969.

26. Ley B, Ryerson CJ, Vittinghoff E, *et al.* A multidimensional index and staging system for idiopathic pulmonary fibrosis. *Ann Intern Med* 2012; 156: 684–691.

27. Ley B, Elicker BM, Hartman TE, *et al.* Idiopathic pulmonary fibrosis: CT and risk of death. *Radiology* 2014; 273: 570–579.

28. Egan JJ, Martinez FJ, Wells AU, *et al.* Lung function estimates in idiopathic pulmonary fibrosis: the potential for a simple classification. *Thorax* 2005; 60: 270–273.

29. Watters LC, King TE, Schwarz MI, *et al.* A clinical, radiographic, and physiologic scoring system for the longitudinal assessment of patients with idiopathic pulmonary fibrosis. *Am Rev Respir Dis* 1986; 133: 97–103.

30. Gay SE, Kazerooni EA, Toews GB, *et al.* Idiopathic pulmonary fibrosis: predicting response to therapy and survival. *Am J Respir Crit Care Med* 1998; 157: 1063–1072.

31. Doherty MJ, Pearson MG, O'Grady EA, *et al.* Cryptogenic fibrosing alveolitis with preserved lung volumes. *Thorax* 1997; 52: 998–1002.

32. Wells AU, King AD, Rubens MB, *et al.* Lone cryptogenic fibrosing alveolitis: a functional-morphologic correlation based on extent of disease on thin-section computed tomography. *Am J Respir Crit Care Med* 1997; 155: 1367–1375.

33. Rozanski C, Mura M. Multi-dimensional indices to stage idiopathic pulmonary fibrosis: a systematic review. *Sarcoidosis Vasc Diffuse Lung Dis* 2014; 31: 8–18.

34. Ryerson CJ, Vittinghoff E, Ley B, *et al.* Predicting survival across chronic interstitial lung disease: the ILD-GAP model. *Chest* 2014; 145: 723–728.

35. Macintyre N, Crapo RO, Viegi G, *et al.* Standardisation of the single-breath determination of carbon monoxide uptake in the lung. *Eur Respir J* 2005; 26: 720–735.

36. O'Connell OJ, Kennedy MP, Henry MT. Idiopathic pulmonary fibrosis: treatment update. *Adv Ther* 2011; 28: 986–999.

37. Kolb M, Collard HR. Staging of idiopathic pulmonary fibrosis: past, present and future. *Eur Respir Rev* 2014; 23: 220–224.

38. O'Dwyer DN, Armstrong ME, Trujillo G, *et al.* The Toll-like receptor 3 L412F polymorphism and disease progression in idiopathic pulmonary fibrosis. *Am J Respir Crit Care Med* 2013; 188: 1442–1450.

Disclosures: None declared.

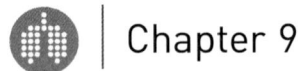

Chapter 9

Monitoring

Katrin Milger[1] and Jürgen Behr[1,2]

Monitoring patients with IPF is crucial to proactively identify those with progressive disease and determine the development of comorbidities to initiate appropriate and timely treatment. Variables whose longitudinal changes predict survival and that are established surrogate markers of disease progression comprise: clinical symptoms (most prominently dyspnoea), PFT (especially D_{LCO} and FVC), and exercise tolerance assessed by 6MWD. Other valuable measures of progression include arterial blood gas exchange measures at rest and during exercise as well as HRCT, but their longitudinal validity and minimal clinically important difference have yet to be fully established. Molecular biomarkers and the composition of the lung microbiome are newly identified, promising predictors that need further investigation. Additionally, acute exacerbations and hospital admission are marker events correlating with mortality. Several composite scoring systems that integrate some of these variables have been developed for a more reliable and valid assessment of disease progression. As the individual disease course and treatment response is variable, so must be the monitoring schedule.

Even though the overall prognosis of IPF is poor, its natural disease history is highly variable and difficult to predict in an individual patient. The clinical course may range from stable disease with only slow lung function decline to rapid progression with respiratory failure, whereas in some patients periods of stability alternate with periods of acute respiratory decline (figure 1a) [1].

Patients with rapidly progressive IPF display a shorter survival time than those with slowly progressive disease [2]. Hence, patients with IPF need to be monitored closely to ensure early detection of disease progression. This regular evaluation helps to appreciate the individual disease course and facilitates timely initiation of appropriate therapeutic interventions, including lung transplantation. Additionally, monitoring for worsening of symptoms and possible complications of treatment is important to optimally preserve QoL [3].

While the baseline parameters used for staging and prognosis at the time of diagnosis have been introduced in the previous chapter, this chapter focuses on parameters that can be used for longitudinal monitoring of disease progression as well as their therapeutic and prognostic implications.

[1]Dept of Internal Medicine V, University of Munich, Comprehensive Pneumology Center, Munich, Germany. [2]Dept of Respiratory Medicine, Asklepios Gauting Clinic, Munich, Germany.

Correspondence: Jürgen Behr, Dept of Internal Medicine V, University of Munich Marchioninstr.15, 81377 Munich, Germany.
E-mail: Juergen.Behr@med.uni-muenchen.de

ERS Monogr 2016; 71: 106–121. DOI: 10.1183/2312508X.10008715

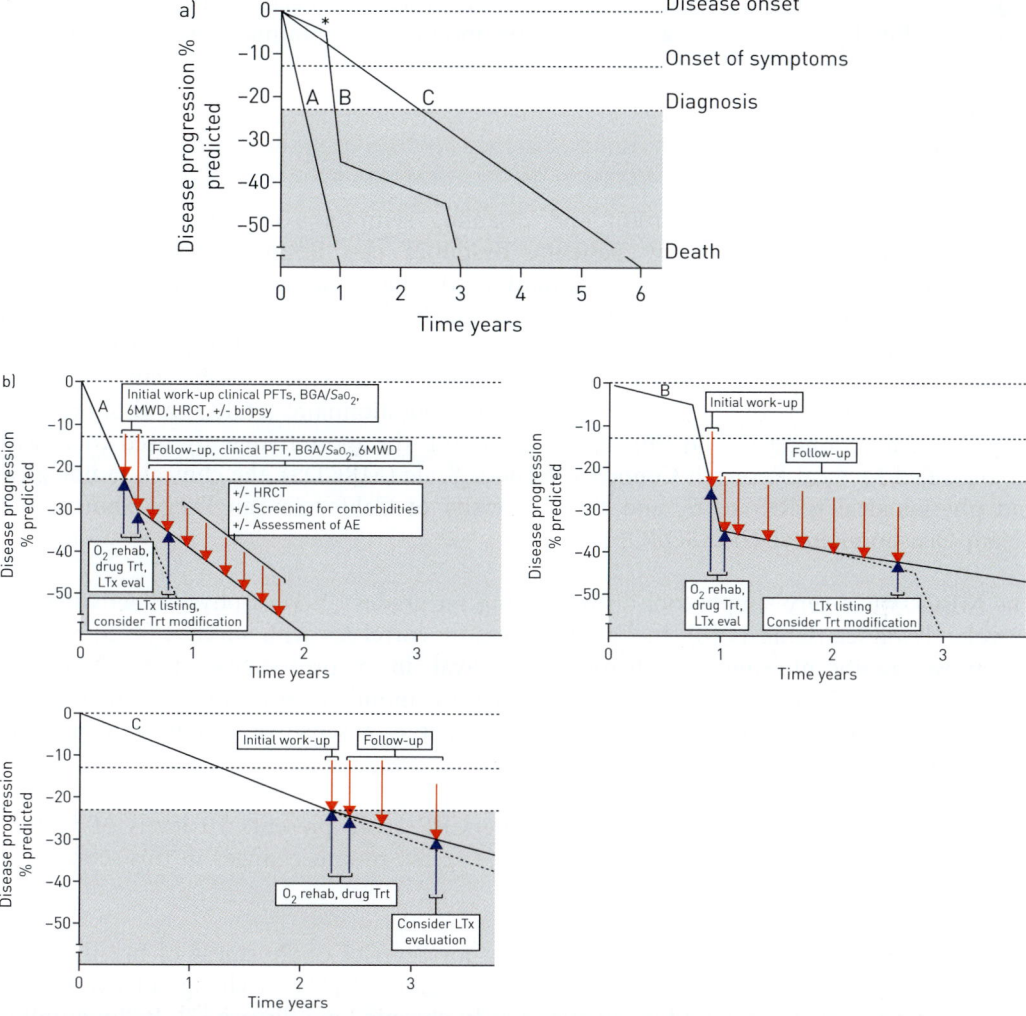

Figure 1. Schematic representation of a) potential clinical courses of IPF and b) examples of individualised monitoring schedule. a). As disease progresses, there is a subclinical period in which only radiographic findings of disease may be present, followed by a symptomatic period consisting of both pre-diagnosis and post-diagnosis clinical phases. The rate of decline and progression to death may be rapid (A), mixed (B) or slow (C), with periods of relative stability interposed with periods of acute decline (*). b) At diagnosis, the work-up should include clinical examination, PFT, blood gas analysis (BGA) or arterial oxygen saturation (S_{aO_2}), 6MWD, HRCT, and potentially lung biopsy. At the follow-up visit, clinical status, PFTs (especially D_{LCO} and FVC), 6MWD, and S_{aO_2} should be assessed. While pharmacological therapy should be offered to all patients with a confident IPF diagnosis, follow-up schedules and management may vary according to the severity and the observed or anticipated clinical course of the disease. In case of rapid progression (top left and top right panels in b), short follow-up intervals and early consideration of modification of drug treatment including participation in clinical trials, evaluation for comorbidities which may influence disease progression, and evaluation for lung transplantation are indicated. If progression is slow, longer intervals and later consideration of treatment modifications can be chosen (lower panel in b). Rehab: pulmonary rehabilitation; AE: adverse event; Trt: treatment; LTx: lung transplantation; eval: evaluation. Solid lines: potential clinical course with pharmacologic intervention; dashed lines: natural history without pharmacological intervention. Reprinted and adapted with permission of the American Thoracic Society [1].

Established parameters whose longitudinal changes predict survival include dyspnoea, FVC, D_{LCO}, extent of fibrosis on HRCT, and acute exacerbations. These have been derived from the data of prospective clinical studies. Additionally, parameters that have recently been suggested, or derived from retrospective cohort analysis and need further evaluation, are presented. Finally, we discuss a schedule for monitoring, minimal clinically important differences (MCIDs), and future directions.

Clinical symptoms

Dyspnoea and cough are important and disabling symptoms of IPF. Despite being a subjective symptom reported by patients, dyspnoea can be quantified and assessed objectively using validated scales. The extent of dyspnoea at baseline [4, 5], as well as change of dyspnoea over time [6], predict survival. Different measures have been used to assess the severity of dyspnoea, for example, the Borg Rating of Perceived Exertion, Baseline and Transition Dyspnoea Index, and QoL measurement tools with respiratory questionnaires, such as the St George's Respiratory Questionnaire (SGRQ) and Short Form 36-physical functioning (SF-36-PF). However, in IPF the most frequently used tools were the modified Medical Research Council Dyspnoea Scale (MRCDS), the clinical, radiological, and physiological (CRP) score, and the University of California San Diego Shortness of Breath Questionnaire (UCSD SOBQ) [7].

The MRCDS is a very simple tool distinguishing six grades (0–5) of physical activities that provoke dyspnoea (table 1) [8]. Its baseline measure correlates with survival [4, 5] and was the most significant single predictor of survival in a prospective study. Moreover, longitudinal validity was evaluated, showing that a 6-month increase of the MRCDS from 0–3 to 4–5 predicts a poor prognosis, suggesting it is a sensitive tool in detecting IPF progression [9].

Similarly, the dyspnoea score derived from the CRP score presents 10 levels of physical activities resulting in a 20-point scale (table 2) [10]. Six-month changes in this score of $\geqslant 2$ points correlate with differences in survival [6].

The UCSD SOBQ is a 24-item measure asking for severity of shortness of breath during various activities of daily life on a six-point scale (table 3) [11]. A change of five units is considered a reasonable MCID for this measure in chronic lung disease [7]. Its longitudinal validity in IPF was shown by correlation with FVC, 6MWD, SGRQ and SF-36-PF [12]. Estimated to be a precise tool, the UCSD SOBQ has been used as an end-point in a recent clinical trial of pirfenidone. Yet, despite the significant treatment effects on FVC and

Table 1. Modified Medical Research Council Dyspnoea Score

Grade	Description of breathlessness
0	I only get breathless with strenuous exercise.
1	I get short of breath when hurrying on level ground or walking up a slight hill.
2	On level ground, I walk slower than people of the same age because of breathlessness, or have to stop for breath when walking at my own pace.
3	On level ground, I have to stop for breath when walking at my own pace.
4	I stop for breath after walking about 100 yards or after 5 min on level ground.
5	I am too breathless to leave the house or I am breathless when dressing.

Reproduced and modified from [8] with permission from the publisher.

Table 2. Clinical component of the clinical, radiological and physiological scoring system

Points	Level of dyspnoea
0	None (or same as peers) even after 30 min of vigorous activity, such as running. Ability to lift and carry 60 lb for a prolonged period of time.
2	After five flights of stairs or 10 min of vigorous activity, prolonged use of heavy tools.
4	After walking more than 1 mile on level ground or up three flights of stairs, or less than 10 min of vigorous activity, such as running.
6	Upon walking 0.25–1 mile on level ground or up two flights of stairs, dyspnoea with paper hanging.
8	Upon walking 300–1320 feet on level ground; bed making.
10	Upon walking 150–300 feet on level ground or up one flight of stairs, scrubbing, truck driving, assembly line work.
12	Upon walking 50–150 feet on level ground at approximately 3 mph, light janitorial work.
14	Upon walking 20–50 feet on level ground, light steady work at one's own pace, seated operation of heavy equipment.
16	With minor exertion, such as dressing, walking less than 20 feet, prolonged talking.
18	With minimal activity such as eating, defecating, writing, sitting up.
20	At rest.

Reproduced and modified from [10] with permission from the publisher.

Table 3. University of California San Diego Shortness of Breath Questionnaire

How short of breath do you get:			Rating			
1. At rest...	0	1	2	3	4	5
2. Walking on a level at your own pace...	0	1	2	3	4	5
3. Walking on a level with others your age...	0	1	2	3	4	5
4. Walking up a hill...	0	1	2	3	4	5
5. Walking up stairs...	0	1	2	3	4	5
6. While eating...	0	1	2	3	4	5
7. Standing up from a chair...	0	1	2	3	4	5
8. Brushing teeth...	0	1	2	3	4	5
9. Shaving and/or brushing hair...	0	1	2	3	4	5
10. Showering/bathing...	0	1	2	3	4	5
11. Dressing...	0	1	2	3	4	5
12. Picking up and straightening...	0	1	2	3	4	5
13. Doing dishes...	0	1	2	3	4	5
14. Sweeping/vacuuming...	0	1	2	3	4	5

Respondents are asked to rate their breathlessness for each activity on a scale of 0–5, where 0 is not at all breathless and 5 is maximally breathless due to the activity. If the activity is not one that the respondent performs, they are asked to give their best estimate of breathlessness. Reproduced and modified from [11] with permission from the publisher.

progression-free survival in this trial, the differences in dyspnoea score did not reach significance [13].

In sum, while the use of objective dyspnoea scales is clearly recommended in clinical routine and research, a comprehensive study of which measure(s) to use is currently lacking.

Regarding available data and feasibility, the MRCDS and the dyspnoea score from the CRP score seem to be well-suited for routine follow-up in the IPF clinic, while the UCSD SOBS is preferred as a measure in clinical studies. However, subjective classification of dyspnoea by the patient as stable, improved, or worse is most widely used in current clinical practice and may also be a valid parameter during routine follow-up.

Moreover, because dyspnoea is subjective and may be confounded by comorbidities, used alone is not sufficient to diagnose progression and trigger therapeutic measures. It should rather be judged along with other objective parameters as, for example, in composite scores. Yet, change in dyspnoea alone can serve as a sensitive marker that should prompt further diagnostic work-up of disease status and comorbidities.

Apart from being a predictor of disease progression and survival, dyspnoea is an uncomfortable sensation that has an impact on the patient's QoL. Therefore, palliative treatment of dyspnoea may be of benefit in some patients.

Cough can be a symptom attributed to IPF itself after other common causes of cough, such as upper airway syndrome and GERD, have been excluded [14]. Severity of cough may also predict progression and prognosis in IPF [15], but this association has not been studied extensively. Interestingly, one study found an association of cough severity with the *mucin 5B, oligomeric mucus/gel-forming* (*MUC5B*) genotype [16]. Validated tools for the assessment of cough are the Leicester Cough Questionnaire and the Cough-Specific Quality-of-Life Questionnaire [17, 18]. The latter was also validated in patients with IPF.

Amelioration of cough improves QoL and can therefore be used as an end-point in clinical studies. However, it is unknown whether change of cough severity over time outside specific (palliative) cough treatments is predictive of progression or survival in IPF.

Pulmonary function tests

Pulmonary function studies are simple, widely available, and therefore easily obtained during routine follow-up visits of patients with IPF.

Reproducibility of spirometry, especially FVC, is generally excellent with 90% of patients being able to repeat the test with <5% of variation [19]. The variability for D_{LCO} is likely higher [20]. In addition to being predictors of mortality at baseline, half-yearly changes in TLC % predicted, FVC % pred, FEV1 % pred, and D_{LCO} % pred are predictive of survival time [6]. This was most conclusively and reliably shown for FVC and D_{LCO} over a timeframe of 6 but also 12 months, and current guidelines recommend these parameters for monitoring. An annual change in absolute FVC of >10% and/or a change of D_{LCO} of 15% are surrogate markers of disease progression [6, 21–24], and this threshold has been adopted as the end-point in clinical studies [25].

Smaller changes of 5–10% in FVC and 10–15% in D_{LCO} may also be relevant if progressive and sustained [26], but changes in single measurements can also be the result of measurement variability. The suggested MCID for FVC % pred is between 2 and 6% and FVC is considered a valid, reliable, and responsive measure of disease status [27]. However, in patients with concomitant emphysema the baseline FVC has been reported to be better preserved and the annual decline is smaller as emphysema partially "compensates" for the loss of FVC [28, 29].

Yet, a reduction in FVC can also be caused by progressive hyperinflation and must therefore be interpreted in consideration of other lung function test parameters, especially D_{LCO} [28]. A decline in D_{LCO} alone can also be caused by the development of pulmonary vascular disease; monitoring for PH should be performed in this case.

For monitoring patients with CPFE, a longitudinal decline in FEV1 over 12 months was found to be the best predictor of mortality [30], while KISHABA *et al.* [31] showed that FEV1 % pred/FVC % pred >1.2 was an independent predictor of survival in this specific population.

Finally, in recent clinical trials a relationship between FVC and mortality trends was found, confirming its utility as a clinically relevant efficacy measure [32, 33].

Intervals for monitoring PFTs are 3–4 months, but shorter intervals may be indicated if disease progression is suspected. An early study suggested that self-monitoring of FVC in IPF patients with handheld devices is feasible [34]. Whether this might also be a possibility to improve early detection of progression and acute exacerbations needs to be evaluated in further studies.

Arterial blood gases and oxygen saturation

Changes in the arterial oxygen tension (P_{aO_2}), O_2 saturation, and alveolar–arterial oxygen tension difference (P_{A-aO_2}) predict survival even after adjustment for baseline values [6, 35].

A decrease of P_{A-aO_2} of >5 mmHg at 6 and 12 months predicts mortality [6]. However, this parameter was not reliable proof of progression in further studies and a higher threshold of >15 mmHg change may be necessary [22]. Hence, P_{A-aO_2} is not recommended for routine monitoring of progressive disease [3].

Instead, current guidelines recommend the measurement of O_2 saturation by pulse oximetry at rest and during 6MWT at each follow-up visit to detect desaturation below 88% that would necessitate prescription of supplemental O_2 or adaptation of flow rate [3].

Exercise testing: 6MWT and cardiopulmonary exercise testing

The 6MWT is a simple and rapid exercise testing tool that provides prognostic information by the distance walked (6MWD), presence of desaturation below 88%, and delayed heart rate recovery [36–38].

EATON *et al.* [39] investigated the intra-individual reproducibility of the 6MWT by test repetition after an interval of 1 week, and found an excellent reproducibility of the distance walked, while O_2 saturation at the end of the test was highly variable. Moreover, there was a highly significant relationship between maximal O_2 uptake ($V'O_2max$) on maximal exercise testing and 6MWD [39]. Routine use of 6MWT to monitor IPF has been questioned in the past due to a lack of standardisation [3] and reproducibility of some of the measured variables in this patient population [39]. However, recent analyses from large clinical trials, including patients from the placebo arms of the INSPIRE and CAPACITY trials, have confirmed the reliability and validity of 6MWD in patients with IPF [38, 40]. Early smaller studies reported a MCID in 6MWD of 29–34 m and 28 m, respectively [41, 42]. This range was confirmed with a MCID of 24–45 m calculated from the INSPIRE trial and 21–37 m from the CAPACITY trial [38]. Strict adherence to the study protocol is essential because alternative instructions [43] and encouragement influence the distance walked [44].

DU BOIS *et al.* [38] found that a decrease in 6MWD over 6 months is highly predictive of 1-year mortality and can be a sign of disease progression.

In sum, the 6MWD can be used for longitudinal evaluation, while other longitudinal parameters derived from 6MWT, such as change in desaturation, should be interpreted with caution.

Cardiopulmonary exercise testing (CPET) provides comprehensive assessment of the exercise response, reflecting cardiac, respiratory, musculoskeletal, and haematological systems, and allowing for the estimation of severity in patients with cardiovascular and respiratory disease under submaximal and peak exercise performance [45].

Several parameters analysed during CPET were found to be independent prognostic factors, most prominently Pa_{O_2} during CPET [46] and exercise-induced hypoxaemia evaluated by change in Pa_{O_2}/change in V'_{O_2} (Pa_{O_2} slope) [47]. Yet, others have not confirmed that CPET measures of gas exchange provide additional value over respective parameters at rest in patients with IPF [48]. A more recent study of 25 patients found that the slope of relation between minute ventilation and CO_2 production and V'_{O_2} peak/kg were significant predictors of survival [49]. Given the highly significant correlation between V'_{O_2}max/peak and 6MWD [39, 49], it is unclear whether CPET can provide additional prognostic information that cannot be derived from 6MWT.

As prognostic evaluation of longitudinal changes in CPET variables is missing, CPET is currently not recommended when monitoring IPF [3]. However, it can be a useful tool for initial work-up because gas exchange abnormalities not yet seen on routine testing may be uncovered in patients with early disease. Further, it may help identify comorbidities such as cardiovascular diseases.

Hence, for routine clinical use the 6MWT is the examination of choice due to ease of practicality, safety, and longitudinal validity.

High-resolution computed tomography

HRCT is an important component of the diagnostic work-up in IPF. Reticular abnormalities and honeycombing are HRCT features of IPF that correlate with physiological parameters, such as FVC and D_{LCO} [50], and predict survival [51–54]. Moreover, HRCT can be used to monitor the extent of the disease over time. One study found that increases in HRCT changes at follow-up after 1 year, especially in the extent of the honeycombing, were predictive of mortality [55].

In the future, quantification of HRCT changes will be important not only to assess prognosis and progression during clinical routine, but also for use as an end-point in clinical trials [56]. Two different approaches can be used to quantify fibrosis: a visual, semiquantitative approach and an automated, computer-aided one.

BEST *et al.* [52] used a visual, semiquantitative assessment, dividing the lung into three zones; trained observers then scored reticular abnormality and honeycombing . The score was then calculated as the mean of the mean extent of reticular abnormality and honeycombing in each of the six zones. ODA *et al.* [57] used a similar approach, but additionally graded the fibrotic changes on a scale of 1–4 based on the following classification system: 1) normal attenuation; 2) reticular abnormality; 3) traction bronchiectasis; and 4) honeycombing. Employing this approach, the researchers found the increase in fibrosis score over time to be a superior predictor of outcome compared to baseline values [57]. Limitations of these scoring systems include the need for experienced, specifically trained thoracic radiologists and possible inter-observer variations.

To overcome these limitations, automated methods to diagnose and quantify interstitial lung disease (ILD) on HRCT have been developed [58, 59]. Computer-aided systems based on segmentation, histogram, and texture analysis showed a good correlation to severity scoring by an expert radiologist at baseline and for change over time [60–62]. Moreover, automated scores could predict survival [63–65] and assess treatment effect by pirfenidone [66]. Even though pattern recognition software is not prone to human observer variation, bias can still be present by relying on training by human beings [56]. Also, the use of different scanners, software, and algorithms makes comparing different studies difficult.

Summing up, HRCT scoring is useful for longitudinal evaluation of disease extent, but further research is needed to standardise its use, and define assessment intervals and MCID. Thus, regular follow-up with HRCT is currently not recommended in stable patients due to radiation exposure and cost. However, if clinical or physiological parameters indicate worsening, HRCT may help to objectify the extent of fibrotic changes and identify complications, as well as differential diagnoses at the same time.

Composite scoring systems

Composite scores have been developed to improve prognosis prediction and quantification of disease severity. WATTERS *et al.* [10] first introduced the CRP scoring system in 1986 to provide a reproducible and quantifiable means of assessment of the clinical status of patients with IPF. The clinical component quantifies dyspnoea as outlined earlier, while the radiographic component takes into account the extent of fibrotic changes, honeycombing, and the presence of signs of PH. The physiological component comprises D_{LCO}, FEV_1, FVC, P_{A-aO_2} at rest and change in arterial oxygen saturation measured by pulse oximetry at exercise. The original study was performed before the introduction of clear diagnostic criteria for IPF. Researchers assessed patients under corticosteroid treatment that is now obsolete [67]. Hence, transferability to current IPF populations is limited and a new CRP score was developed after survival analysis of 238 patients with IPF. It consists of smoking status and finger clubbing as the clinical component, the extent of profusion of interstitial opacities and evidence of PH as the radiographic component, and TLC % pred and P_{aO_2} during maximal exercise as the physiological measures [46]. Use of the new CRP score in clinical routine to monitor patients is limited due to the complexity and necessity of exercise testing. Moreover, longitudinal validity and MCID need further investigation.

Using physiological variables that were independently related to IPF severity on HRCT, a Composite Physiologic Index (CPI) consisting of D_{LCO}, FEV_1, and FVC has been introduced to predict the extent of fibrosis on HRCT (table 4) [35]. It can be used to estimate the extent of the disease without follow-up CT and to predict survival. Inclusion of the FEV1 also takes into account concomitant emphysema. The CPI has been validated in an external cohort of IPF patients with and without concomitant emphysema and a five-point increase in CPI over 12 months predicted mortality similarly to relative declines of 10% in FVC and 15% in DLCO [30].

An advantage of the CPI is its simplicity; only routinely assessed physiologic variables are used. It has been adopted in other composite scores (Risk stratificatiOn ScorE (ROSE), table 5). However, calculation of the CPI may not be possible in patients with severe disease, as often the DLCO measurement cannot be performed.

The GAP score uses commonly measured clinical and physiological (DLCO, FVC) variables. These are added up into a simple point scoring system that allows the classification of disease severity into three stages based on 1-year mortality. The mortality risk of an individual patient can also be calculated more precisely using the GAP calculator that is based on a regression model with continuous variables [68].

The GAP model was validated using external cohorts for prediction at baseline and in follow-up visits [68–70]. Further, a CT extent score can be included in the GAP model and replace the DLCO measurement without significant change in prognostic accuracy [71]; the score can also be used in other ILDs with little adaptation [69]. Yet, the predictive value of the longitudinal change of GAP score has not been evaluated so far.

DU BOIS et al. [72] developed a 1-year mortality risk score system using data from 1099 patients in the INSPIRE trials. Hence, only patients with mild to moderate physiological impairment were included. The score contains the following variables: age; respiratory

Table 4. Composite Physiologic Index

Extent of disease on CT = 91.0
− (0.65 × DLCO % pred)
− (0.53 × FVC % pred)
+ (0.34 × FEV1 % pred)

Reproduced and modified from [35] with permission from the publisher.

Table 5. Risk stratification ScorE

Low risk (I): all of the below	Intermediate risk (II): one of the below	High risk (II): all of the below
MRCDS <3 6MWD >72% pred CPI <41	MRCDS >3 6MWD <72% pred CPI >41	MRCDS >3 6MWD <72% pred CPI >41

MRCDS: Medical Research Council Dyspnoea Score; CPI: Composite Physiologic Index. Data from [9].

hospitalisation; FVC % pred; 24-week change in FVC; DLCO % pred; and 24-week change in DLCO % pred. Optionally, the 24-week change in health-related QoL can also be included. Even though longitudinal components are inherent to this score, the significance of score changes over time has not been investigated.

The use of hospitalisation for respiratory causes as a predictor of mortality has been criticised in the past, as defining causes for hospitalisation may be difficult. Yet, an association between hospital admission (in general and specifically for respiratory causes) and survival was recently confirmed using data from three large clinical trials (PANTHER-IPF, STEP-IPF, and ACE-IPF) [32].

The most recent composite score has been proposed by MURA et al. [9] who prospectively observed 70 patients with newly diagnosed IPF for 3 years. The score (ROSE) derived from these data predicts a 3-year-mortality based on MRCDS, 6MWD % pred, and CPI and was validated with an independent retrospective cohort (table 2). Using these three independent variables, it may be more specific in predicting survival than one variable, for example, the CPI alone. Importantly, longitudinal analyses found that a 6-month progression of ROSE predicted rapid disease progression and increased the sensitivity of survival prediction.

As most of the composite scores have been developed very recently, it is not clear which score will prove most useful and prevail in the future. At present, the ROSE score appeals when monitoring IPF patients because longitudinal evaluation is available, but confirmation in another large prospective cohort would be useful. The GAP score is striking for its simplicity, the possibility to replace DLCO with an HRCT score, and transferability to other ILDs.

Detection and prediction of acute exacerbations

Patients with IPF may present with acute respiratory worsening characterised by a rapid worsening of symptoms (within <4 weeks) in symptoms, lung function, and radiographic findings [73]. Clinical symptoms include worsening of dyspnoea, cough, and fever, while new bilateral opacities with peripheral, multifocal, or diffuse pattern are found on HRCT. If known identifiable causes, such as infection, thromboembolism, or pneumothorax have been excluded, these periods are called acute exacerbation of IPF. However, it is currently unclear if these "idiopathic" acute exacerbations are pathogenetically and prognostically different from those with known causes [74]. Biologically, an acceleration of the underlying IPF is found [75]. Being associated with a high mortality of up to 50% within 6 months [73], acute exacerbations have recently been used as end-points in clinical trials [76].

Risk factors for AEs comprise internal factors, such as severely impaired baseline lung function, severe dyspnoea, a history of coronary artery disease, and the presence of PH or emphysema [9, 76–79], but also external factors, such as cigarette smoking and air pollution [80]. Additionally, exacerbation frequency was found to be higher in winter than in the other seasons [78, 81], pointing towards a role for infectious causes. Mechanical or chemical stress induced by aspiration, high flow oxygen, pulmonary infection, BAL, mechanical ventilation, and lung surgery has also been linked to AEs. However, the risk of inducing an exacerbation may be low for some of these factors, such as BAL, but this will be discussed in more detail in another chapter of this Monograph [82]. Finally, a history of acute exacerbations is a predictor of future acute exacerbation, suggesting a distinct phenotype or persisting cause in affected patients [80].

Identifying acute exacerbations but also other, "non-idiopathic" acute worsening is important due to high morbidity and mortality. Scoring of fibrosis extent on HRCT during exacerbation may predict mortality in IPF [83]. Monitoring must rely on the patient and his primary physician to inform the IPF centre in case of any acute clinical deterioration or hospitalisation.

Even though therapeutic options for acute exacerbations, such as anti-infective drugs and corticosteroids are of questionable effectiveness, their identification must lead to reconsideration of the individual IPF treatment approach and prompt a close follow-up schedule afterwards. Continuous antireflux therapy may reduce exacerbations in patients with gastro-oesophageal reflux [67, 84]. Moreover, nintedanib therapy can be considered as it has shown promise in reducing exacerbation frequency [85]; lung transplantation may be indicated in eligible patients.

Detection of comorbidities and complications

IPF is associated with multiple comorbidities including GERD, venous thromboembolism, coronary artery disease, obesity, sleep-disordered breathing, depression, emphysema, PH, and lung cancer. Development of these comorbidities may increase morbidity and worsen prognosis of the affected patient; they will be discussed in more detail in the following chapters of this *Monograph* [86]. However, data on the role of routine screening by instrumental diagnostic methods for identification of comorbidities are mostly lacking [87]. Consequently, clinicians must exhibit a high level of suspicion and awareness for these comorbidities, looking for clinical signs and symptoms at regular follow-up visits and in case of clinical deterioration.

Solely screening for PH is currently recommended in patients with IPF who are eligible for lung transplantation [3], and presence of PH is implemented in the lung allocation score. As echocardiography is not a reliable screening tool in patients with IPF and other prediction models have not been thoroughly validated, right heart catheterisation is indicated in these patients. However, *N*-terminal pro-brain natriuretic peptide has a high negative predictive value and in case of normal value further invasive evaluation might not be necessary [88].

Monitoring schedule and future directions

Monitoring patients with IPF is crucial to proactively identify those with progressive disease and to determine the development of comorbidities to initiate appropriate and timely treatment. To answer the question at which intervals to monitor, we must take into account the patient's disease history, MCIDs of the variables measured, and treatment tolerability and efficacy. Current guidelines recommend follow-up visits with clinical and physiological assessment every 3–6 months. Earlier follow-up is indicated if the patient recognises a change in clinical status or has recently experienced progression or acute exacerbation. Further examinations, such as radiographic studies, may be useful in this case. Thus the monitoring schedule must be individualised and adapted according to the individual disease course, as illustrated in figure 1b.

The MCID is the smallest difference in a measure that patients perceive to be important, either beneficial or harmful, and that would lead a clinician to consider a change in a patient's therapy [89]. In addition to providing a therapeutic threshold for an outcome measure in clinical routine, the MCID impacts the design of clinical trials in terms of the selection of end-points and the determination of sample size [90]. There are two main approaches to determine the MCID: 1) the anchor-based method links the change in the outcome variable to a meaningful external anchor accounting for the patient's perspective, generally a QoL measurement tool like the SF-36; and 2) distribution-based methods are derived from statistical measures of spread of data, like standard deviation, standard error of the mean and effect size [91]. A meaningful range for the MCID can be estimated by combining both methods. So far, IPF-specific MCIDs have been calculated for FVC [27] and 6MWD [38], while available estimates for dyspnoea scales, for example, UCSD SOBQ [7], are derived from other chronic lung diseases. Further studies of MCID are needed to fully establish the implementation of new outcome variables, such as HRCT scores, into clinical routine and trials. The estimated MCID for FVC is 2–6%. As patients with rapidly progressive disease may exceed this threshold within a quarterly follow-up, frequent FVC monitoring with handheld devices and telemonitoring might become interesting options.

Recently two drugs, nintedanib and pirfenidone, have been approved for the treatment of IPF as they are effective at reducing lung function decline. However, studies have suggested that both can have substantial adverse effects (AEs) leading to discontinuation of treatment in approximately 15–19% of patients [92–94]. These AEs include photosensitivity reaction, rash, and nausea for pirfenidone, and gastrointestinal side effects, especially diarrhoea for nintedanib. They can be managed with symptomatic treatment and dose reduction or discontinuation. Moreover, response to therapy is variable and rapid progression can occur in some patients despite treatment [95]. In those patients, an alternative agent, participation in clinical trials that include combination therapies, or non-medical therapy with lung transplantation may be considered. Thus, after treatment initiation closer monitoring is advisable for timely recognition of adverse events and consecutive treatment adaptation.

Despite sputum cultures taken during acute exacerbation being negative, analysis of BAL with culture-independent methods found a distinct microbiome in IPF lungs compared to healthy ones [96, 97]. Importantly, progression of IPF was associated with the presence of specific members within the *Staphylococcus* and *Streptococcus* genera [97]. In experimental lung fibrosis, streptococcal pneumolysin induced progression even in the absence of infection [98]. Furthermore, treating IPF patients with co-trimoxazole continuously was found to reduce mortality [99]. These data suggest a role for microorganisms in acute exacerbation and disease progression. However, the exact pathogenesis with interplay of microbiome and host responses is not well characterised as yet. The field being still in its infancy, monitoring of BAL microbiome is currently only useful within studies.

At present, IPF monitoring relies on clinical biomarkers that reflect the result, rather than ongoing pathobiological processes of the disease. Therefore, there is a great need for molecular biomarkers derived from biological tissue or fluids that inform about the underlying biological disease mechanisms. They could not only be used for the monitoring of disease activity and prognosis, but possibly also for subphenotyping and predicting treatment response. At this time, the most promising prognostic markers for translation into clinical use are MUC5B, matrix metalloproteinase 7, and Krebs von den Lungen-6 (KL-6)/Mucin 1 (MUC1). A detailed overview of this field will be presented in another chapter of this *Monograph* [100].

Conclusion

The IPF field has seen major advances in recent years with refinement of diagnostic criteria, observation of natural history, the establishment of prognostic factors for baseline and longitudinal evaluation, and the introduction of the first two effective drug treatments. Thus, monitoring for progressive disease, comorbidities, and treatment response is becoming increasingly important and defined. In addition to established criteria such as clinical, physiological, and exercise variables, radiographic quantification of fibrosis extent is becoming more standardised and objective. Composite scores allow for the integration of different variables into a more accurate estimate of prognosis. Biological biomarkers based on genetic analysis, serum, or BAL proteins are currently being developed. Their integration into staging and monitoring will be another important milestone in IPF care. Recent findings of microbial dysbiosis in IPF hold promise not only for monitoring, but also to gain novel insights into pathobiology and guide therapeutic directions.

References

1. Ley B, Collard HR, King TE Jr. Clinical course and prediction of survival in idiopathic pulmonary fibrosis. *Am J Respir Crit Care Med* 2011; 183: 431–440.
2. Selman M, Carrillo G, Estrada A, *et al.* Accelerated variant of idiopathic pulmonary fibrosis: clinical behavior and gene expression pattern. *PLoS One* 2007; 2: e482.
3. Raghu G, Collard HR, Egan JJ, *et al.* An official ATS/ERS/JRS/ALAT statement: idiopathic pulmonary fibrosis: evidence-based guidelines for diagnosis and management. *Am J Respir Crit Care Med* 2011; 183: 788–824.
4. Manali ED, Stathopoulos GT, Kollintza A, *et al.* The Medical Research Council chronic dyspnea score predicts the survival of patients with idiopathic pulmonary fibrosis. *Respir Med* 2008; 102: 586–592.
5. Nishiyama O, Taniguchi H, Kondoh Y, *et al.* A simple assessment of dyspnoea as a prognostic indicator in idiopathic pulmonary fibrosis. *Eur Respir J* 2010; 36: 1067–1072.
6. Collard HR, King TE Jr, Bartelson BB, *et al.* Changes in clinical and physiologic variables predict survival in idiopathic pulmonary fibrosis. *Am J Respir Crit Care Med* 2003; 168: 538–542.
7. Kupferberg DH, Kaplan RM, Slymen DJ, *et al.* Minimal clinically important difference for the UCSD Shortness of Breath Questionnaire. *J Cardiopulm Rehabil* 2005; 25: 370–377.
8. Murciano D, Pichot MH, Boczkowski J, *et al.* Expiratory flow limitation in COPD patients after single lung transplantation. *Am J Respir Crit Care Med* 1997; 155: 1036–1041.
9. Mura M, Porretta MA, Bargagli E, *et al.* Predicting survival in newly diagnosed idiopathic pulmonary fibrosis: a 3-year prospective study. *Eur Respir J* 2012; 40: 101–109.
10. Watters LC, King TE, Schwarz MI, *et al.* A clinical, radiographic, and physiologic scoring system for the longitudinal assessment of patients with idiopathic pulmonary fibrosis. *Am Rev Respir Dis* 1986; 133: 97–103.
11. Eakin EG. Validation of a new dyspnea measure: the UCSD Shortness of Breath Questionnaire. University of California, San Diego. *Chest* 1998; 113: 619–624.
12. Swigris JJ, Han M, Vij R, *et al.* The UCSD shortness of breath questionnaire has longitudinal construct validity in idiopathic pulmonary fibrosis. *Respir Med* 2012; 106: 1447–1455.
13. King TE Jr, Bradford WZ, Castro-Bernardini S, *et al.* A phase 3 trial of pirfenidone in patients with idiopathic pulmonary fibrosis. *N Engl J Med* 2014; 370: 2083–2092.
14. Brown KK. Chronic cough due to chronic interstitial pulmonary diseases: ACCP evidence-based clinical practice guidelines. *Chest* 2006; 129: Suppl. 1, 180–185.
15. Ryerson CJ, Abbritti M, Ley B, *et al.* Cough predicts prognosis in idiopathic pulmonary fibrosis. *Respirology* 2011; 16: 969–975.
16. Scholand MB, Wolff R, Crossno PF, *et al.* Severity of cough in idiopathic pulmonary fibrosis is associated with MUC5 B genotype. *Cough* 2014; 10: 3.
17. Lechtzin N, Hilliard ME, Horton MR. Validation of the Cough Quality-of-Life Questionnaire in patients with idiopathic pulmonary fibrosis. *Chest* 2013; 143: 1745–1749.
18. Boulet LP, Coeytaux RR, McCrory DC, *et al.* Tools for assessing outcomes in studies of chronic cough: CHEST guideline and expert panel report. *Chest* 2015; 147: 804–814.
19. Enright PL, Beck KC, Sherrill DL. Repeatability of spirometry in 18 000 adult patients. *Am J Respir Crit Care Med* 2004; 169: 235–238.
20. Pellegrino R, Viegi G, Brusasco V, *et al.* Interpretative strategies for lung function tests. *Eur Respir J* 2005; 26: 948–968.
21. Jegal Y, Kim DS, Shim TS, *et al.* Physiology is a stronger predictor of survival than pathology in fibrotic interstitial pneumonia. *Am J Respir Crit Care Med* 2005; 171: 639–644.
22. King TE Jr, Safrin S, Starko KM, *et al.* Analyses of efficacy end points in a controlled trial of interferon-gamma1b for idiopathic pulmonary fibrosis. *Chest* 2005; 127: 171–177.

23. Latsi PI, du Bois RM, Nicholson AG, *et al.* Fibrotic idiopathic interstitial pneumonia: the prognostic value of longitudinal functional trends. *Am J Respir Crit Care Med* 2003; 168: 531–537.

24. Flaherty KR, Mumford JA, Murray S, *et al.* Prognostic implications of physiologic and radiographic changes in idiopathic interstitial pneumonia. *Am J Respir Crit Care Med* 2003; 168: 543–548.

25. Richeldi L, Cottin V, Flaherty KR, *et al.* Design of the INPULSIS^{TM} trials: two phase 3 trials of nintedanib in patients with idiopathic pulmonary fibrosis. *Respir Med* 2014; 108: 1023–1030.

26. Zappala CJ, Latsi PI, Nicholson AG, *et al.* Marginal decline in forced vital capacity is associated with a poor outcome in idiopathic pulmonary fibrosis. *Eur Respir J* 2010; 35: 830–836.

27. du Bois RM, Weycker D, Albera C, *et al.* Forced vital capacity in patients with idiopathic pulmonary fibrosis: test properties and minimal clinically important difference. *Am J Respir Crit Care Med* 2011; 184: 1382–1389.

28. Akagi T, Matsumoto T, Harada T, *et al.* Coexistent emphysema delays the decrease of vital capacity in idiopathic pulmonary fibrosis. *Respir Med* 2009; 103: 1209–1215.

29. Aduen JF, Zisman DA, Mobin SI, *et al.* Retrospective study of pulmonary function tests in patients presenting with isolated reduction in single-breath diffusion capacity: implications for the diagnosis of combined obstructive and restrictive lung disease. *Mayo Clin Proc* 2007; 82: 48–54.

30. Schmidt SL, Nambiar AM, Tayob N, *et al.* Pulmonary function measures predict mortality differently in IPF *versus* combined pulmonary fibrosis and emphysema. *Eur Respir J* 2011; 38: 176–183.

31. Kishaba T, Shimaoka Y, Fukuyama H, *et al.* A cohort study of mortality predictors and characteristics of patients with combined pulmonary fibrosis and emphysema. *BMJ Open* 2012; 2: e000988.

32. Durheim MT, Collard HR, Roberts RS, *et al.* Association of hospital admission and forced vital capacity endpoints with survival in patients with idiopathic pulmonary fibrosis: analysis of a pooled cohort from three clinical trials. *Lancet Respir Med* 2015; 3: 388–396.

33. Karimi-Shah BA, Chowdhury BA. Forced vital capacity in idiopathic pulmonary fibrosis – FDA review of pirfenidone and nintedanib. *N Engl J Med* 2015; 372: 1189–1191.

34. Russell A-M, Lukey P, Fraser U, *et al.* Daily hand-held spirometry for the monitoring of patients with idiopathic pulmonary fibrosis. *Eur Respir J* 2011; 38: Suppl. 55, 655.

35. Wells AU, Desai SR, Rubens MB, *et al.* Idiopathic pulmonary fibrosis: a composite physiologic index derived from disease extent observed by computed tomography. *Am J Respir Crit Care Med* 2003; 167: 962–969.

36. Enright PL. The six-minute walk test. *Respir Care* 2003; 48: 783–785.

37. Lama VN, Flaherty KR, Toews GB, *et al.* Prognostic value of desaturation during a 6-minute walk test in idiopathic interstitial pneumonia. *Am J Respir Crit Care Med* 2003; 168: 1084–1090.

38. du Bois RM, Weycker D, Albera C, *et al.* Six-minute-walk test in idiopathic pulmonary fibrosis: test validation and minimal clinically important difference. *Am J Respir Crit Care Med* 2011; 183: 1231–1237.

39. Eaton T, Young P, Milne D, *et al.* Six-minute walk, maximal exercise tests: reproducibility in fibrotic interstitial pneumonia. *Am J Respir Crit Care Med* 2005; 171: 1150–1157.

40. Nathan SD, du Bois RM, Albera C, *et al.* Validation of test performance characteristics and minimal clinically important difference of the 6-minute walk test in patients with idiopathic pulmonary fibrosis. *Respir Med* 2015; 109: 914–922.

41. Holland AE, Hill CJ, Conron M, *et al.* Small changes in six-minute walk distance are important in diffuse parenchymal lung disease. *Respir Med* 2009; 103: 1430–1435.

42. Swigris JJ, Wamboldt FS, Behr J, *et al.* The 6 minute walk in idiopathic pulmonary fibrosis: longitudinal changes and minimum important difference. *Thorax* 2010; 65: 173–177.

43. Weir NA, Brown AW, Shlobin OA, *et al.* The influence of alternative instruction on 6-min walk test distance. *Chest* 2013; 144: 1900–1905.

44. ATS Committee on Proficiency Standards for Clinical Pulmonary Function Laboratories. ATS statement: guidelines for the six-minute walk test. *Am J Respir Crit Care Med* 2002; 166: 111–117.

45. American Thoracic Society, American College of Chest Physicians. ATS/ACCP Statement on cardiopulmonary exercise testing. *Am J Respir Crit Care Med* 2003; 167: 211–277.

46. King TE Jr, Tooze JA, Schwarz MI, *et al.* Predicting survival in idiopathic pulmonary fibrosis: scoring system and survival model. *Am J Respir Crit Care Med* 2001; 164: 1171–1181.

47. Miki K, Maekura R, Hiraga T, *et al.* Impairments and prognostic factors for survival in patients with idiopathic pulmonary fibrosis. *Respir Med* 2003; 97: 482–490.

48. Erbes R, Schaberg T, Loddenkemper R. Lung function tests in patients with idiopathic pulmonary fibrosis. Are they helpful for predicting outcome? *Chest* 1997; 111: 51–57.

49. Triantafillidou C, Manali E, Lyberopoulos P, *et al.* The role of cardiopulmonary exercise test in IPF prognosis. *Pulm Med* 2013; 2013: 4–7.

50. Lynch DA, Godwin JD, Safrin S, *et al.* High-resolution computed tomography in idiopathic pulmonary fibrosis: diagnosis and prognosis. *Am J Respir Crit Care Med* 2005; 172: 488–493.

51. Jeong YJ, Lee KS, Müller NL, *et al.* Usual interstitial pneumonia and non-specific interstitial pneumonia: serial thin-section CT findings correlated with pulmonary function. *Korean J Radiol* 2005; 6: 143–152.

52. Best AC, Meng J, Lynch AM, *et al.* Idiopathic pulmonary fibrosis: physiologic tests, quantitative CT indexes, and CT visual scores as predictors of mortality. *Radiology* 2008; 246: 935–940.

53. Shin KM, Lee KS, Chung MP, *et al.* Prognostic determinants among clinical, thin-section CT, and histopathologic findings for fibrotic idiopathic interstitial pneumonias: tertiary hospital study. *Radiology* 2008; 249: 328–337.

54. Sumikawa H, Johkoh T, Colby TV, *et al.* Computed tomography findings in pathological usual interstitial pneumonia: relationship to survival. *Am J Respir Crit Care Med* 2008; 177: 433–439.

55. Hwang JH, Misumi S, Curran-Everett D, *et al.* Longitudinal follow-up of fibrosing interstitial pneumonia: relationship between physiologic testing, computed tomography changes, and survival rate. *J Thorac Imaging* 2011; 26: 209–217.

56. Hansell DM, Goldin JG, King TE Jr, *et al.* CT staging and monitoring of fibrotic interstitial lung diseases in clinical practice and treatment trials: a position paper from the Fleischner Society. *Lancet Respir Med* 2015; 3: 483–496.

57. Oda K, Ishimoto H, Yatera K, *et al.* High-resolution CT scoring system-based grading scale predicts the clinical outcomes in patients with idiopathic pulmonary fibrosis. *Respir Res* 2014; 15: 10.

58. Rodriguez LH, Vargas PF, Raff U, *et al.* Automated discrimination and quantification of idiopathic pulmonary fibrosis from normal lung parenchyma using generalized fractal dimensions in high-resolution computed tomography images. *Acad Radiol* 1995; 2: 10–18.

59. Zavaletta VA, Bartholmai BJ, Robb RA. High resolution multidetector CT-aided tissue analysis and quantification of lung fibrosis. *Acad Radiol* 2007; 14: 772–787.

60. Park SO, Seo JB, Kim N, *et al.* Comparison of usual interstitial pneumonia and nonspecific interstitial pneumonia: quantification of disease severity and discrimination between two diseases on HRCT using a texture-based automated system. *Korean J Radiol* 2011; 12: 297–307.

61. Yoon RG, Seo JB, Kim N, *et al.* Quantitative assessment of change in regional disease patterns on serial HRCT of fibrotic interstitial pneumonia with texture-based automated quantification system. *Eur Radiol* 2013; 23: 692–701.

62. Rosas IO, Yao J, Avila NA, *et al.* Automated quantification of high-resolution CT scan findings in individuals at risk for pulmonary fibrosis. *Chest* 2011; 140: 1590–1597.

63. Maldonado F, Moua T, Rajagopalan S, *et al.* Automated quantification of radiological patterns predicts survival in idiopathic pulmonary fibrosis. *Eur Respir J* 2014; 43: 204–212.

64. Iwasawa T, Asakura A, Sakai F, *et al.* Assessment of prognosis of patients with idiopathic pulmonary fibrosis by computer-aided analysis of CT images. *J Thorac Imaging* 2009; 24: 216–222.

65. Colombi D, Dinkel J, Weinheimer O, *et al.* Visual *vs* fully automatic histogram-based assessment of idiopathic pulmonary fibrosis (IPF) progression using sequential multidetector computed tomography (MDCT). *PLoS One* 2015; 10: e0130653.

66. Iwasawa T, Ogura T, Sakai F, *et al.* CT analysis of the effect of pirfenidone in patients with idiopathic pulmonary fibrosis. *Eur J Radiol* 2014; 83: 32–38.

67. Raghu G, Rochwerg B, Zhang Y, *et al.* An official ATS/ERS/JRS/ALAT clinical practice guideline: treatment of idiopathic pulmonary fibrosis. An update of the 2011 clinical practice guideline. *Am J Respir Crit Care Med* 2015; 192: e3–19.

68. Ley B, Ryerson CJ, Vittinghoff E, *et al.* A multidimensional index and staging system for idiopathic pulmonary fibrosis. *Ann Intern Med* 2012; 156: 684–691.

69. Ryerson CJ, Vittinghoff E, Ley B, *et al.* Predicting survival across chronic interstitial lung disease: the ILD-GAP model. *Chest* 2014; 145: 723–728.

70. Kim HJ, Perlman D, Tomic R. Natural history of idiopathic pulmonary fibrosis. *Respir Med* 2015; 109: 661–670.

71. Ley B, Elicker BM, Hartman TE, *et al.* Idiopathic pulmonary fibrosis: CT and risk of death. *Radiology* 2014; 273: 570–579.

72. du Bois RM, Weycker D, Albera C, *et al.* Ascertainment of individual risk of mortality for patients with idiopathic pulmonary fibrosis. *Am J Respir Crit Care Med* 2011; 184: 459–466.

73. Collard HR, Moore BB, Flaherty KR, *et al.* Acute exacerbations of idiopathic pulmonary fibrosis. *Am J Respir Crit Care Med* 2007; 176: 636–643.

74. Johannson K, Collard HR. Acute exacerbation of idiopathic pulmonary fibrosis: a proposal. *Curr Respir Care Rep* 2013; 2: DOI: 10.1007/s13665-013-0065-x.

75. Konishi K, Gibson KF, Lindell KO, *et al.* Gene expression profiles of acute exacerbations of idiopathic pulmonary fibrosis. *Am J Respir Crit Care Med* 2009; 180: 167–175.

76. Collard HR, Yow E, Richeldi L, *et al.* Suspected acute exacerbation of idiopathic pulmonary fibrosis as an outcome measure in clinical trials. *Respir Res* 2013; 14: 73.

77. Judge EP, Fabre A, Adamali HI, *et al.* Acute exacerbations and pulmonary hypertension in advanced idiopathic pulmonary fibrosis. *Eur Respir J* 2012; 40: 93–100.

78. Simon-Blancal V, Freynet O, Nunes H, *et al.* Acute exacerbation of idiopathic pulmonary fibrosis: outcome and prognostic factors. *Respiration* 2012; 83: 28–35.

79. Song JW, Hong SB, Lim CM, *et al.* Acute exacerbation of idiopathic pulmonary fibrosis: incidence, risk factors and outcome. *Eur Respir J* 2011; 37: 356–363.

80. Johannson KA, Vittinghoff E, Lee K, *et al.* Acute exacerbation of idiopathic pulmonary fibrosis associated with air pollution exposure. *Eur Respir J* 2014; 43: 1124–1131.

81. Olson AL, Swigris JJ, Raghu G, *et al.* Seasonal variation: mortality from pulmonary fibrosis is greatest in the winter. *Chest* 2009; 136: 16–22.

82. Prasse A. Acute exacerbations. *In*: Costabel U, Crestani B, Wells AU, eds. Idiopathic Pulmonary Fibrosis (ERS Monograph). Sheffield, European Respiratory Society, 2016; pp. 143–150.

83. Fujimoto K, Taniguchi H, Johkoh T, *et al.* Acute exacerbation of idiopathic pulmonary fibrosis: high-resolution CT scores predict mortality. *Eur Radiol* 2012; 22: 83–92.

84. Raghu G, Meyer KC. Silent gastro-oesophageal reflux and microaspiration in IPF: mounting evidence for anti-reflux therapy? *Eur Respir J* 2012; 39: 242–245.

85. Richeldi L, du Bois RM, Raghu G, *et al.* Efficacy and safety of nintedanib in idiopathic pulmonary fibrosis. *N Engl J Med* 2014; 370: 2071–2082.

86. Kreuter M, Brunnemer E, Ehlers-Tenenbaum S, *et al.* Other comorbidities. *In*: Costabel U, Crestani B, Wells AU, eds. Idiopathic Pulmonary Fibrosis (ERS Monograph). Sheffield, European Respiratory Society, 2016; pp. 186–195.

87. Martinez FJ, Safrin S, Weycker D, *et al.* The clinical course of patients with idiopathic pulmonary fibrosis. *Ann Intern Med* 2005; 142: 963–967.

88. Andersen CU, Mellemkjær S, Hilberg O, *et al.* Pulmonary hypertension in interstitial lung disease: prevalence, prognosis and 6 min walk test. *Respir Med* 2012; 106: 875–882.

89. Jaeschke R, Singer J, Guyatt GH. Measurement of health status. Ascertaining the minimal clinically important difference. *Control Clin Trials* 1989; 10: 407–415.

90. Man-Son-Hing M, Laupacis A, O'Rourke K, *et al.* Determination of the clinical importance of study results. *J Gen Intern Med* 2002; 17: 469–476.

91. Wright A, Hannon J, Hegedus EJ, *et al.* Clinimetrics corner: a closer look at the minimal clinically important difference (MCID). *J Man Manip Ther* 2012; 20: 160–166.

92. Noble PW, Albera C, Bradford WZ, *et al.* Pirfenidone in patients with idiopathic pulmonary fibrosis (CAPACITY): two randomised trials. *Lancet* 2011; 377: 1760–1769.

93. Richeldi L, Costabel U, Selman M, *et al.* Efficacy of a tyrosine kinase inhibitor in idiopathic pulmonary fibrosis. *N Engl J Med* 2011; 365: 1079–1087.

94. King TE Jr, Bradford WZ, Castro-Bernardini S, *et al.* A phase 3 trial of pirfenidone in patients with idiopathic pulmonary fibrosis. *N Engl J Med* 2014; 370: 2083–2092.

95. Loeh B, Drakopanagiotakis F, Bandelli GP, *et al.* Intraindividual response to treatment with pirfenidone in idiopathic pulmonary fibrosis. *Am J Respir Crit Care Med* 2015; 191: 110–113.

96. Molyneaux PL, Cox MJ, Willis-Owen SA, *et al.* The role of bacteria in the pathogenesis and progression of idiopathic pulmonary fibrosis. *Am J Respir Crit Care Med* 2014; 190: 906–913.

97. Han MK, Zhou Y, Murray S, *et al.* Lung microbiome and disease progression in idiopathic pulmonary fibrosis: an analysis of the COMET study. *Lancet Respir Med* 2014; 2: 548–556.

98. Knippenberg S, Ueberberg B, Maus R, *et al. Streptococcus pneumoniae* triggers progression of pulmonary fibrosis through pneumolysin. *Thorax* 2015; 70: 636–646.

99. Shulgina L, Cahn AP, Chilvers ER, *et al.* Treating idiopathic pulmonary fibrosis with the addition of co-trimoxazole: a randomised controlled trial. *Thorax* 2013; 68: 155–162.

100. Kokosi MA, Renzoni E, Bonella F. Biomarkers. *In*: Costabel U, Crestani B, Wells AU, eds. Idiopathic Pulmonary Fibrosis (ERS Monograph). Sheffield, European Respiratory Society, 2016; pp. 122–142.

Disclosures: J. Behr reports receiving the following outside the submitted work: grants and personal fees from Boehringer-Ingelheim for steering committee activities, lecturing and consulting; a grant from Boehringer-Ingelheim; and grants and personal fees from Actelion, Bayer, Gilead, GSK and Pfizer for lecturing and consulting.

Chapter 10

Biomarkers

Maria A. Kokosi[1], Elisabetta Renzoni[1] and Francesco Bonella[2]

IPF is characterised by a complex pathobiology, which progressively leads to irreversible architectural distortion of the lungs and impaired respiratory function. The management of IPF patients is difficult and still inadequate. Existing assessment tools, including PFTs, are poorly predictive of disease progression and response to treatment. In the last decade, biomarker research in IPF has grown consistently. The multiple pathways involved in the pathogenesis of IPF provide a plethora of molecules, some of which appear to play a role in biological processes rather than simply representing epiphenomena, and could have a role as biomarkers. Selected biomarkers appear to be repeatable, easy to detect and correlated with prognosis, but inter- and intra-individual variability, including variation linked to genetic polymorphisms, has been observed. A number of promising, although not yet fully validated, circulating biomarkers are close to utilisation in routine clinical practice, and encouraging data are emerging from genetic and epigenetic investigations. Confirmation of the results of potential genetic variants linked to prognosis and/or response to treatment should lead to their inclusion into future clinical trials and to their use in clinical practice in the near future.

The aetiology of IPF is unknown, although several risk factors have been implicated, including cigarette smoke [1]. The development of IPF involves dysregulation of multiple pathways and phenotypic abnormalities of a variety of cell types. Pulmonary fibrogenesis is thought to result from recurrent injury to alveolar epithelial cells caused by a variety of exposures, with subsequent activation of aberrant repair processes, including fibroblast proliferation, and accumulation of extracellular matrix (ECM), with failed resolution of the wound-healing response and fibrosis [2, 3].

Clinicians managing patients with IPF are faced with multiple challenges. The need for accurate diagnosis of IPF has never been so crucial, particularly since the finding that immunosuppression is not effective in IPF and that specific antifibrotic treatments for IPF are now available [4]. Although HRCT represents the cornerstone in the diagnosis of ILD in association with supportive clinical data, almost half of the IPF patients present with atypical imaging. Furthermore, histology is not always helpful. There is considerable overlap in the histological appearances of the different IIPs and poor inter-observer agreement [5, 6]. Given the morbidity and mortality associated with surgical lung biopsy, there is a pressing need for better, minimally invasive and reliable diagnostic tests to reach confident diagnostic and prognostic statements [1], although more recently, cryobiopsy has

[1]Interstitial Lung Disease Unit, Royal Brompton Hospital and National Heart and Lung Institute, Imperial College London, London, UK.
[2]Interstitial and Rare Lung Disease Unit, Ruhrlandklinik, Universitiy of Duisburg-Essen, Essen, Germany.

Correspondence: Francesco Bonella, Interstitial and Rare Lung Disease Unit, Ruhrlandklinik, Tüschener Weg 40, 45239, Essen, Germany. E-mail: francesco.bonella@ruhrlandklinik.uk-essen.de

Copyright ©ERS 2016. Print ISBN: 978-1-84984-067-5. Online ISBN: 978-1-84984-068-2. Print ISSN: 2312-508X. Online ISSN: 2312-5098.

demonstrated a promising role in the diagnostic algorithm of IPF [7, 8]. Moreover, we are unable to adequately subphenotype patients with IPF who may have different biological mechanisms responsible for their underlying disease, disease behaviour, rate of progression and response to treatment. Given the complexity of the molecular processes involved in IPF, the potential therapeutic targets are numerous, and it is extremely difficult to identify and select the most promising ones.

Biomarkers could have a cardinal role in the management of IPF and could, in combination with clinical information, address several of the above-mentioned dilemmas. The role of biomarkers in IPF could include: improved understanding of underlying pathogenic mechanisms, identification of individuals at risk of developing IPF, noninvasive and more accurate diagnosis of IPF, prediction of disease behaviour to allow optimal timing of transplant referral, choice of treatment, monitoring of treatment response, clinical trial design and identification of potential therapeutic targets. The ideal biomarker should have high sensitivity and specificity, and be easy to measure, reproducible, technically accurate and cost-effective [9]. Therefore, measurement from easily obtainable body fluids or tissues is preferred (e.g. blood/serum, exhaled breath condensate, BALF) compared with invasive procedures such as a surgical lung biopsy.

This chapter focuses on validated or potential biomarkers in the serum, BALF or tissue in IPF patients.

Circulating biomarkers in IPF

Candidate biomarkers will be presented according to key pathogenic pathways and cell types (table 1).

Alveolar epithelial cell dysfunction

Repetitive injuries to alveolar epithelial cells result in an exaggerated wound-healing response, including hyperplastic epithelial changes, augmented permeability of the air–blood membrane and, subsequently, extensive scar formation. These phenomena are associated with augmented protein production and spillover to the systemic circulation [10].

KL-6/mucin 1 (MUC-1) is a circulating glycoprotein belonging to the MUC-1 class and is expressed on alveolar epithelial cells and bronchiolar epithelial cells. KL-6 exerts antifibrotic and antiapoptotic effects on lung fibroblasts [11]. KL-6 is probably the most extensively studied serum biomarker in ILD, at least in Japan, where it has been used to assess patients in the clinical routine [12]. Serum KL-6 shows good correlation with disease severity, although it does not discriminate between different ILD patterns. Serum levels of KL-6 are significantly elevated in IPF and are associated with increased mortality. A serum cut-off value of $\geqslant 1000$ U·mL^{-1} has been associated with poor prognosis [13]. The presence of the MUC1 568 adenosine to guanine polymorphism (rs4072037) has been found to influence serum KL-6 levels in Caucasian and Japanese subjects, and may need to be considered in the calculation of normal upper limits and cut-off values [14, 15].

Surfactant proteins (SPs) are synthesised and secreted by type II alveolar epithelial cells and facilitate surfactant function/transport and innate host defence. Abnormalities in SPs seem to increase alveolar epithelial endoplasmic reticulum stress and trigger the unfolded protein response [16]. Serum levels of SP-A and SP-D are elevated in IPF [17, 18] and, specifically,

Table 1. Circulating biomarkers in IPF

Biomarker(s)	Diagnosis of lung fibrosis	Prognosis	Treatment	Significance	Cohort n	[Ref.]
Alveolar epithelial cell dysfunction						
KL-6	++	+++	−	Association with disease severity and mortality	98	[11–13, 45, 47]
SP-A and SP-D	++	+++	−	Predictor of acute exacerbation	47 and 20	[17, 18]
				When included in predictor model was predictive of mortality	118	
				Correlation of SP-A levels with early mortality	82	
CK18	+	−	−	Elevated in IPF compared with healthy controls but no association with disease severity or outcome	84	[20]
Immune dysregulation and inflammation						
CCL18	+	+	−	Elevated in IPF compared with healthy controls	21	[21, 22]
				Correlation with IPF progression and survival	72	
S100A12	+/−	+	−	Association with poor survival	140 and 101	[23]
YKL-40	+	+	−	Elevated in IPF compared with healthy controls	63	[24, 25]
				Association with survival	85	
CXCL13	+	++	−	Association with worse outcome	95	[26, 27]
				Association with disease severity and outcome	80	
HSP-70	+/−	+	−	Association with survival	122	[28]
T-cells	−	+	−	Association with disease severity and survival	51	[29, 30]
				Correlation with progressive disease	45 and 75	

Continued

Table 1. Continued

Biomarker(s)	Diagnosis of lung fibrosis	Prognosis	Treatment	Significance	Cohort n	[Ref.]
Tregs/semaphorin 7a	+	+	−	Association with disease progression	21	[31, 32]
				Association with rapidly progressive disease	5	
IL-2, IL-4, IL-6, IL-13	+	−	+/−	Elevated in IPF patients	72 and 58	[33–35]
α-defensins	+	+	−	Elevated in IPF patients and association with disease severity	30 and 130	[36, 37, 48]
				Elevated in AEIPF	16	
ECM remodelling and fibroproliferation						
MMP-7	++	+++	−	Correlation with disease severity	74	[17, 23, 39]
				When included in predictor model was predictive of mortality	118	
MMP-3	+/−	+	−	Association with poor prognosis	140 and 101	[27]
LOXL	+	++	+/−	Association with rapid decline	80	[41]
				Association with IPF progression	Two IPF groups, 70 and 69	
Periostin	+	+	−	Association with IPF progression	54	[42–44]
				Inverse correlation with PFTs	37	
				Association with increase of fibrosis on CT and outcome	29	
Fibrocytes	+	+	−	Association with early mortality in stable IPF and acute exacerbation of IPF	Stable IPF [51] and acute exacerbation [7]	[29]
Osteopontin	++	−	−	Association with presence of fibrosis	7	[125–128]

SP: surfactant protein; CK: cytokeratin; HSP: heat shock protein; Treg: regulatory T-cells; IL: interleukin; ECM: extracellular matrix; MMP: matrix metalloproteinase; LOXL: lysyl oxidase-like; AEIPF: acute exacerbation of IPF.

SP-A levels correlate strongly with early mortality in IPF [18]. Polymorphisms in the SP-D gene (*SFTPD*) affect the serum levels of SP-D [19].

Cytokeratin-18 (CK18) is a cytoskeletal protein primarily found in pseudostratified and simple epithelia such as alveolar epithelial cells. During apoptosis, CK18 is catabolised to an 18 kDa fragment "cleaved CK18". Serum levels of cleaved CK18 seemed to differentiate IPF from other ILDs and healthy controls but were not associated with disease severity or outcome [20].

Immune dysregulation and inflammation

Innate immunity

Toll-interacting protein (TOLLIP) and Toll-like receptors (TLRs) are included under genetic biomarkers.

CCL18 is a chemotactic cytokine produced by alveolar macrophages, which stimulates fibroblast proliferation and collagen production. In IPF patients, serum CCL18 concentrations are elevated compared with normal controls [21] and CCL18 levels >150 ng·mL^{-1} are strongly predictive of functional decline and survival [22].

S100A12 is a calcium-binding protein, which binds to the receptor for advanced glycation-end products (RAGE) and activates innate and adaptive immunity in response to tissue injury and inflammation. High serum levels have recently been associated with poor survival in a relatively large IPF cohort [23].

Chitinase-like protein (YKL-40) is produced by activated macrophages and type II pneumocytes and seems to have a role in the release of fibrotic and inflammatory mediators from alveolar macrophages. YKL-40 serum levels are increased in IPF patients compared with controls [24] and were associated with survival in a small single-centre study [25].

Adaptive immunity

There is possibly a role for B-cells in the pathogenesis of IPF supported by the presence of lymphoid aggregates in IPF lungs along with evidence of antibody dysregulation in IPF patients. CXCL13, a specific mediator of B-cell trafficking to lymphoid aggregates and inflammatory foci, is overexpressed in the lungs and serum of patients with IPF compared with healthy controls. Serum levels of CXCL13 are higher in IPF patients with PH or acute exacerbations and are therefore related to a worse outcome [26]. Both lung tissue and serum CXCL13 levels were correlated with lymphoid infiltration in IPF and were predictive of subsequent IPF progression independent of disease severity [27].

Serum autoantibodies to heat-shock protein 70 (HSP-70) have been found in 25% of patients with IPF (compared with 3% in healthy controls). HSP-70 autoantibodies were also associated with worse pulmonary physiology and survival, independent of disease severity at baseline [28].

T-cells are the predominant mononuclear cells in IPF lungs and have been associated with disease severity and survival [29]. Increased CD8+ T-cell density in the lungs and decreased serum CD28+ T-cells both correlate with progressive disease. Furthermore, the level of gene expression associated with the co-stimulatory signal during T-cell activation has shown a prognostic role in IPF patients [30].

CD4+ CD25+ FOXP3+ regulatory T-cells (Tregs) control innate immunity and exert an important role in self-tolerance. Their dysfunction is associated with the development of autoimmune diseases. Tregs have been found to be reduced in the blood of patients with IPF compared with healthy controls and other ILDs in a small study and were associated with disease progression when semaphorin was expressed on the cell membrane [31]. Expression of semaphorin 7A on Tregs is increased in the lung and peripheral blood of patients with IPF, and serum semaphorin 7a+ Tregs are elevated in patients with rapidly progressive disease [32].

Interleukin (IL)-13 is a Th2 cytokine produced by immune cell types such as T-lymphocytes and activated macrophages. It has been found to promote fibrosis in animal models in synergy with IL-4 [33]. Blockage of IL-13 alone (by lebrikizumab) and of both IL-13 and IL-4 (by SAR156597) are being used as therapeutic strategies in clinical trials in IPF. In addition, serum IL-6 and soluble IL-2 receptor have been found to be elevated in IPF patients [34, 35].

α-defensins are cationic proteins with antimicrobial activity, four of which are exclusive to neutrophils. Serum α-defensin levels have been found to be elevated in IPF patients, to correlate with physiological parameters [36] and to predict DLCO deterioration in IPF [37].

ECM remodelling and fibroproliferation

Matrix metalloproteinases (MMPs), a large family of endopeptidases that degrade multiple components of the ECM, are upregulated during the wound-healing response. MMP-7 represents one of the most extensively studied biomarkers in IPF and is among the most highly upregulated mRNA in IPF lungs [38]. Higher plasma MMP-7 levels correlate significantly with disease severity, as measured by FVC and DLCO [39], and predicted survival in a large IPF cohort [17]. Furthermore, MMP-7 is a marker of poor prognosis, even after adjustment for disease severity [23], as further detailed in the later section on Circulating and genetic biomarkers in clinical predictor models.

MMP-7 plasma levels in IPF have been associated with two single-nucleotide polymorphisms (SNPs) in the gene's promoter region, thus providing a potential genetic contribution to MMP-7 upregulation [23]. MMP-3 is highly upregulated in the bronchiolised areas in IPF, and peripheral blood MMP-3 levels are predictive of a more rapid decline, independent of disease severity [27]. Recently, analysis of data from the PROFILE study has shown that concentrations of protein fragments generated by MMP activity are increased in the serum of IPF patients compared with healthy controls. Increased neoepitope concentrations were associated with disease progression, and the rate of this increase predicted survival [40].

The lysyl oxidase-like (LOXL) proteins are a group of enzymes that promote collagen accumulation and deposition, stabilising the ECM. In two independent IPF cohorts, baseline serum LOXL2 levels were increased in patients with IPF compared with healthy controls. Furthermore, higher levels of LOXL2 among IPF patients were strongly associated with the risk of progression and mortality [41]. A phase II clinical trial with simtuzumab, a monoclonal antibody targeting soluble LOXL2, is currently ongoing in IPF subjects (NCT01769196, clinicaltrials.gov).

Periostin is an ECM and intracellular protein localised in fibroblasts, and is upregulated in fibroblastic foci in IPF. IL-13 leads to production of periostin by bronchial epithelial cells. Periostin promotes ECM deposition, mesenchymal cell proliferation and fibrosis.

Lung tissue and serum periostin levels are elevated in IPF and correlate with physiological progression [42–44].

Fibrocytes are mesenchymal progenitor cells that can produce ECM, and differentiate into fibroblasts and myofibroblasts. In one study, circulating fibrocytes were higher in IPF patients compared with healthy controls [29]. A proportion of circulating fibrocytes >5% was associated with worse survival, although there was no correlation with clinical parameters [29].

Circulating biomarkers in acute exacerbation of IPF

The pathobiology of acute exacerbation of IPF (AEIPF) is not fully understood. Only a few studies on circulating biomarkers have focused on the prediction of AEIPF and its differentiation from stable IPF. The serum biomarker profile of AEIPF was compared with that of stable IPF and acute lung injury. KL-6, SP-D, RAGE, IL-6 and coagulation markers were significantly elevated in the AEIPF group compared with stable IPF and acute lung injury [45]. Serum levels of HSP-47 above 559 pg·mL^{-1} had a sensitivity of 94% and a specificity of 96% for AEIPF compared with stable disease [46]. Baseline levels of KL-6 were shown to be predictive of AEIPF at a cut-off value of $\geqslant$1300 U·mL^{-1} after adjustment for disease severity [47]. Patients with AEIPF had a significantly higher concentration of serum CXCL13 compared with those with stable IPF [26]. Circulating fibrocytes were elevated in AEIPF compared with stable IPF in one study [29]. Interestingly, in three patients who recovered from AEIPF, circulating fibrocytes returned to the pre-exacerbation levels [29]. Finally, α-defensins were increased in the peripheral blood of patients with AEIPF compared with stable IPF [48].

BAL as a source of biomarkers

BAL is a minimally invasive technique used to obtain cells, inhaled particles, infectious organisms and solutes from the lower respiratory tract and, in particular, from the alveolar spaces of the lung [49]. In the last two decades, BAL has been profiled as a pivotal method to obtain alveolar space and airway specimens for research [49]. However, insufficient standardisation of BAL procedures among different centres as well as technical issues related to sampling and storage of BAL fluid, which can influence the stability of soluble molecules, represent major limitations to the reproducibility and generalisability of the results.

Although almost all investigated candidate biomarkers for ILD/IPF in the last several years have been measured both in serum and BALF, the majority of studies have focused on the correlation between serum levels and disease activity or outcome [50].

In addition to the known utility of BAL cell counts in the diagnosis of IPF, mainly in terms of exclusion of other diagnoses [51], it is unclear whether BAL cellularity is useful for assessing the activity of disease processes with respect to obtaining prognostic information. In IPF, an increased BAL neutrophil percentage was found to correlate with early mortality [52], although another study did not find that BAL neutrophils predicted survival at 1 year [53]. Fibrocytes have been described in the BAL of about half of IPF patients [54]. Fibrocytes are circulating precursors for fibroblasts, and blood fibrocytes are increased in the blood of patients with IPF [29]. In a study by BORIE et al. [54], the number of alveolar fibrocytes was correlated with the number of alveolar macrophages and was associated with a less severe disease but poor outcome.

It is not proven that BAL or serial BAL is useful to guide therapy or predict treatment response. Larger prospective studies are required to shed light on this issue. At present, BAL cannot be routinely recommended for this purpose.

A number of molecules have been investigated in BAL supernatant and have been found in abnormal concentrations in IPF. Most of these proteins are of epithelial origin [50, 55]. The mucin 1 KL-6 is increased in BALF in 70% of IPF patients [47], but data on a correlation between BALF levels and disease severity/outcome are lacking. With regard to SPs, the BALF concentration of SP-A in IPF patients was not found to be different from healthy controls, but SP-D levels seemed to be lower in IPF [50, 55]. An association between SP-A BALF levels and survival has been described in a small single-centre IPF cohort [56].

CCL18 levels are elevated in the BALF of IPF patients in comparison with healthy controls but are not significantly different from the levels found in other ILDs [21, 57], and correlate inversely with TLC and DLCO [57].

In a recent study on the chitinase-like protein YKL-40 in IPF, KORTHAGEN et al. [25] found that BALF YKL-40 levels were significantly higher in patients than in healthy controls and that the −329 A/G polymorphism can influence BALF YKL-40 levels. IPF patients with high BALF YKL-40 levels (>17 ng·mL^{-1}) have significantly shorter survival times than those with low YKL-40 levels in serum or BAL.

Within the MMP family, only MMP-7, MMP-8 and MMP-9 show higher BALF levels in IPF patients when compared with control subjects [58, 59], although only MMP-9 is higher in IPF than in other ILDs [60].

Recent proteomic-approach studies have demonstrated that the application of two-dimensional electrophoresis to BAL samples is extremely useful for detailed analysis of the pathogenic mechanisms of ILD [60–63]. Differentially expressed protein spots, found by image analysis of gel electrophoresis, can be identified successfully by mass spectrometry (generally Matrix-Assisted Laser Desorption/Ionisation Time-of-Flight Mass Spectrometry or Liquid Chromatography Tandem Mass Spectrometry) and further processed by pathway analysis. Using this process, it is possible to build hypothetical networks between the experimental proteins and the existing protein databases. In a recent study, LANDI et al. [62] performed proteomic analysis on BALF from seven IPF patients and highlighted specific proteins, the expression of which distinguished IPF from healthy smoker and nonsmoker controls. Interestingly, transcriptional factors (nuclear factor-κB, peroxisome proliferator-activated receptor-γ and c-myc), together with several protein hubs, including angiotensin system maturation, the coagulation system and oxidative stress, emerged from the integrated analysis. Plastin 2, implicated in cytoskeleton rearrangement and epithelial–mesenchymal transition, was significantly downregulated in IPF. Although promising, these results need to be validated in adequate numbers of patients before definitive conclusions can be drawn.

The microbiome

Global screening of microbial communities has revealed the existence of a healthy microbiome (defined as the entire set of microbes in a particular environment) in normal lungs. MOLYNEAUX et al. [64] found clear differences in the BAL microbiome composition in patients with IPF compared with healthy and COPD lungs, suggesting fibrosis-specific changes. BAL from IPF patients was characterised by a higher bacterial burden and a loss of bacterial species diversity compared with controls. Patients with the highest BAL bacterial burden had the worse survival, independent of disease severity, although no specific microbe was associated with rate of progression [64]. Conversely, HAN *et al.* [65] reported that specific *Streptococcus* or *Staphylococcus* spp. were associated with more rapid disease progression in patients with IPF, while a relationship between overall bacterial burden and disease progression was not assessed. Although further studies are required to conclude whether microbial organisms could be driving IPF progression, these studies suggest that bacterial burden could be a useful marker of more progressive disease and that modification of bacterial populations in the lungs may be of benefit to IPF patients.

Genetic biomarkers in IPF

A genetic basis for pulmonary fibrosis is supported by a number of findings, including familial clustering and the occurrence of lung fibrosis in genetic multisystem disorders [66–69]. Recent findings indicate that both sporadic and familial presentations of IPF have similar genetic risk factors [70, 71], although familial forms tend to present earlier and have more diverse morphological patterns [72–74]. In table 2, the genes involved in the pathogenesis of IPF with a potential role as biomarkers are presented.

The identification of gene variants associated with pulmonary fibrosis has drawn from the study of rare variants in familial disease, gene linkage studies in familial disease and, more recently, the use of genome-wide association studies (GWASs) to identify more common variants associated with sporadic and familial pulmonary fibrosis. The first rare variants to be identified were the mutations in surfactant genes C and A in familial disease [75–78], followed by the rare variants of the genes involved in stabilisation of telomeres, including *TERT* and *TERC* [79, 80], ultimately found in approximately 15% of familial cases and 1–2% of sporadic IPF cases [81].

In 2011, SEIBOLD *et al.* [82], through a genome-wide linkage analysis performed initially in families with pulmonary fibrosis, demonstrated that a variant (rs35705950) in the promoter region of the *MUC5B* gene on chromosome 11 was strongly associated with familial pulmonary fibrosis and sporadic IIPs. The *MUC5B* variant minor allele was present in 34% of patients with familial pulmonary fibrosis, 37.5% of patients with IPF and 9% of healthy controls. This variant appears to be specific to the IIPs, as it is not associated with scleroderma-associated lung fibrosis, fibrotic sarcoidosis or asbestosis [83, 84]. The fact that approximately 10% of the general population carries the *MUC5B* variant indicates that it is not sufficient on its own to cause disease, although interstitial lung abnormalities were found more frequently in healthy carriers of the variant allele in a population study [52]. The frequency with which these could develop into full-blown IPF is not known and will require further study, although it is possible that this gene variant will be used as a biomarker of the likelihood of developing disease in the future [85].

Two recently performed large GWASs confirmed the strong association with *MUC5B* and revealed a number of additional variants associated with increased risk of pulmonary fibrosis. These include confirmation of loci close to the *TERT* and *TERC* genes, as well as novel associations such as *FAM13A*, *DSP*, *OBFC1*, *ATP11A*, *DPP9* and chromosomal regions 7q22 and 15q14–15. The GWAS by NOTH *et al.* [86] also identified associations with

Table 2. Genetic biomarkers in IPF

Gene	Chromosome	Protein	Mechanism	[Ref.]
MUC5B	11p15	Mucin 5B	Encodes glycoproteins in airway mucus	[82–85, 87, 88, 90–92]
MUC1	1q21	KL-6	Transmembrane mucin involved in the protection of secretory epithelial cells	[14]
TOLLIP	11p15	Toll-interacting protein	Regulates innate immunity through Toll-like receptors	[86, 97]
TLR3	4q35	Toll-like receptor 3	Regulates innate immunity	[99]
TERT	5p15.33	Telomerase reverse transcriptase	Maintains telomere length	[71, 79, 103]
TERC	3q26	Telomerase RNA component	Maintains telomere length	[103]
SFTPC	8p21	Surfactant protein C	Facilitates surfactant function and transport and innate defence	[76, 129]
SFTPA2	10q22.3	Surfactant protein A	Facilitates surfactant function and transport and innate defence	[78]
ABCA3	16p13.3	ATP-binding cassette member A3	Involved in surfactant production	[130, 131]
ELMOD2	4q31.1	ELMO/CED12 domain-containing protein 2	GTPase-activating protein and antiviral response	[132, 133]
DKC1	Xq28	Dyskerin	Decreases telomerase activity	[71, 134]
DSP	6p24	Desmoplakin	Associated with epithelial cell adhesion and maintenance of its cytoskeleton	[71]
DPP9	19p13	Dipeptidyl peptidase 9	Associated with epithelial cell adhesion and maintenance of its cytoskeleton	[71]
OBFC1	10q24	Oligonucleotide/oligosaccharide-binding fold containing 1	Maintains telomere length	[71]
FAM13A	4q22	Family with sequence similarity 13, member A	IPF susceptibility	[71]
ATP11A	13q34	ATPase, class VI, type 11A	IPF susceptibility	[71]
SPPL2C	17q21	Signal peptide peptidase-like 2C	IPF susceptibility	[86]

additional variants in the *TOLLIP* and signal peptide peptidase-like 2C (*SPPL2C*) genes. Detailing the rare and common gene variants that have been associated with IIPs is outside the scope of this chapter [87], but the genetic polymorphisms with prognostic significance and/or associated with phenotypic differences will be discussed in the following section.

Gene variants with prognostic significance and/or phenotypic differences

MUC5B

As discussed above, the association between the *MUC5B* promoter variant and pulmonary fibrosis is the most consistently reproducible genetic finding in pulmonary fibrosis [71, 83, 86–91]. Interestingly, the *MUC5B* variant is associated with slower progression of IPF once disease severity is taken into account [83] and has been associated with better survival in two separate cohorts of IPF patients, independent of disease severity [92]. The intriguing finding of a gene that is highly associated with the disease but that marks a more benign outcome suggests that different subsets of IPF are identified by this variant [83, 92]. MUC5B is overexpressed in IPF lungs and is seen mainly in terminal bronchioles and areas of microscopic honeycombing in IPF [93]. CONTI *et al.* [94] reported that, on immunohistochemistry, the overexpression of MUC5B was most evident in the distal airways of IPF and was specific to the disease, as it was not observed in patients with idiopathic and systemic sclerosis-associated fibrotic NSIP. Interestingly, NAKANO *et al.* [95] reported in abstract form an association between the *MUC5B* variant and overexpression of MUC5B in the distal airways but not in honeycomb cysts of IPF lungs. Whether distal airway expression levels are linked to survival is not currently known. Interestingly, MOLYNEAUX *et al.* [64] found that the *MUC5B* variant was associated with a lower pulmonary bacterial burden, in turn associated with a better survival. If this finding is replicated, it suggests that the more benign disease course associated with MUC5B could be related to an antimicrobial effect of MUC5B, as this mucin has a protective impact on bacterial-induced infections and inflammation in animal models [96].

TOLLIP

TOLLIP is an innate immunity adapter protein that modulates TLRs, IL-1 and TGF-β signalling through receptor trafficking and degradation. A recent GWAS reported the association of three *TOLLIP* SNPs with pulmonary fibrosis, again implicating innate immunity processes in IPF pathogenesis. Intriguingly, the minor allele rs5743890_G appeared to protect from the development of IPF but was associated with increased mortality [86]. A different SNP, rs3750920, within the *TOLLIP* gene was found to be associated with a differential response to NAC treatment in a retrospective analysis of subjects in the PANTHER-IPF (Prednisone, Azathioprine, and *N*-Acetylcysteine: A Study That Evaluates Response in Idiopathic Pulmonary Fibrosis) trial. While NAC treatment was associated with a significant reduction in a composite endpoint (defined as death, transplant, hospitalisation or ⩾10% FVC decline) in patients with an rs3750920 TT genotype, a trend towards an increase in endpoint risk was seen in patients with a CC genotype [97]. Although retrospective in design, this study is the first to suggest that the response to specific treatments may differ according to genotype in patients with IPF, and strongly supports the need to stratify for known key genetic risk variants in future IPF trials.

TLR3

TLR3 acts as a sensor of tissue necrosis during acute inflammation, recognises virus-associated molecular patterns and activates proinflammatory cascades [98]. Recently, a specific variant in the *TLR3* gene (L412F) was found to be associated with decreased TLR3 activity in primary fibroblasts from IPF patients. Fibroblasts homozygous for the variant allele had an impaired interferon-β response. The variant was associated with early mortality and accelerated lung function decline in IPF [99].

Telomeres

Telomeres are repetitive nucleotide structures that protect chromosome ends from degradation. The telomerase complex is a multiunit enzyme that extends telomere lengths, counteracting the shortening that occurs at each cell division. Once a critical length is reached, cell senescence or apoptosis is triggered. Telomere length shortens progressively with age, and telomere dysfunction may be involved in a number of age-related degenerative disorders [100]. IPF affects older individuals, and telomerase gene variants have been associated with familial and sporadic pulmonary fibrosis. As the telomerase defect affects all tissues, carriers of telomerase mutations can suffer from a number of extrapulmonary manifestations, including bone marrow complications, and skin and haematological malignancies. Of note, special attention to post-transplantation complications is needed in patients with IPF and telomerase mutations, as they can develop a number of complications, most frequently haematological, in response to routinely used immunosuppressive drugs, requiring treatment adjustments and/or transfusion support for significant cytopenias [101].

Interestingly, shorter telomeres are also seen in a proportion of IPF patients, even in the absence of identifiable telomerase variants, and "sporadic" IPF patients can manifest extrapulmonary features of telomere-mediated disease [102]. These findings suggest that telomere defects may play a role in IPF pathogenesis, even outside the setting of telomerase mutations.

Recent data suggest that peripheral blood leukocyte telomere lengths may be a useful prognostic marker. Shorter telomere lengths were associated with worse survival, independent of baseline disease severity, in three separate IPF cohorts from the USA [80] and were replicated in a Chinese cohort of IPF patients [103]. On aggregate, these studies suggest that telomere length could be a useful prognostic indicator and that its measurement should be included in future clinical trials to assess potentially different responses to treatment [80].

Epigenetic biomarkers in IPF

IPF is likely to result from the complex interaction of genes and environmental exposures. Epigenetic processes, defined as relatively stable modifications to gene expression that do not involve changes to the DNA sequence, are influenced by a number of factors, including age, environmental exposures and genetic variants [69]. Global gene expression profiles have consistently shown differential regulation of gene families in IPF lungs, with consistent findings across different studies [104, 105]. Such coordinated changes in gene expression are likely to be regulated by epigenetic processes. Two highly significant risk factors for IPF, age and cigarette smoking, are themselves strongly associated with marked epigenetic changes [106]. Epigenetic processes, including DNA methylation, histone modifications and noncoding RNAs, could represent the link between environmental exposures and genetics in IPF, and could be a source of biomarkers to aid in early diagnosis, prognosis and identification of new treatment targets in IPF. Currently, noncoding RNAs, and specifically miRNAs, are the most promising and easy-to-detect molecules with a near-future perspective as biomarkers in ILD. As such, the following section will focus on noncoding RNAs as potential biomarkers; data on DNA methylation and histone modification in IPF will not be covered in this chapter.

Noncoding RNAs (miRNAs and long noncoding RNAs)

Noncoding RNAs are functional RNA molecules that are not translated into proteins; the two most well-described types are miRNAs and long noncoding RNAs (lncRNAs). Both types are involved in a number of transcriptional and post-transcriptional mechanisms. miRNAs are small single-stranded RNAs of 18–24 nt that negatively regulate gene expression by binding to the 3′-untranslated regions of mRNA, leading to either silencing or degradation of the mRNA. lncRNAs represent noncoding transcripts of more than 200 nt. Diverse functions have been suggested for lncRNAs, including roles in regulating DNA metabolism, chromatin structure and gene expression [107].

miRNAs, released into the extracellular environment mostly as a by-product of cell death, are measurable in significant amounts in body fluids, including plasma and urine [70]. Extracellular miRNAs are potentially excellent biomarkers due to their stability, as the majority are protected from nuclease/protease digestion by forming complexes with argonaute proteins [108]. Published studies on miRNAs are listed in table 3.

In IPF lung tissue, approximately 10% of miRNAs are differentially expressed compared with control lung tissue [109–111]. Consistently downregulated miRNAs in IPF lungs include let-7d, miR-29 and the miR-200 family, while upregulated miRNAs include miR-155, miR-21, miR-199 and miR-154 [104, 105]. OAK et al. [110] identified a panel of miRNAs (miR-302c, miR-423, miR-210, miR-376C and miR-185) in lung biopsies from patients with IPF that could differentiate rapid from slow progressors.

Circulating miRNAs are also differentially expressed in IPF patients, suggesting their potential utility as repeatable/accessible biomarkers. YANG et al. [112] recently described the differential expression of 46 miRNAs in IPF patients compared with controls, with significant enrichment in the Wnt, TGF-β, mitogen-activated protein kinase and phosphatidylinositol 3-kinase–Akt pathways. Selected miRNAs were validated in independent cohorts and appeared to differentiate slow *versus* rapid progressors. Compared with slow progressors, and in turn with controls, rapid progressors displayed higher circulating miR-21, miR-199a-5p and miR-200c, and lower levels of miR-31, let-7a and let-7d.

A number of targeted studies have sought to consider in more detail the role played by miRNAs in IPF. miR-29 and let-7d have so far been the most studied. miR-29 is involved in the regulation of fibroblast activation, and its inhibition has been shown to induce a coordinated increase of ECM genes in fibroblasts. Based on previous observations showing downregulation of miR-29 following bleomycin treatment [113], XIAO et al. [114] demonstrated a beneficial effect of intravenously administered miR-29 in a mouse model of pulmonary fibrosis. Genes regulated by the antifibrotic miR-29 were significantly downregulated in normal fibroblasts following culture with ECM components derived from patients with IPF [115]. Recently, an miR-29 mimic has been suggested as a potential IPF treatment in view of its ability to inhibit fibroblast production of ECM [116].

The miRNA let-7d, which is consistently downregulated in IPF lungs, is believed to play a crucial role in inhibiting epithelial–mesenchymal transdifferentiation. It is inhibited by TGF-β and has a protective role in a murine model of lung fibrosis, through inhibition of SMAD3-dependent epithelial–mesenchymal transition [109]. Inhibition of the let-7d family resulted in upregulation of mesenchymal and downregulation of epithelial markers in alveolar epithelial cell lines [117]. Expression of the miR-17–92 cluster is reduced in lung

Table 3. miRNAs in IPF

miRNA	Tissue	Mechanism	[Ref.]
Downregulated			
miR-29	HLT, HLF, MLF, serum	Regulated by TGF-β–SMAD3–CTGF pathway	[114, 115, 135]
miR let-7a/d	HLT, HLF, MLF, MLT	HMGA2 (fibroblast proliferation/migration, EMT regulation)	[109, 117]
miR-26a	HLT and MLT	CTGF and HMGA2 (fibroblast proliferation/migration, EMT regulation)	
miR-17~92	MLT	DNMT1	[118]
miR-200	HLF, MLT	Not clear	[136]
miR-326	HLT and MLT	TGF-β (fibroblast proliferation)	[137]
Upregulated			
miR-21	HLF and MLF	SMAD7/SMAD2 (fibroblast proliferation)	[110, 138, 139]
miR-154	HLT	P15 and Wnt/β-catenin pathway (fibroblast proliferation/migration)	[111]
miR-145	MLF, MLT	KLF4/α-SMA (fibroblast proliferation/differentiation)	[140]
miR-199a-5p	HLT and MLT	CAV1 (fibroblast proliferation/migration/invasion)	[141]
miR-96	MLT	Fox03a (fibroblast proliferation)	[142]
miR-302c, -423, -210, -376, -185	MLT	EMT-associated genes	[110]
miR-31	HLF, MLF, MLT	Integrin-α/RhoA (fibroblast proliferation)	[136]
miR-375	MLT	Frizzled–Wnt/β-catenin pathway	[143]
lncRNA MRAK088388, lncRNA MRAK081523	MLT	Not clear	[119]

HLT: human lung tissue; HLF: human lung fibroblasts; MLF: mouse lung fibroblasts; CTGF: connective tissue growth factor; MLT: mouse lung tissue; EMT: epithelial–mesenchymal transition; HMGA2: high-mobility group AT-hook 2; DNMT1: DNA methyltransferase 1; α-SMA: alpha smooth muscle actin; CAV1: caveolin 1; lncRNA: long noncoding RNA.

biopsies and in lung fibroblasts from patients with IPF, whereas DNA methyltransferase (DNMT)-1 expression and methylation of the miR-17–92 cluster promoter are increased, thus resulting in a negative-feedback loop. Moreover, treatment with 5′-aza-2′-deoxycytidine in a murine bleomycin-induced pulmonary fibrosis model reduced fibrotic gene and *DNMT-1* expression, enhanced miR-17–92 cluster expression and attenuated pulmonary fibrosis [118].

Only a small number of studies have so far investigated the contribution of lncRNAs in the pathogenesis of lung fibrosis. Distinct lncRNA profiles between normal and fibrotic rat lungs following bleomycin treatment were observed by Cao *et al.* [120]. Two of the most upregulated lncRNAs (AJ005396 and S69206) were localised in the fibrotic interstitium, suggesting their role as potential therapeutic targets [120]. HUANG *et al.* [121] identified two lncRNAs (CD99P1and n341773) that may be involved in the regulation of lung fibroblast proliferation and differentiation.

Circulating and genetic biomarkers in clinical predictor models

The clinical utility of a single predictive biomarker can be limited, while a combination of clinical and molecular markers is more likely to increase the accuracy of outcome prediction. A model including sex, FVC %, D_{LCO} % and serum levels of MMP-7 was strongly predictive of mortality [23]. In a separate IPF cohort, a combination of three serum biomarkers (MMP-7, SP-A and KL-6) with clinical data provided a stronger prediction of outcome than clinical markers alone [17]. The addition of the *MUC5B* promoter genotype (rs35705950) to a model containing clinical parameters and serum MMP-7 levels significantly increased the accuracy of the model [92]. KINDER *et al.* [18] reported a significant improvement in their 1-year mortality predictive model in IPF when serum levels of SP-A and SP-D were added to the clinical predictors. Decreased peripheral blood mononuclear cell (PBMC) expression of genes involved in the "co-stimulatory signal during T-cell activation" (including *CD28*, *ICOS*, *LCK* and *ITK*) was associated with a shorter transplant-free survival. The addition of the gene expression levels of these four genes increased the predictive capacity of a prognostic model compared with one containing solely clinical data (age, sex and FVC %) [30]. A gene set that included downregulation of genes involved in T-cell immune responses was predictive of poor prognosis, even after adjusting for the composite physiologic index [122].

Limits and perspective of biomarker research in IPF

Although recent findings from biomarker research are promising, huge limits remain in their application in clinical practice in IPF. Major discrepancies across different studies arise from collection protocols and matrices (*e.g.* serum, plasma, BALF, lung tissue and PBMCs), as well as from tools applied for validating and refining genomic findings (*e.g.* large-scale exact replication, fine mapping and resequencing, and improved phenotype mapping of the implicated genetic effects) [123, 124]. Many of the published reports are based on single-centre retrospective studies, thus failing to provide data on reliability and reproducibility. Consequently, we do not yet have sufficiently robust evidence to choose the most reliable diagnostic and prognostic biomarkers for IPF.

In the future, introducing biomarker collections in large multicentre cohort clinical trials will allow the collection of more data on reliability/reproducibility of several candidate molecules as well as identification of subgroups of patients with distinct pathogenic profiles [123].

As discussed above and shown by OLDHAM *et al.* [97] in their study on NAC responses and TOLLIP SNPs, identifying genetic variants that correlate with treatment response raises awareness of the urgent need for "targeted therapy" and "personalised medicine" in IPF.

An understanding of which molecular pathways play key roles in individual patients should lead to more precise outcome prediction, timely prevention of complications and delivery of the appropriate treatments, including lung transplantation. In addition to the two recently approved antifibrotic drugs (nintedanib and pirfenidone), several new molecules are likely to become available for IPF treatment in the near future. The ability to predict individual responses to different drugs will shift the focus of IPF management to a much more tailored approach to an individual patient. Biomarkers could represent a strategic tool for optimising the cost/benefit ratio of IPF treatment.

Conclusion

Significant advances in the pathogenesis of IPF have occurred over the last two decades, leading to the identification of a large number of candidate biomarkers. Circulating biomarkers are preferred in routine clinical practice as they are easier to obtain. Of these, KL-6 and MMP-7 are the most studied. Interestingly, it is a genetic variant, the *MUC5B* polymorphism, that appears to be the most powerful prognostic determinant identified so far for IPF, highlighting its potential use for routine clinical practice. Furthermore, a *TOLLIP* variant was the first genetic variant to be recently associated with a differential response to a specific treatment, albeit in a retrospective series. In light of these findings, it will be crucial for future IPF clinical trials to genotype patients for these variants, to assess differential responses to treatment prospectively. In conclusion, IPF is a highly heterogeneous disease with multiple pathobiological pathways. Biomarkers could potentially aid in phenotyping IPF patients in the future and lead to the stratification of IPF patients in terms of molecular pathways, prognosis and response treatment, and therefore to a more targeted approach to IPF management.

References

1. Raghu G, Collard HR, Egan JJ, *et al.* An official ATS/ERS/JRS/ALAT statement: idiopathic pulmonary fibrosis: evidence-based guidelines for diagnosis and management. *Am J Respir Crit Care Med* 2011; 183: 788–824.
2. Selman M, Pardo A. Revealing the pathogenic and aging-related mechanisms of the enigmatic idiopathic pulmonary fibrosis. an integral model. *Am J Respir Crit Care Med* 2014; 189: 1161–1172.
3. Renzoni E, Srihari V, Sestini P. Pathogenesis of idiopathic pulmonary fibrosis: review of recent findings. *F1000Prime Rep* 2014; 6: 69.
4. Raghu G, Rochwerg B, Zhang Y, *et al.* An Official ATS/ERS/JRS/ALAT Clinical Practice Guideline: Treatment of Idiopathic Pulmonary Fibrosis. An Update of the 2011 Clinical Practice Guideline. *Am J Respir Crit Care Med* 2015; 192: e3–e19.
5. Nicholson AG, Addis BJ, Bharucha H, *et al.* Inter-observer variation between pathologists in diffuse parenchymal lung disease. *Thorax* 2004; 59: 500–505.
6. Monaghan H, Wells AU, Colby TV, *et al.* Prognostic implications of histologic patterns in multiple surgical lung biopsies from patients with idiopathic interstitial pneumonias. *Chest* 2004; 125: 522–526.
7. Casoni GL, Tomassetti S, Cavazza A, *et al.* Transbronchial lung cryobiopsy in the diagnosis of fibrotic interstitial lung diseases. *PloS One* 2014; 9: e86716.
8. Hetzel J, Eberhardt R, Herth FJ, *et al.* Cryobiopsy increases the diagnostic yield of endobronchial biopsy: a multicentre trial. *Eur Respir J* 2012; 39: 685–690.
9. Biomarkers Definitions Working Group. Biomarkers and surrogate endpoints: preferred definitions and conceptual framework. *Clin Pharmacol Ther* 2001; 69: 89–95.
10. Prasse A, Muller-Quernheim J. Non-invasive biomarkers in pulmonary fibrosis. *Respirology* 2009; 14: 788–795.
11. Ohshimo S, Yokoyama A, Hattori N, *et al.* KL-6, a human MUC1 mucin, promotes proliferation and survival of lung fibroblasts. *Biochem Biophys Res Commun* 2005; 338: 1845–1852.
12. Ishikawa N, Hattori N, Yokoyama A, *et al.* Utility of KL-6/MUC1 in the clinical management of interstitial lung diseases. *Respir Investig* 2012; 50: 3–13.
13. Satoh H, Kurishima K, Ishikawa H, *et al.* Increased levels of KL-6 and subsequent mortality in patients with interstitial lung diseases. *J Intern Med* 2006; 260: 429–434.
14. Horimasu Y, Hattori N, Ishikawa N, *et al.* Different *MUC1* gene polymorphisms in German and Japanese ethnicities affect serum KL-6 levels. *Respir Med* 2012; 106: 1756–1764.
15. Janssen R, Kruit A, Grutters JC, *et al.* The mucin-1 568 adenosine to guanine polymorphism influences serum Krebs von den Lungen-6 levels. *Am J Respir Cell Mol Biol* 2006; 34: 496–499.
16. Tanjore H, Blackwell TS, Lawson WE. Emerging evidence for endoplasmic reticulum stress in the pathogenesis of idiopathic pulmonary fibrosis. *Am J Physiol Lung Cell Mol Physiol* 2012; 302: L721–L729.

17. Song JW, Do KH, Jang SJ, *et al.* Blood biomarkers MMP-7 and SP-A: predictors of outcome in idiopathic pulmonary fibrosis. *Chest* 2013; 143: 1422–1429.

18. Kinder BW, Brown KK, McCormack FX, *et al.* Serum surfactant protein-A is a strong predictor of early mortality in idiopathic pulmonary fibrosis. *Chest* 2009; 135: 1557–1563.

19. Horimasu Y, Hattori N, Ishikawa N, *et al.* Differences in serum SP-D levels between German and Japanese subjects are associated with *SFTPD* gene polymorphisms. *BMC Med Genet* 2014; 15: 4.

20. Cha SI, Ryerson CJ, Lee JS, *et al.* Cleaved cytokeratin-18 is a mechanistically informative biomarker in idiopathic pulmonary fibrosis. *Respir Res* 2012; 13: 105.

21. Prasse A, Pechkovsky DV, Toews GB, *et al.* CCL18 as an indicator of pulmonary fibrotic activity in idiopathic interstitial pneumonias and systemic sclerosis. *Arthritis Rheum* 2007; 56: 1685–1693.

22. Prasse A, Probst C, Bargagli E, *et al.* Serum CC-chemokine ligand 18 concentration predicts outcome in idiopathic pulmonary fibrosis. *Am J Respir Crit Care Med* 2009; 179: 717–723.

23. Richards TJ, Kaminski N, Baribaud F, *et al.* Peripheral blood proteins predict mortality in idiopathic pulmonary fibrosis. *Am J Respir Crit Care Med* 2012; 185: 67–76.

24. Furuhashi K, Suda T, Nakamura Y, *et al.* Increased expression of YKL-40, a chitinase-like protein, in serum and lung of patients with idiopathic pulmonary fibrosis. *Respir Med* 2010; 104: 1204–1210.

25. Korthagen NM, van Moorsel CH, Barlo NP, *et al.* Serum and BALF YKL-40 levels are predictors of survival in idiopathic pulmonary fibrosis. *Respir Med* 2011; 105: 106–113.

26. Vuga LJ, Tedrow JR, Pandit KV, *et al.* C-X-C motif chemokine 13 (CXCL13) is a prognostic biomarker of idiopathic pulmonary fibrosis. *Am J Respir Crit Care Med* 2014; 189: 966–974.

27. DePianto DJ, Chandriani S, Abbas AR, *et al.* Heterogeneous gene expression signatures correspond to distinct lung pathologies and biomarkers of disease severity in idiopathic pulmonary fibrosis. *Thorax* 2015; 70: 48–56.

28. Kahloon RA, Xue J, Bhargava A, *et al.* Patients with idiopathic pulmonary fibrosis with antibodies to heat shock protein 70 have poor prognoses. *Am J Respir Crit Care Med* 2013; 187: 768–775.

29. Moeller A, Gilpin SE, Ask K, *et al.* Circulating fibrocytes are an indicator of poor prognosis in idiopathic pulmonary fibrosis. *Am J Respir Crit Care Med* 2009; 179: 588–594.

30. Herazo-Maya JD, Noth I, Duncan SR, *et al.* Peripheral blood mononuclear cell gene expression profiles predict poor outcome in idiopathic pulmonary fibrosis. *Sci Transl Med* 2013; 5: 205ra136.

31. Kotsianidis I, Nakou E, Bouchliou I, *et al.* Global impairment of $CD4^+CD25^+FOXP3^+$ regulatory T cells in idiopathic pulmonary fibrosis. *Am J Respir Crit Care Med* 2009; 179: 1121–1130.

32. Reilkoff RA, Peng H, Murray LA, *et al.* Semaphorin $7a^+$ regulatory T cells are associated with progressive idiopathic pulmonary fibrosis and are implicated in transforming growth factor-β1-induced pulmonary fibrosis. *Am J Respir Crit Care Med* 2013; 187: 180–188.

33. Belperio JA, Dy M, Burdick MD, *et al.* Interaction of IL-13 and C10 in the pathogenesis of bleomycin-induced pulmonary fibrosis. *Am J Respir Cell Mol Biol* 2002; 27: 419–427.

34. Homolka J, Ziegenhagen MW, Gaede KI, *et al.* Systemic immune cell activation in a subgroup of patients with idiopathic pulmonary fibrosis. *Respiration* 2003; 70: 262–269.

35. De Lauretis A, Sestini P, Pantelidis P, *et al.* Serum interleukin 6 is predictive of early functional decline and mortality in interstitial lung disease associated with systemic sclerosis. *J Rheumatol* 2013; 40: 435–446.

36. Mukae H, Iiboshi H, Nakazato M, *et al.* Raised plasma concentrations of α-defensins in patients with idiopathic pulmonary fibrosis. *Thorax* 2002; 57: 623–628.

37. Yang IV, Luna LG, Cotter J, *et al.* The peripheral blood transcriptome identifies the presence and extent of disease in idiopathic pulmonary fibrosis. *PLoS One* 2012; 7: e37708.

38. Zuo F, Kaminski N, Eugui E, *et al.* Gene expression analysis reveals matrilysin as a key regulator of pulmonary fibrosis in mice and humans. *Proc Natl Acad Sci U S A* 2002; 99: 6292–6297.

39. Rosas IO, Richards TJ, Konishi K, *et al.* MMP1 and MMP7 as potential peripheral blood biomarkers in idiopathic pulmonary fibrosis. *PLoS Med* 2008; 5: e93.

40. Jenkins RG, Simpson JK, Saini G, *et al.* Longitudinal change in collagen degradation biomarkers in idiopathic pulmonary fibrosis: an analysis from the prospective, multicentre PROFILE study. *Lancet Respir Med* 2015; 3: 462–472.

41. Chien JW, Richards TJ, Gibson KF, *et al.* Serum lysyl oxidase-like 2 levels and idiopathic pulmonary fibrosis disease progression. *Eur Respir J* 2014; 43: 1430–1438.

42. Naik PK, Bozyk PD, Bentley JK, *et al.* Periostin promotes fibrosis and predicts progression in patients with idiopathic pulmonary fibrosis. *Am J Physiol Lung Cell Mol Physiol* 2012; 303: L1046–L1056.

43. Okamoto M, Hoshino T, Kitasato Y, *et al.* Periostin, a matrix protein, is a novel biomarker for idiopathic interstitial pneumonias. *Eur Respir J* 2011; 37: 1119–1127.

44. Tajiri M, Okamoto M, Fujimoto K, *et al.* Serum level of periostin can predict long-term outcome of idiopathic pulmonary fibrosis. *Respir Investig* 2015; 53: 73–81.

45. Collard HR, Calfee CS, Wolters PJ, *et al.* Plasma biomarker profiles in acute exacerbation of idiopathic pulmonary fibrosis. *Am J Physiol Lung Cell Mol Physiol* 2010; 299: L3–L7.

46. Kakugawa T, Yokota S, Ishimatsu Y, *et al.* Serum heat shock protein 47 levels are elevated in acute exacerbation of idiopathic pulmonary fibrosis. *Cell Stress Chaperones* 2013; 18: 581–590.

47. Ohshimo S, Ishikawa N, Horimasu Y, *et al.* Baseline KL-6 predicts increased risk for acute exacerbation of idiopathic pulmonary fibrosis. *Respir Med* 2014; 108: 1031–1039.

48. Konishi K, Gibson KF, Lindell KO, *et al.* Gene expression profiles of acute exacerbations of idiopathic pulmonary fibrosis. *Am J Respir Crit Care Med* 2009; 180: 167–175.

49. Bonella F, Ohshimo S, Bauer P, *et al.* Bronchoalveolar lavage. *In*: Strausz J, Bolliger CT, eds. Interventional Pulmonology (ERS Monograph). Sheffield, European Respiratory Society, 2010; pp. 59–72.

50. Campo I, Zorzetto M, Bonella F. Facts and promises on lung biomarkers in interstitial lung diseases. *Expert Rev Respir Med* 2015: 1–21.

51. Kohno N, Awaya Y, Oyama T, *et al.* KL-6, a mucin-like glycoprotein, in bronchoalveolar lavage fluid from patients with interstitial lung disease. *Am Rev Respir Dis* 1993; 148: 637–642.

52. Kinder BW, Brown KK, Schwarz MI, *et al.* Baseline BAL neutrophilia predicts early mortality in idiopathic pulmonary fibrosis. *Chest* 2008; 133: 226–232.

53. Veeraraghavan S, Latsi PI, Wells AU, *et al.* BAL findings in idiopathic nonspecific interstitial pneumonia and usual interstitial pneumonia. *Eur Respir J* 2003; 22: 239–244.

54. Borie R, Quesnel C, Phin S, *et al.* Detection of alveolar fibrocytes in idiopathic pulmonary fibrosis and systemic sclerosis. *PLoS One* 2013; 8: e53736.

55. De Lauretis A, Renzoni EA. Molecular biomarkers in interstitial lung diseases. *Mol Diagn Ther* 2014; 18: 505–522.

56. McCormack FX, King TE Jr, Bucher BL, *et al.* Surfactant protein A predicts survival in idiopathic pulmonary fibrosis. *Am J Respir Crit Care Med* 1995; 152: 751–759.

57. Cai M, Bonella F, He X, *et al.* CCL18 in serum, BAL fluid and alveolar macrophage culture supernatant in interstitial lung diseases. *Respir Med* 2013; 107: 1444–1452.

58. Huh JW, Kim DS, Oh YM, *et al.* Is metalloproteinase-7 specific for idiopathic pulmonary fibrosis? *Chest* 2008; 133: 1101–1106.

59. Willems S, Verleden SE, Vanaudenaerde BM, *et al.* Multiplex protein profiling of bronchoalveolar lavage in idiopathic pulmonary fibrosis and hypersensitivity pneumonitis. *Ann Thorac Med* 2013; 8: 38–45.

60. Magi B, Bargagli E, Bini L, *et al.* Proteome analysis of bronchoalveolar lavage in lung diseases. *Proteomics* 2006; 6: 6354–6369.

61. Landi C, Bargagli E, Magi B, *et al.* Proteome analysis of bronchoalveolar lavage in pulmonary Langerhans cell histiocytosis. *J Clin Bioinforma* 2011; 1: 31.

62. Landi C, Bargagli E, Carleo A, *et al.* A system biology study of BALF from patients affected by idiopathic pulmonary fibrosis (IPF) and healthy controls. *Proteomics Clin Appl* 2014; 8: 932–950.

63. Rottoli P, Magi B, Perari MG, *et al.* Cytokine profile and proteome analysis in bronchoalveolar lavage of patients with sarcoidosis, pulmonary fibrosis associated with systemic sclerosis and idiopathic pulmonary fibrosis. *Proteomics* 2005; 5: 1423–1430.

64. Molyneaux PL, Cox MJ, Willis-Owen SA, *et al.* The role of bacteria in the pathogenesis and progression of idiopathic pulmonary fibrosis. *Am J Respir Crit Care Med* 2014; 190: 906–913.

65. Han MK, Zhou Y, Murray S, *et al.* Lung microbiome and disease progression in idiopathic pulmonary fibrosis: an analysis of the COMET study. *Lancet Respir Med* 2014; 2: 548–556.

66. Javaheri S, Lederer DH, Pella JA, *et al.* Idiopathic pulmonary fibrosis in monozygotic twins. The importance of genetic predisposition. *Chest* 1980; 78: 591–594.

67. Bonanni PP, Frymoyer JW, Jacox RF. A family study of idiopathic pulmonary fibrosis. A possible dysproteinemic and genetically determined disease. *Am J Med* 1965; 39: 411–421.

68. Solliday NH, Williams JA, Gaensler EA, *et al.* Familial chronic interstitial pneumonia. *Am Rev Respir Dis* 1973; 108: 193–204.

69. Bitterman PB, Rennard SI, Keogh BA, *et al.* Familial idiopathic pulmonary fibrosis. Evidence of lung inflammation in unaffected family members. *N Engl J Med* 1986; 314: 1343–1347.

70. Mathai SK, Schwartz DA, Warg LA. Genetic susceptibility and pulmonary fibrosis. *Curr Opin Pulm Med* 2014; 20: 429–435.

71. Fingerlin TE, Murphy E, Zhang W, *et al.* Genome-wide association study identifies multiple susceptibility loci for pulmonary fibrosis. *Nat Genet* 2013; 45: 613–620.

72. Lee HL, Ryu JH, Wittmer MH, *et al.* Familial idiopathic pulmonary fibrosis: clinical features and outcome. *Chest* 2005; 127: 2034–2041.

73. Lee HY, Seo JB, Steele MP, *et al.* High-resolution CT scan findings in familial interstitial pneumonia do not conform to those of idiopathic interstitial pneumonia. *Chest* 2012; 142: 1577–1583.

74. Kropski JA, Blackwell TS, Loyd JE. The genetic basis of idiopathic pulmonary fibrosis. *Eur Respir J* 2015; 45: 1717–1727.

75. Borie R, Kannengiesser C, Nathan N, *et al.* Familial pulmonary fibrosis. *Rev Mal Respir* 2015; 32: 413–434.

76. Thomas AQ, Lane K, Phillips J III, *et al.* Heterozygosity for a surfactant protein C gene mutation associated with usual interstitial pneumonitis and cellular nonspecific interstitial pneumonitis in one kindred. *Am J Respir Crit Care Med* 2002; 165: 1322–1328.

77. Lawson WE, Loyd JE, Degryse AL. Genetics in pulmonary fibrosis – familial cases provide clues to the pathogenesis of idiopathic pulmonary fibrosis. *Am J Med Sci* 2011; 341: 439–443.

78. Wang Y, Kuan PJ, Xing C, *et al.* Genetic defects in surfactant protein A2 are associated with pulmonary fibrosis and lung cancer. *Am J Hum Genet* 2009; 84: 52–59.

79. Diaz de Leon A, Cronkhite JT, Katzenstein AL, *et al.* Telomere lengths, pulmonary fibrosis and telomerase (*TERT*) mutations. *PloS One* 2010; 5: e10680.

80. Stuart BD, Lee JS, Kozlitina J, *et al.* Effect of telomere length on survival in patients with idiopathic pulmonary fibrosis: an observational cohort study with independent validation. *Lancet Respir Med* 2014; 2: 557–565.

81. Tsakiri KD, Cronkhite JT, Kuan PJ, *et al.* Adult-onset pulmonary fibrosis caused by mutations in telomerase. *Proc Natl Acad Sci U S A* 2007; 104: 7552–7557.

82. Seibold MA, Wise AL, Speer MC, *et al.* A common *MUC5B* promoter polymorphism and pulmonary fibrosis. *N Engl J Med* 2011; 364: 1503–1512.

83. Stock CJ, Sato H, Fonseca C, *et al.* Mucin 5B promoter polymorphism is associated with idiopathic pulmonary fibrosis but not with development of lung fibrosis in systemic sclerosis or sarcoidosis. *Thorax* 2013; 68: 436–441.

84. Borie R, Crestani B, Dieude P, *et al.* The *MUC5B* variant is associated with idiopathic pulmonary fibrosis but not with systemic sclerosis interstitial lung disease in the European Caucasian population. *PloS One* 2013; 8: e70621.

85. Hunninghake GM, Hatabu H, Okajima Y, *et al.* MUC5B promoter polymorphism and interstitial lung abnormalities. *N Engl J Med* 2013; 368: 2192–2200.

86. Noth I, Zhang Y, Ma SF, *et al.* Genetic variants associated with idiopathic pulmonary fibrosis susceptibility and mortality: a genome-wide association study. *Lancet Respir Med* 2013; 1: 309–317.

87. Zhang GY, Liao T, Gao WY. *MUC5B* promoter polymorphism and pulmonary fibrosis. *N Engl J Med* 2011; 365: 178.

88. Zhang Y, Noth I, Garcia JG, *et al.* A variant in the promoter of *MUC5B* and idiopathic pulmonary fibrosis. *N Engl J Med* 2011; 364: 1576–1577.

89. Peljto AL, Selman M, Kim DS, *et al.* The *MUC5B* promoter polymorphism is associated with idiopathic pulmonary fibrosis in a Mexican cohort but is rare among Asian ancestries. *Chest* 2015; 147: 460–464.

90. Horimasu Y, Ohshimo S, Bonella F, *et al.* *MUC5B* promoter polymorphism in Japanese patients with idiopathic pulmonary fibrosis. *Respirology* 2015; 20: 439–444.

91. Wei R, Li C, Zhang M, *et al.* Association between *MUC5B* and *TERT* polymorphisms and different interstitial lung disease phenotypes. *Transl Res* 2014; 163: 494–502.

92. Peljto AL, Zhang Y, Fingerlin TE, *et al.* Association between the *MUC5B* promoter polymorphism and survival in patients with idiopathic pulmonary fibrosis. *JAMA* 2013; 309: 2232–2239.

93. Seibold MA, Smith RW, Urbanek C, *et al.* The idiopathic pulmonary fibrosis honeycomb cyst contains a mucocilary pseudostratified epithelium. *PloS One* 2013; 8: e58658.

94. Conti CM-FA, Nicholson AG, Osadolor T, *et al.* Distribution of mucins MUC5B and MUC5AC in distal airways and honeycomb spaces: a comparison between UIP and other ILD patterns. *Am J Respir Crit Care Med* 2015; 191: A2161.

95. Nakano Y, Evans CM, Yang MI, *et al.* *MUC5B* promoter variant rs35705950 affects *MUC5B* expression and this effect is localized to the distal airways in IPF. *Am J Respir Crit Care Med* 2015; 191: A3446.

96. Roy MG, Livraghi-Butrico A, Fletcher AA, *et al.* Muc5b is required for airway defence. *Nature* 2014; 505: 412–416.

97. Oldham JM, Ma SF, Martinez FJ, *et al.* TOLLIP, MUC5B and the response to N-acetylcysteine among individuals with idiopathic pulmonary fibrosis. *Am J Respir Crit Care Med* 2015; 192: 1475–1482.

98. Kawai T, Akira S. The role of pattern-recognition receptors in innate immunity: update on Toll-like receptors. *Nat Immunol* 2010; 11: 373–384.

99. O'Dwyer DN, Armstrong ME, Trujillo G, *et al.* The Toll-like receptor 3 L412F polymorphism and disease progression in idiopathic pulmonary fibrosis. *Am J Respir Crit Care Med* 2013; 188: 1442–1450.

100. Armanios M, Blackburn EH. The telomere syndromes. *Nat Rev Genet* 2012; 13: 693–704.

101. Silhan LL, Shah PD, Chambers DC, *et al.* Lung transplantation in telomerase mutation carriers with pulmonary fibrosis. *Eur Respir J* 2014; 44: 178–187.

102. Alder JK, Chen JJ, Lancaster L, *et al.* Short telomeres are a risk factor for idiopathic pulmonary fibrosis. *Proc Natl Acad Sci U S A* 2008; 105: 13051–13056.

103. Dai J, Cai H, Li H, *et al.* Association between telomere length and survival in patients with idiopathic pulmonary fibrosis. *Respirology* 2015; 20: 947–952.

104. Yang IV, Schwartz DA. Epigenetics of idiopathic pulmonary fibrosis. *Transl Res* 2015; 165: 48–60.

105. Tzouvelekis A, Kaminski N. Epigenetics in idiopathic pulmonary fibrosis. *Biochem Cell Biol* 2015; 93: 159–170.

106. Yang IV. Epigenomics of idiopathic pulmonary fibrosis. *Epigenomics* 2012; 4: 195–203.

107. Yang IV, Schwartz DA. Epigenetic control of gene expression in the lung. *Am J Respir Crit Care Med* 2011; 183: 1295–1301.

108. Turchinovich A, Weiz L, Langheinz A, *et al.* Characterization of extracellular circulating microRNA. *Nucleic Acids Res* 2011; 39: 7223–7233.

109. Pandit KV, Corcoran D, Yousef H, *et al.* Inhibition and role of let-7d in idiopathic pulmonary fibrosis. *Am J Respir Crit Care Med* 2010; 182: 220–229.

110. Oak SR, Murray L, Herath A, *et al.* A micro RNA processing defect in rapidly progressing idiopathic pulmonary fibrosis. *PloS One* 2011; 6: e21253.

111. Milosevic J, Pandit K, Magister M, *et al.* Profibrotic role of miR-154 in pulmonary fibrosis. *Am J Respir Cell Mol Biol* 2012; 47: 879–887.

112. Yang G, Yang L, Wang W, *et al.* Discovery and validation of extracellular/circulating microRNAs during idiopathic pulmonary fibrosis disease progression. *Gene* 2015; 562: 138–144.

113. Cushing L, Kuang PP, Qian J, *et al.* miR-29 is a major regulator of genes associated with pulmonary fibrosis. *Am J Respir Cell Mol Biol* 2011; 45: 287–294.

114. Xiao J, Meng XM, Huang XR, *et al.* miR-29 inhibits bleomycin-induced pulmonary fibrosis in mice. *Mol Ther* 2012; 20: 1251–1260.

115. Parker MW, Rossi D, Peterson M, *et al.* Fibrotic extracellular matrix activates a profibrotic positive feedback loop. *J Clin Invest* 2014; 124: 1622–1635.

116. Montgomery RL, Yu G, Latimer PA, *et al.* MicroRNA mimicry blocks pulmonary fibrosis. *EMBO Mol Med* 2014; 6: 1347–1356.

117. Huleihel L, Ben-Yehudah A, Milosevic J, *et al.* Let-7d microRNA affects mesenchymal phenotypic properties of lung fibroblasts. *Am J Physiol Lung Cell Mol Physiol* 2014; 306: L534–L542.

118. Dakhlallah D, Batte K, Wang Y, *et al.* Epigenetic regulation of miR-17~92 contributes to the pathogenesis of pulmonary fibrosis. *Am J Respir Crit Care Med* 2013; 187: 397–405.

119. Song X, Cao G, Jing L, *et al.* Analysing the relationship between lncRNA and protein-coding gene and the role of lncRNA as ceRNA in pulmonary fibrosis. *J Cell Mol Med* 2014; 18: 991–1003.

120. Cao G, Zhang J, Wang M, *et al.* Differential expression of long non-coding RNAs in bleomycin-induced lung fibrosis. *Int J Mol Med* 2013; 32: 355–364.

121. Huang C, Yang Y, Liu L. Interaction of long non-coding RNAs and microRNAs in the pathogenesis of idiopathic pulmonary fibrosis. *Physiol Genomics* 2015; 47: 463–469.

122. Huang Y, Ma SF, Vij R, *et al.* A functional genomic model for predicting prognosis in idiopathic pulmonary fibrosis. *BMC Pulm Med* 2015; 15: 147.

123. Spagnolo P, Tzouvelekis A, Maher TM. Personalized medicine in idiopathic pulmonary fibrosis: facts and promises. *Curr Opin Pulm Med* 2015; 21: 470–478.

124. Ioannidis JP, Thomas G, Daly MJ. Validating, augmenting and refining genome-wide association signals. *Nat Rev Genet* 2009; 10: 318–329.

125. Takahashi F, Takahashi K, Okazaki T, *et al.* Role of osteopontin in the pathogenesis of bleomycin-induced pulmonary fibrosis. *Am J Respir Cell Mol Biol* 2001; 24: 264–271.

126. Pardo A, Gibson K, Cisneros J, *et al.* Up-regulation and profibrotic role of osteopontin in human idiopathic pulmonary fibrosis. *PLoS Med* 2005; 2: e251.

127. Agnihotri R, Crawford HC, Haro H, *et al.* Osteopontin, a novel substrate for matrix metalloproteinase-3 (stromelysin-1) and matrix metalloproteinase-7 (matrilysin). *J Biol Chem* 2001; 276: 28261–28267.

128. Kadota J, Mizunoe S, Mito K, *et al.* High plasma concentrations of osteopontin in patients with interstitial pneumonia. *Respir Med* 2005; 99: 111–117.

129. Lawson WE, Grant SW, Ambrosini V, *et al.* Genetic mutations in surfactant protein C are a rare cause of sporadic cases of IPF. *Thorax* 2004; 59: 977–980.

130. Young LR, Nogee LM, Barnett B, *et al.* Usual interstitial pneumonia in an adolescent with *ABCA3* mutations. *Chest* 2008; 134: 192–195.

131. Campo I, Zorzetto M, Mariani F, *et al.* A large kindred of pulmonary fibrosis associated with a novel *ABCA3* gene variant. *Respir Res* 2014; 15: 43.

132. Hodgson U, Pulkkinen V, Dixon M, *et al.* ELMOD2 is a candidate gene for familial idiopathic pulmonary fibrosis. *Am J Hum Genet* 2006; 79: 149–154.

133. Pulkkinen V, Bruce S, Rintahaka J, *et al.* ELMOD2, a candidate gene for idiopathic pulmonary fibrosis, regulates antiviral responses. *FASEB J* 2010; 24: 1167–1177.

134. Kropski JA, Mitchell DB, Markin C, *et al.* A novel dyskerin (*DKC1*) mutation is associated with familial interstitial pneumonia. *Chest* 2014; 146: e1–e7.

135. Cushing L, Kuang P, Lu J. The role of miR-29 in pulmonary fibrosis. *Biochem Cell Biol* 2015; 93: 109–118.

136. Yang S, Banerjee S, de Freitas A, *et al.* Participation of miR-200 in pulmonary fibrosis. *Am J Pathol* 2012; 180: 484–493.

137. Das S, Kumar M, Negi V, *et al.* MicroRNA-326 regulates profibrotic functions of transforming growth factor-β in pulmonary fibrosis. *Am J Respir Cell Mol Biol* 2014; 50: 882–892.

138. Liu G, Friggeri A, Yang Y, *et al.* miR-21 mediates fibrogenic activation of pulmonary fibroblasts and lung fibrosis. *J Exp Med* 2010; 207: 1589–1597.

139. Yamada M, Kubo H, Ota C, *et al.* The increase of microRNA-21 during lung fibrosis and its contribution to epithelial-mesenchymal transition in pulmonary epithelial cells. *Respir Res* 2013; 14: 95.

140. Yang S, Cui H, Xie N, *et al.* miR-145 regulates myofibroblast differentiation and lung fibrosis. *FASEB J* 2013; 27: 2382–2391.

141. Lino Cardenas CL, Henaoui IS, Courcot E, *et al.* miR-199a-5p is upregulated during fibrogenic response to tissue injury and mediates TGFβ-induced lung fibroblast activation by targeting caveolin-1. *PLoS Genet* 2013; 9: e1003291.

142. Nho RS, Im J, Ho YY, *et al.* MicroRNA-96 inhibits FoxO3a function in IPF fibroblasts on type I collagen matrix. *Am J Physiol Lung Cell Mol Physiol* 2014; 307: L632–L642.

143. Wang Y, Huang C, Reddy Chintagari N, *et al.* miR-375 regulates rat alveolar epithelial cell trans-differentiation by inhibiting Wnt/β-catenin pathway. *Nucleic Acids Res* 2013; 41: 3833–3844.

Disclosures: None declared.

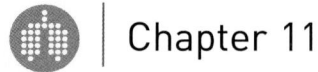
Acute exacerbations

Antje Prasse

This chapter summarises recent advances regarding definition, clinical features, underlying mechanisms, and management of acute exacerbation of IPF. Whilst recent studies suggest risk modulation for acute exacerbations may become feasible with treatment, shortcomings in the current definition and a need for standardised diagnostic algorithms have become apparent.

IPF is a heterogeneous disease with different courses. Median survival remains poor at 3 years, with acute exacerbation being a leading cause of mortality [1–3]. 2007, a perspective paper was published in the *American Journal of Respiratory and Critical Care Medicine* by a group of authors endorsed by the Idiopathic Pulmonary Fibrosis Clinical Research Network, which defined consensus criteria for acute exacerbation of IPF as any acute worsening in respiratory symptoms within 30 days accompanying new opacities on HRCT (figure 1) in the absence of other identifiable causes [4]. Typical clinical features include acute increase in dyspnoea, worsening cough, fatigue and occasionally sub-febrile temperatures or fever. Current Japanese criteria for acute exacerbation include the additional criterion of a decrease of arterial oxygen tension by more than 10 Torr [5].

Given its nature, the consensus definition of 2007 requires active exclusion of alternative causes, such as acute infection, pneumothorax, pulmonary embolism and congestive heart failure [4]. The basis for this recommendation stems from the assumption that decompensation resulting from such identifiable causes may be pathobiologically different. In practice however, implementing this approach has proved difficult, with some of the underlying assumptions being called into question. Distinguishing between an acute infection and changes in microbiome, for example, can prove extremely challenging, whilst having limited implications for treatment [6–8]. Compounding these difficulties, no recommendations exist regarding how rigorous physicians should be, in assessing for identifiable causes. Currently, there is no standardised diagnostic work-up for IPF acute exacerbations worldwide. BAL for example, is an accepted gold standard for detecting infectious diseases, particularly viral infections. However, currently the majority of IPF specialists fear further acceleration of acute exacerbation as a consequence of the manoeuvre [7], with many considering bronchoscopy as being more harmful to patients than the potential benefit of changing treatment. Furthermore, advances in viral detection

Dept of Respiratory Medicine, Hanover Medical School, Hanover, Germany. Fraunhofer Institute ITEM, Hanover, Germany. Biomedical Research in End-Stage and Obstructive Lung Disease (BREATH), German Centre for Lung Research (DZL), Hanover, Germany.

Correspondence: Antje Prasse, Dept of Respiratory Medicine, Hanover Medical School, Carl-Neuberg-Strasse 1, 30625 Hanover, Germany. E-mail: prasse.antje@mh-hannover.de

Copyright ©ERS 2016. Print ISBN: 978-1-84984-067-5. Online ISBN: 978-1-84984-068-2. Print ISSN: 2312-508X. Online ISSN: 2312-5098.

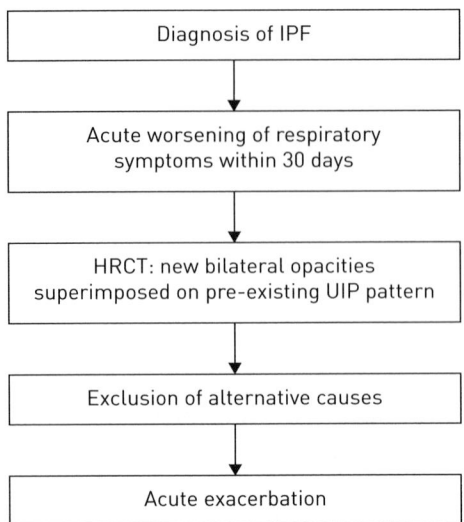

Figure 1. Diagnostic algorithm for acute exacerbation of IPF based on the criteria defined by the perspective paper in 2007 [4]. Data from [4].

techniques increasingly result in positive BAL findings that remain of unclear clinical significance for IPF patients [9].

Given these inherent limitations, reappraisal of available data has suggested broadening the existing definition to include any acute worsening of dyspnoea within 30 days after excluding non-pulmonary causes, such as heart failure [10, 11]. COLLARD *et al.* [12] retrospectively analysed the data of the STEP trial, which tested originally the effect of sildenafil, using different sets of criteria defining acute exacerbation. Suspected acute exacerbation was defined as an idiopathic acute respiratory worsening that could not be classified as a definite acute exacerbation due to missing data or criteria. The authors found no clinical differences between suspected and definite acute exacerbations. The broadening of the existing definition of acute exacerbation would allow its easier implementation as a useable endpoint in clinical trials, but may come with less precision. The existence of this debate reflects again the variable nature of IPF acute exacerbations and the inevitable challenge of assigning a suitable definition. The aim of simplifying the definition remains better standardisation of cohorts between centres, improving comparability of outcomes [13].

Incidence and outcome

Given this variable interpretation of the current, the true incidence of IPF acute exacerbation remains unclear. Considerable variations in incidence between centres have been reported, most likely reflecting both regional differences and local appraisal of the recommendations [14]. Rough estimates suggest a yearly incidence approximating 5–10% [3, 14, 15]. The incidence of acute exacerbations appears higher in winter and among patients receiving corticosteroids or other immunosuppressants. Retrospective studies in Asian cohorts suggested a possibly higher incidence of acute exacerbation compared with non-Asian patients, but a recent global clinical trial did not show any difference [2, 3, 9, 14–16]. Risk appears higher in patients with severe disease, with particularly poor outcomes among ventilated patients [17–23]. Reported outcomes also vary, with median survival of approximately 3 months [16, 24, 25].

HRCT in acute exacerbation of IPF

Current diagnostic criteria for HRCT require the presence of new bilateral opacities superimposed on pre-existing UIP patterns (figure 2) in an acute exacerbation [3, 4]. Such patients usually present with predominately ground glass lesions, some with additional minor consolidations [24, 26, 27]. There is an HRCT-based score available predictive of mortality in IPF patients presenting with acute exacerbation [27].

Histology of acute exacerbation of IPF and parallels to acute respiratory distress syndrome

Autopsy studies and lung biopsies taken during acute exacerbations typically reveal acute lung injury (*e.g.* diffuse alveolar damage) including the presence of hyaline membranes, ruptured basement membranes and loss of alveolar epithelial as well as endothelial cells [21–23, 28]. In contrast to stable IPF, not only the alveolar epithelium but also the endothelium and basement membrane are commonly injured [23]. Another hallmark is the influx of neutrophils and macrophages. All these findings are very similar to those

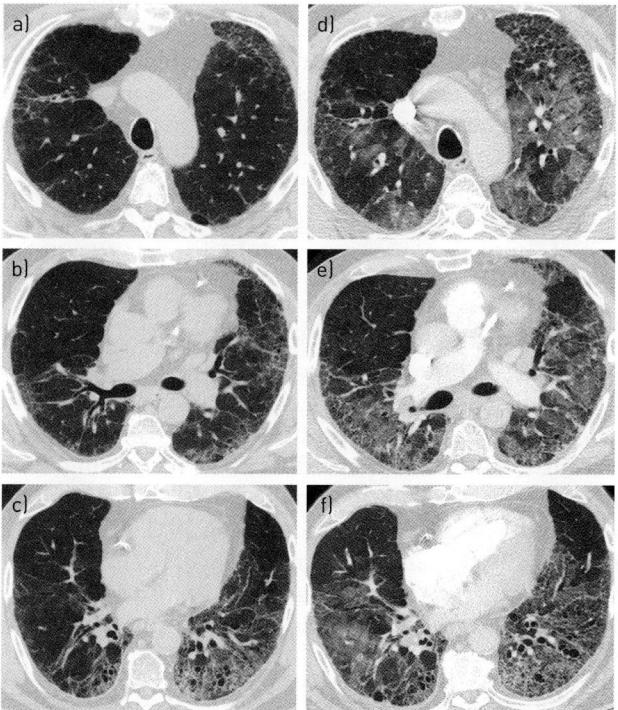

Figure 2. HRCT of a patient with IPF a–c) 3 months prior to acute exacerbation and d–f) at the time of acute exacerbation. At the time of acute exacerbation, there were new, bilateral ground-glass lesions superimposed on the pre-existing possible UIP pattern. The patient was diagnosed 3 years earlier including a video-assisted thoracoscopic surgery-derived biopsy showing definite UIP and was treated with pirfenidone. The patient died 16 h after the HRCT was performed.

described in acute respiratory distress syndrome (ARDS) [29]. A recent autopsy study has also reported that one-third of patients had signs of alveolar haemorrhage, not related to anticoagulation [30]. Furthermore, several studies have shown that a minority of cases also exhibit other histopathological patterns such as organising pneumonia [23, 30]. It was recently proposed to limit the term IPF acute exacerbation to patients with signs of diffuse acute damage only [10]. Although the presence of hyaline membranes and signs of acute lung injury represent indisputable evidence of diffuse alveolar damage and acute exacerbation of IPF, it is not recommended to perform lung biopsies during suspected acute exacerbation because of the instability of patients and the high mortality [31].

BAL findings in acute exacerbation

As part of the current diagnostic work–up for acute exacerbations, only a few centres support performing a BAL. Previously, in the era of immunosuppressive triple therapy, the incidence of infectious diseases was considered high and BAL was necessary to exclude opportunistic infections, such as *Pneumocystis jirovecii*, viruses or fungi [4, 9]. Differential cell counts during acute exacerbation of IPF often show an increased neutrophilia and hyperplastic type II cells similarly to ARDS and acute lung injury [21, 22, 32].

Pathogenesis and risk factors

Histology changes during IPF acute exacerbations clearly demonstrate triggering by acute injury to the alveolar epithelium and endothelium (also called acute lung injury). Known trigger factors for IPF acute exacerbations include any trauma to the chest/lung, mechanical ventilation, thoracic surgery including video-assisted thoracic surgery, environmental pollution, aspiration and lung toxic substances [33–38]. In addition, infectious diseases that injure alveolar tissue are similarly capable of triggering IPF acute exacerbations [9]. Clearly, all these factors can also induce ARDS in healthy individuals. In IPF however, lungs appear more sensitive to these trigger factors than normal. In particular, the risk of acute lung injury due to mechanical ventilation appears much higher in IPF patients [39, 40].

Underlying cellular and molecular mechanisms

Only a minority of IPF patients will experience an acute exacerbation during the course of their disease and the risk for developing an acute exacerbation appears to differ between patients. Recent molecular studies support this view, identifying biomarkers capable of predicting IPF acute exacerbations. Firstly, high levels in baseline serum KL-6 appear associated with an increased risk for acute exacerbation [41]. KL-6 is a cleaved glycoprotein derived from mucin-1, produced mainly by lung epithelial cells. The increased serum KL-6 levels in IPF may be due to an increase in KL-6 expression by regenerating type II pneumocytes in IPF [42]. Injury to the alveolar–capillary unit and increases in permeability also raise KL-6 levels [43]. Thus, KL-6 serum levels reflect alveolar damage and alveolar type II hyperplasia. In various ILDs, including ARDS, serum KL-6 are high. COLLARD *et al.* [44] have previously demonstrated a broad overlap in cytokine up-regulation in both ARDS and IPF acute exacerbations. Secondly, it has been shown that CCL18 levels, produced by alveolar macrophages, are predictive of IPF acute exacerbations [32]. Similar to KL-6, CCL18 appears related to disease activity and injury to alveolar tissues. It is highly up-regulated by "wound healing" M2 macrophages, which are induced by tissue injury, facilitating its role as a surrogate marker [45]. Collectively, there is strong evidence that acute exacerbation is induced by alveolar tissue injury and that baseline levels of alveolar damage appear related to the risk of development of severe alveolar damage, which is seen in acute exacerbation [46, 47].

As mentioned above, IPF itself is induced by alveolar epithelial cell injury, resulting in aberrant wound healing responses and leading to fibrotic remodelling of the alveolar compartment [48]. Also in mice, damage to the alveolar epithelial cells induces fibrosis [49]. Alveolar epithelium in pulmonary fibrosis does appear to be more susceptible to injury [50–53]. Normal wound healing responses of the alveolar epithelium fail as a result of genetic and/or environmental (re-)programming [48, 52, 53]. Hence, IPF acute exacerbations are intertwined with the dysregulatory mechanisms underpinning IPF and these same mechanisms seem to propagate acute exacerbations.

Treatment strategies

Currently, no validated treatment strategies exist for patients with established IPF developing an acute exacerbation. Given the serious prognostic implications, most clinicians adopt a pragmatic approach consisting of high-dose intravenous corticosteroids and empirical antibiotics. A minority of patients receiving corticosteroids may respond; usually as a result of underlying autoimmunity and/or histologic pattern suggestive of organising pneumonia. At least half of patients diagnosed with acute exacerbation will die within a matter of days. Treatment with haemoperfusion using polymyxin B-immobilised fibre columns or with thrombomodulin has been recently shown to be beneficial in Japanese populations [54–56]. The role of these treatments in non-Japanese populations remains unclear and warrants urgent assessment.

Given current treatment limitations, prevention of acute exacerbations is of outmost importance, with recent data are still conflicting. A *post hoc* analysis of the placebo arms of three National Institutes of Health studies has revealed that anti-acidic treatments, especially proton pump inhibitors, significantly reduced hospitalisation and the incidence of IPF acute exacerbations [57]. It remains unclear if this effect is dependent on the presence of gastro-oesophageal reflux or not. Gastro-oesophageal reflux is common among IPF patients with rates of up to 70% [58, 59]. Most of the patients receiving treatment in the National Institutes of Health trials had reported gastro-oesophageal reflux. In contrast, in the *post hoc* analyses of data of two recently published multicentre clinical trials, this effect of anti-acidic treatment upon acute exacerbation was not evident [60, 61].

In a phase II trial (To Improve Pulmonary Fibrosis with BIBF-1120 (TOMORROW)), nintedanib was associated with a significant reduction in acute exacerbation rates [62]. The subsequent phase III trial (Safety and Efficacy of BIBF 1120 at High Dose in Idiopathic Pulmonary Fibrosis (INPULSIS)) confirmed this result in only one study arm however, while in the other the incidence of acute exacerbation was low and underpowered [18]. If both study arms of INPULSIS were analysed together a statistically significant risk reduction with nintedanib for adjudicated acute exacerbations by an external board was reported confirming the signal of the TOMORROW trial. These trial data suggest a beneficial effect of nintedanib on risk reduction of acute exacerbation.

Regarding pirfenidone, the first multicentre phase II trial, involving exclusively Japanese patients, was stopped because of a lower incidence of acute exacerbation in the pirfenidone group compared with placebo [63]. Subsequent Japanese phase III and global phase III

(Safety and Efficacy of Pirfenidone in Patients with Idiopathic pulmonary Fibrosis (CAPACITY) I and II) trials have demonstrated a low incidence of acute exacerbations in patients with FVC >50% pred [5, 17, 64]. As a result, none of the later trials could demonstrate a significant effect of pirfenidone on acute exacerbation.

Conclusion

Acute exacerbation of IPF is an often fatal event, characterised by the development of diffuse alveolar damage on background of pre-existing interstitial fibrosis. Avoidance of acute exacerbations is important in improving mortality in IPF. Use of nintedanib appears to lower the risk of acute exacerbations. A consensus on feasible, unequivocal diagnostic criteria as well as algorithmic approach to work-up is urgently warranted to optimise comparability of future trials studying the effect of new treatment concepts in this profoundly life-limiting disease.

References

1. Panos RJ, Mortenson RL, Niccoli SA, et al. Clinical deterioration in patients with idiopathic pulmonary fibrosis: causes and assessment. Am J Med 1990; 88: 396–404.
2. Jeon K, Chung MP, Lee KS, et al. Prognostic factors and causes of death in Korean patients with idiopathic pulmonary fibrosis. Respir Med 2006; 100: 451–457.
3. Natsuizaka M, Chiba H, Kuronuma K, et al. Epidemiologic survey of Japanese patients with idiopathic pulmonary fibrosis and investigation of ethnic differences. Am J Respir Crit Care Med 2014; 190: 773–779.
4. Collard HR, Moore BB, Flaherty KR, et al. Acute exacerbations of idiopathic pulmonary fibrosis. Am J Respir Crit Care Med 2007; 176: 636–643.
5. Taniguchi H, Ebina M, Kondoh Y, et al. Pirfenidone in idiopathic pulmonary fibrosis. Eur Respir J 2010; 35: 821–829.
6. Molyneaux PL, Cox MJ, Willis-Owen SA, et al. The role of bacteria in the pathogenesis and progression of idiopathic pulmonary fibrosis. Am J Respir Crit Care Med 2014; 190: 906–913.
7. Petrosyan F, Culver DA, Reddy AJ. Role of bronchoalveolar lavage in the diagnosis of acute exacerbations of idiopathic pulmonary fibrosis: a retrospective study. BMC Pulm Med 2015; 15: 70.
8. Han MK, Zhou Y, Murray S, et al. Lung microbiome and disease progression in idiopathic pulmonary fibrosis: an analysis of the COMET study. Lancet Respir Med 2014; 2: 548–556.
9. Wootton SC, Kim DS, Kondoh Y, et al. Viral infection in acute exacerbation of idiopathic pulmonary fibrosis. Am J Respir Crit Care Med 2011; 183: 1698–1702.
10. Ryerson CJ, Cottin V, Brown KK, et al. Acute exacerbation of idiopathic pulmonary fibrosis: shifting the paradigm. Eur Respir J 2015; 46: 512–520.
11. Johannson K, Collard HR. Acute exacerbation of idiopathic pulmonary fibrosis: a proposal. Curr Respir Care Rep 2013; 2.
12. Collard HR, Yow E, Richeldi L, et al. Suspected acute exacerbation of idiopathic pulmonary fibrosis as an outcome measure in clinical trials. Respir Res 2013; 14: 73.
13. Raghu G, Rochwerg B, Zhang Y, et al. An Official ATS/ERS/JRS/ALAT Clinical Practice Guideline: Treatment of Idiopathic Pulmonary Fibrosis. An Update of the 2011 Clinical Practice Guideline. Am J Respir Crit Care Med 2015; 192: e3–e19.
14. Kim DS, Park JH, Park BK, et al. Acute exacerbation of idiopathic pulmonary fibrosis: frequency and clinical features. Eur Respir J 2006; 27: 143–150.
15. Kim DS. Acute exacerbation of idiopathic pulmonary fibrosis. Clin Chest Med 2012; 33: 59–68.
16. Song JW, Hong SB, Lim CM, et al. Acute exacerbation of idiopathic pulmonary fibrosis: incidence, risk factors and outcome. Eur Respir J 2011; 37: 356–363.
17. Noble PW, Albera C, Bradford WZ, et al. Pirfenidone in patients with idiopathic pulmonary fibrosis (CAPACITY): two randomised trials. Lancet 2011; 377: 1760–1769.
18. Richeldi L, du Bois RM, Raghu G, et al. Efficacy and safety of nintedanib in idiopathic pulmonary fibrosis. N Engl J Med 2014; 370: 2071–2082.
19. Zisman DA, Schwarz M, Anstrom KJ, et al. A controlled trial of sildenafil in advanced idiopathic pulmonary fibrosis. N Engl J Med 2010; 363: 620–628.

20. Akira M, Hamada H, Sakatani M, *et al.* CT findings during phase of accelerated deterioration in patients with idiopathic pulmonary fibrosis. *AJR Am J Roentgenol* 1997; 168: 79–83.

21. Kondoh Y, Taniguchi H, Kawabata Y, *et al.* Acute exacerbation in idiopathic pulmonary fibrosis. Analysis of clinical and pathologic findings in three cases. *Chest* 1993; 103: 1808–1812.

22. Ambrosini V, Cancellieri A, Chilosi M, *et al.* Acute exacerbation of idiopathic pulmonary fibrosis: report of a series. *Eur Respir J* 2003; 22: 821–826.

23. Parambil JG, Myers JL, Ryu JH. Histopathologic features and outcome of patients with acute exacerbation of idiopathic pulmonary fibrosis undergoing surgical lung biopsy. *Chest* 2005; 128: 3310–3315.

24. Kishaba T, Tamaki H, Shimaoka Y, *et al.* Staging of acute exacerbation in patients with idiopathic pulmonary fibrosis. *Lung* 2014; 192: 141–149.

25. Huie TJ, Olson AL, Cosgrove GP, *et al.* A detailed evaluation of acute respiratory decline in patients with fibrotic lung disease: aetiology and outcomes. *Respirology* 2010; 15: 909–917.

26. Akira M, Kozuka T, Yamamoto S, *et al.* Computed tomography findings in acute exacerbation of idiopathic pulmonary fibrosis. *Am J Respir Crit Care Med* 2008; 178: 372–378.

27. Fujimoto K, Taniguchi H, Johkoh T, *et al.* Acute exacerbation of idiopathic pulmonary fibrosis: high-resolution CT scores predict mortality. *Eur Radiol* 2012; 22: 83–92.

28. Konishi K, Gibson KF, Lindell KO, *et al.* Gene expression profiles of acute exacerbations of idiopathic pulmonary fibrosis. *Am J Respir Crit Care Med* 2009; 180: 167–175.

29. Jantz MA. Acute exacerbation of idiopathic pulmonary fibrosis and fibroproliferative acute respiratory distress syndrome: similar disease, similar treatment? *Respir Care* 2001; 46: 664–665.

30. Oda K, Ishimoto H, Yamada S, *et al.* Autopsy analyses in acute exacerbation of idiopathic pulmonary fibrosis. *Respir Res* 2014; 15: 109.

31. Al-Hameed FM, Sharma S. Outcome of patients admitted to the intensive care unit for acute exacerbation of idiopathic pulmonary fibrosis. *Can Respir J* 2004; 11: 117–122.

32. Schupp JC, Binder H, Jager B, *et al.* Macrophage activation in acute exacerbation of idiopathic pulmonary fibrosis. *PLoS One* 2015; 10: e0116775.

33. Sakamoto K, Taniguchi H, Kondoh Y, *et al.* Acute exacerbation of IPF following diagnostic bronchoalveolar lavage procedures. *Respir Med* 2012; 106: 436–442.

34. Kondoh Y, Taniguchi H, Katsuta T, *et al.* Risk factors of acute exacerbation of idiopathic pulmonary fibrosis. *Sarcoidosis Vasc Diffuse Lung Dis* 2010; 27: 103–110.

35. Lee JS, Song JW, Wolters PJ, *et al.* Bronchoalveolar lavage pepsin in acute exacerbation of idiopathic pulmonary fibrosis. *Eur Respir J* 2012; 39: 352–358.

36. Johannson KA, Vittinghoff E, Lee K, *et al.* Acute exacerbation of idiopathic pulmonary fibrosis associated with air pollution exposure. *Eur Respir J* 2014; 43: 1124–1131.

37. Kim DS. Acute exacerbations in patients with idiopathic pulmonary fibrosis. *Respir Res* 2013; 14: 86.

38. Bennett D, Bargagli E, Refini RM, *et al.* Acute exacerbation of idiopathic pulmonary fibrosis after inhalation of a water repellent. *Int J Occup Med Environ Health* 2015; 28: 775–779.

39. Gaudry S, Vincent F, Rabbat A, *et al.* Invasive mechanical ventilation in patients with fibrosing interstitial pneumonia. *J Thorac Cardiovasc Surg* 2014; 147: 47–53.

40. Stern JB, Mal H, Groussard O, *et al.* Prognosis of patients with advanced idiopathic pulmonary fibrosis requiring mechanical ventilation for acute respiratory failure. *Chest* 2001; 120: 213–219.

41. Ohshimo S, Ishikawa N, Horimasu Y, *et al.* Baseline KL-6 predicts increased risk for acute exacerbation of idiopathic pulmonary fibrosis. *Respir Med* 2014; 108: 1031–1039.

42. Ishikawa N, Hattori N, Yokoyama A, *et al.* Utility of KL-6/MUC1 in the clinical management of interstitial lung diseases. *Respir Investig* 2012; 50: 3–13.

43. Inoue Y, Barker E, Daniloff E, *et al.* Pulmonary epithelial cell injury and alveolar-capillary permeability in berylliosis. *Am J Respir Crit Care Med* 1997; 156: 109–115.

44. Collard HR, Calfee CS, Wolters PJ, *et al.* Plasma biomarker profiles in acute exacerbation of idiopathic pulmonary fibrosis. *Am J Physiol Lung Cell Mol Physiol* 2010; 299: L3–L7.

45. Sica A, Mantovani A. Macrophage plasticity and polarization: in vivo veritas. *J Clin Invest* 2012; 122: 787–795.

46. Li LF, Liu YY, Kao KC, *et al.* Mechanical ventilation augments bleomycin-induced epithelial-mesenchymal transition through the Src pathway. *Lab Invest* 2014; 94: 1017–1029.

47. Xu J, Mora AL, LaVoy J, *et al.* Increased bleomycin-induced lung injury in mice deficient in the transcription factor T-bet. *Am J Physiol Lung Cell Mol Physiol* 2006; 291: L658–L667.

48. King TE Jr, Pardo A, Selman M. Idiopathic pulmonary fibrosis. *Lancet* 2011; 378: 1949–1961.

49. Sisson TH, Mendez M, Choi K, *et al.* Targeted injury of type II alveolar epithelial cells induces pulmonary fibrosis. *Am J Respir Crit Care Med* 2010; 181: 254–263.

50. Korfei M, Ruppert C, Mahavadi P, *et al.* Epithelial endoplasmic reticulum stress and apoptosis in sporadic idiopathic pulmonary fibrosis. *Am J Respir Crit Care Med* 2008; 178: 838–846.

51. van Moorsel CH, Hoffman TW, van Batenburg AA, *et al.* Understanding Idiopathic Interstitial Pneumonia: A Gene-Based Review of Stressed Lungs. *Biomed Res Int* 2015; 2015: 304186.

52. Chilosi M, Carloni A, Rossi A, *et al.* Premature lung aging and cellular senescence in the pathogenesis of idiopathic pulmonary fibrosis and COPD/emphysema. *Transl Res* 2013; 162: 156–173.

53. Chilosi M, Doglioni C, Murer B, *et al.* Epithelial stem cell exhaustion in the pathogenesis of idiopathic pulmonary fibrosis. *Sarcoidosis Vasc Diffuse Lung Dis* 2010; 27: 7–18.

54. Enomoto N, Mikamo M, Oyama Y, *et al.* Treatment of acute exacerbation of idiopathic pulmonary fibrosis with direct hemoperfusion using a polymyxin B-immobilized fiber column improves survival. *BMC Pulm Med* 2015; 15: 15.

55. Kataoka K, Taniguchi H, Kondoh Y, *et al.* Recombinant human thrombomodulin in acute exacerbation of idiopathic pulmonary fibrosis. *Chest* 2015; 148: 436–443.

56. Tachibana K, Inoue Y, Nishiyama A, *et al.* Polymyxin-B hemoperfusion for acute exacerbation of idiopathic pulmonary fibrosis: serum IL-7 as a prognostic marker. *Sarcoidosis Vasc Diffuse Lung Dis* 2011; 28: 113–122.

57. Lee JS, Collard HR, Anstrom KJ, *et al.* Anti-acid treatment and disease progression in idiopathic pulmonary fibrosis: an analysis of data from three randomised controlled trials. *Lancet Respir Med* 2013; 1: 369–376.

58. Raghu G, Freudenberger TD, Yang S, *et al.* High prevalence of abnormal acid gastro-oesophageal reflux in idiopathic pulmonary fibrosis. *Eur Respir J* 2006; 27: 136–142.

59. Tobin RW, Pope CE II, Pellegrini CA, *et al.* Increased prevalence of gastroesophageal reflux in patients with idiopathic pulmonary fibrosis. *Am J Respir Crit Care Med* 1998; 158: 1804–1808.

60. Kreuter M, Wuyts W, Renzoni E, *et al.* Antiacid therapy and progression free survival in idiopathic pulmonary fibrosis (IPF). *Eur Respir J* 2015; 46: Suppl. 56, OA3478.

61. Raghu G, Crestani B, Bailes Z, *et al.* Effect of anti-acid medication on reduction in FVC decline with nintedanib. *Eur Respir J* 2015; 46: Suppl. 56, OA4502.

62. Richeldi L, Costabel U, Selman M, *et al.* Efficacy of a tyrosine kinase inhibitor in idiopathic pulmonary fibrosis. *N Engl J Med* 2011; 365: 1079–1087.

63. Azuma A, Nukiwa T, Tsuboi E, *et al.* Double-blind, placebo-controlled trial of pirfenidone in patients with idiopathic pulmonary fibrosis. *Am J Respir Crit Care Med* 2005; 171: 1040–1047.

64. King TE Jr, Bradford WZ, Castro-Bernardini S, *et al.* A phase 3 trial of pirfenidone in patients with idiopathic pulmonary fibrosis. *N Engl J Med* 2014; 370: 2083–2092.

Disclosures: A. Prasse reports personal fees and other fees from Boehringer Ingelheim and Intermune/ Roche during the conduct of the study; and personal fees from Boehringer Ingelheim Pharma, Pirfenidone, Bayer, Sanofi Aventis and GlaxoSmithKline, and grants from Biogen Idec outside the submitted work.

Acknowledgements: The author would like to thank Mark Greer (Hanover Medical School, Hanover, Germany) for detailed editing of the manuscript.

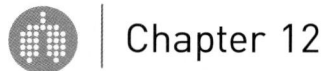
Cancer

Carlo Vancheri

IPF and cancer share similar risk factors and have a number of pathogenic mechanisms in common, which makes the two diseases very similar. This aetiopathogenic commonality may explain the relative frequency of the occurrence of lung cancer in IPF patients. Both diseases find their origin in the continuous exposure of alveolar and bronchiolar epithelial cells to microinjuries caused by exogenous agents that, depending on individual susceptibility, may lead to fibrosis and/or cancer. Based on that, lung cancer can be considered a true comorbidity for patients with IPF in which a proper screening programme based on annual HRCT might be helpful in disclosing lung cancer at early stages. However, the presence of IPF, even if an early diagnosis of lung cancer is made, virtually precludes the possibility of an effective treatment of cancer. The lack of effective and safe therapeutic options for patients with IPF and lung cancer, and the poor prognosis that characterises this association of diseases makes the therapeutic strategy extremely complicated. The best approach is to treat these patients on a case-by-case basis, trying to find a balance between the possibility of cure or practising palliation on one hand, and the potential complications that may be induced by diagnostic procedures and therapeutic approaches on the other hand.

In the lung, as in other organs, the activity of specific risk factors, associated with a genetic background that establish the degree of individual susceptibility, may determine the appearance of different diseases. In particular, risk factors are the reason of recurrent microinjuries and chronic damage to lung cells. According to the level of genetic susceptibility, chronic tissue damage may be followed by tissue destruction, as happens in emphysema, or cellular degenerative processes, as in lung cancer [1]. In the case of IPF, an excessive and redundant repair process creates progressive and irreversible fibrosis of the lung. In some other individuals, risk factors such as cigarette smoke may favour the appearance of both emphysema and fibrosis, as in the CPFE syndrome, not that rarely followed by the appearance of lung cancer [2]. A number of epidemiological studies have established a consistent association between smoking, GERD, viral infections, occupational and environmental exposures, and these pulmonary diseases [3–5]. The mechanisms through which these risk factors can act are unclear, and several studies have been undertaken aimed at explaining and identifying these mechanisms. Risk factors may affect the activity of respiratory cells through multiple mechanisms. They induce cellular oxidative stress, DNA damage, epigenetic alterations, protein misfolding and the unfolded protein response. Some risk factors may also impair proteasome activity leading to endoplasmic

Regional Referral Centre for Rare Lung Diseases, University Hospital "Policlinico – Vittorio Emanuele", Dept of Clinical and Experimental Medicine, University of Catania, Catania, Italy.

Correspondence: Carlo Vancheri, Regional Referral Centre for Rare Lung Diseases, University Hospital "Policlinico – Vittorio Emanuele", Dept of Clinical and Experimental Medicine, University of Catania, Sofia 78, Catania 95123, Italy. E-mail: vancheri@unict.it reticulum stress and cellular apoptosis, making the lung into either a proinflammatory or a profibrotic milieu [6, 7]. In this context, ageing plays an additional and important role, acting as an endogenous risk factor. This is a process characterised by progressive loss of physiological functions that in cancer or in other diseases such as IPF, is expressed by a number of genetic and epigenetic mutations that affect the behaviour of lung cells, altering their normal response to chronic damage [8, 9]. Indeed, incidence and prevalence of IPF increases with each decade of life, as in the common age-related diseases. Moreover, the relatively frequent finding, in individuals >75 years old, of ILD features at HRCT, seems to further support this hypothesis [10]. Cancer, in general, is also related to ageing and cell senescence, and similarly to IPF, affects susceptible individuals, sharing with IPF similar risk factors such as smoking, environmental or occupational exposure and viral infections. Apart from this obvious and circumstantial evidence, IPF and cancer have an incredible number of pathogenic mechanisms in common that make the two diseases very similar. Epigenetic and genetic alterations, abnormal expression of miRNAs, cellular and molecular aberrances such as the altered response to regulatory signals, and delayed apoptosis or reduced cell-to-cell communication along with the activation of specific signalling transduction pathways are all features that characterise the pathogenesis of both diseases [11–13]. This pathogenic commonality between IPF and cancer has a further and even more dramatic consequence for IPF patients: the increased incidence of lung cancer. In this chapter, the relationship between IPF and cancer will be reviewed from two different points of view. First, the underlying pathogenic mechanisms favouring the development of lung cancer in IPF patients will be explored. Secondly, the clinical association between these two diseases will be thoroughly analysed, highlighting the diagnostic and therapeutic problems that this deadly association may present.

How and why

The presence in cancer of similar risk factors as in IPF and the appearance of similar genetic/epigenetic alterations, together with the activation of a number of signalling pathways strictly related to cell proliferation and differentiation as well as to the regulation of apoptosis, may easily explain the relative frequency of the occurrence of lung cancer in IPF patients. Indeed, the inception of both IPF and IPF-associated lung cancer (I-ALC) finds its origin in the continuous exposure of alveolar and bronchiolar epithelial cells to microinjuries, such as those caused by smoking, viral infections, traction injury, and environmental and/or occupational exposures such as asbestosis [14, 15]. These chronic insults may damage the epithelium, causing aberrant activation of these cells and loss of epithelial integrity. In susceptible individuals, it may also activate incorrect repair mechanisms and stress response pathways, including endoplasmic reticulum stress and epithelial–mesenchymal transition, causing further dysfunction of alveolar epithelial cells (AECs) that may, on one hand, lead to fibrosis and, on the other hand, to uncontrolled cell proliferation and possibly to cancer [16–18]. Indeed, it has been recently demonstrated that type II AECs are damaged in IPF and that these cells may be found adjacent to myofbroblasts, suggesting their involvement in the abnormal tissue repair that characterises lung fibrosis. In addition, it has been observed that metaplastic epithelium is more common in IPF patients with lung cancer than in those without cancer [19]. It is evident that over time, these epithelial abnormalities, in more susceptible individuals, may represent the starting point for the development of I-ALC. Indeed, a number of epigenetic and genetic disorders have been identified in IPF affecting specific cellular mechanisms related to the regulation of cell cycle, cell differentiation and apoptosis that may predispose some patients to lung cancer. For instance, the reduced expression of the Thy-1 glycoprotein in IPF, due to the hypermethylation of the promoter region of the gene coding for this glycoprotein, is related to the differentiation of fibroblasts into myofibroblasts, whereas in cancer, it is associated with more invasive behaviour of cancer cells [20, 21]. Mutations of p53 and FHIT (fragile histidine triad), as well as microsatellite instability and loss of gene heterozygosity, are very often distinctive of many cancers. Interestingly, in IPF, these alterations are present in about 50% of IPF patients and, in most of the cases observed, in the parenchymal areas of honeycombing, the paradigmatic lesion of IPF [22–24]. Another common feature of cancer is the altered expression of telomerase and the subsequent shortening of telomeres. Recently, a lower expression of two subunits of telomerase (human telomerase reverse transcriptase and RNA component mRNA) has been also demonstrated in lung tissue from IPF patients compared with lung tissue of controls [25, 26]. The aberrant expression of miRNAs is an alteration linked to initiation and progression of cancer, and interestingly, is largely present in patients with IPF [27, 28]. A wide variety of signal transduction pathways are also activated both in cancer and IPF, and many studies have demonstrated their involvement in the pathogenesis of these two diseases. The alteration of the Wnt/β-catenin pathway has pathogenic and clinical relevance in diseases such as lung cancer, mesothelioma and desmoid tumours. Interestingly, this pathway is strongly activated in IPF lung tissue, as evidenced by extensive nuclear accumulation of β-catenin at different involved sites such as bronchiolar proliferative lesions, damaged alveolar structures and fibroblast foci. The Wnt/β-catenin signalling pathway regulates the expression of specific molecules involved in tissue invasion and proliferation, such as matrilysin, laminin and cyclin D1 [29–31]. Failure of cell apoptosis represents another key process in carcinogenesis and in establishing chemotherapy resistance mechanisms in cancer, but is also present in IPF. In this regard, the phosphatidylinositol 3-kinase (PI3K)/AKT signalling pathway is involved in the regulation of cell growth, proliferation and survival in both IPF and cancer. PI3K stimulates the synthesis of phosphatidylinositol 3,4,5-triphosphate that causes the activation of AKT, which in turn regulates cellular processes such as protection from apoptosis [32–34]. Another key signalling pathway strongly activated in many cancers, but also in IPF, is the tyrosine kinase pathways through the activation of tyrosine kinase receptors such as the VEGF, platelet-derived growth factor (PDGF) and fibroblast growth factor (FGF) receptors. They are involved in cell growth, differentiation, adhesion, motility and regulation of cell death. Indeed, mutations of tyrosine kinases may lead to initiation or progression of cancer and, more recently, this pathway has been also studied in wound healing and, most importantly, during fibrogenesis. PDGF signalling plays an important role in tissue homeostasis and repair, and specifically promotes wound closure, scar formation and vascular remodelling [35]. VEGF is better known for its activity on endothelial cells, although recent studies have shown that this growth factor influences the activity of mesenchymal cells, and may regulate epithelial cell proliferation and apoptosis [36]. FGF, however, is fully involved in the wound healing process, specifically regulating fibroblast proliferation and collagen production [37].

Tyrosine kinase receptor inhibitors have been widely used in non-small cell lung carcinoma and other cancers, and more recently in IPF. The contemporary inhibition of more receptors seems to be associated to an increased antifibrotic effect [38–41]. On this basis, nintedanib, a triple kinase inhibitor with potent suppressing effects on the VEGF, PDGF and FGF receptors, was evaluated in IPF, demonstrating that treatment with this drug may reduce the decline in lung function of IPF patients by about 50%. Based on these results, nintedanib has been approved as a new and additional therapeutic opportunity together with pirfenidone in patients with IPF [42, 43]. The use of nintedanib in IPF is a classical example of "drug repositioning" of an existing molecule already approved for a different disease [44]. Interestingly, nintedanib was first approved as second-line therapy for lung cancer in combination with docetaxel and, at least in theory, could be useful not just for slowing down the progression of IPF but also for "preventing" or "treating" I-ALC [45]. There is also some evidence showing that patients with IPF treated with pirfenidone may have a lower incidence of lung cancer and some protection towards acute exacerbations triggered by surgery in patients with I-ALC [46, 47].

When and where

The incidence of I-ALC ranges from 4.4% to 48%. Interestingly, its cumulative incidence increases strikingly over time, from around 3.3% at 1 year after IPF diagnosis to 15.4% at 5 years and 54.7% at 10 years of follow-up [48–51]. I-ALC is more frequent in males, smokers and patients with CPFE. The association between IPF and lung cancer significantly increases the risk of death compared to IPF alone [52]. The majority of patients die because of respiratory failure due to IPF, although a high number of adverse events strictly related to the diagnostic procedures and treatment of lung cancer have been described. In a recent study, TOMASSETTI et al. [53] studied 23 patients with I-ALC out of 181 patients with IPF (13%). In seven (30%) of these patients, the diagnosis of I-ALC was made at the time of the identification of IPF, whereas the other 16 (70%) patients were diagnosed in a period of time ranging from 27.4 to 84.1 months. According to their findings, the most frequent histological subtype is represented by peripheral squamous cell carcinoma and adenocarcinoma, often showing a similar anatomical distribution to the lung fibrosis. I-ALC is typically localised at a subpleural or peripheral level, close to or within honeycomb and fibrotic areas. Less often, the appearance is of isolated areas of ground glass [54, 55]. This can make radiological diagnosis of I-ALC arduous, especially at the time of the first HRCT scan. To make things even more complicated, the vast majority of patients do not present cancer-related symptoms and the diagnosis of lung cancer is an incidental finding during the follow-up for IPF [53]. Old or relatively old age of IPF patients reduces the radiological risk for these patients; thus, it may be considered appropriate to repeat HRCT every year (figure 1).

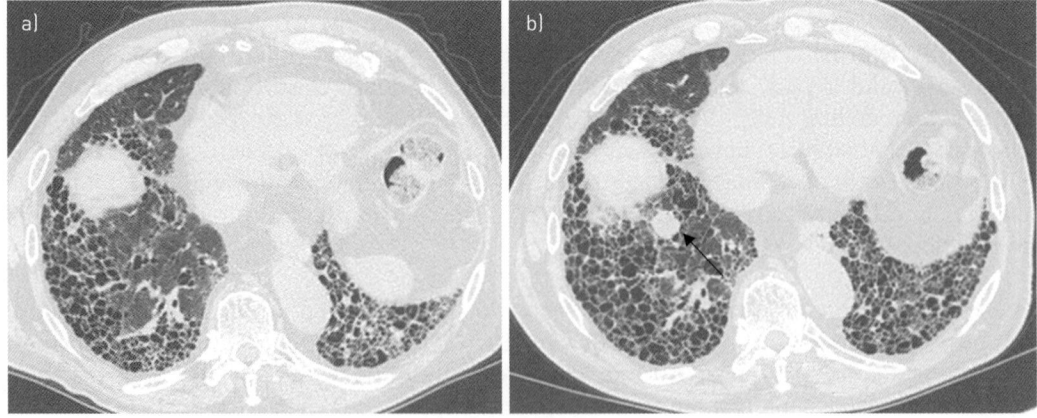

Figure 1. a) Thoracic CT scan of a patient with IPF. b) The same patient about 12 months later. Arrow: nodular lesion with a well-defined and irregular margin. The histological examination confirmed the diagnosis of adenocarcinoma.

This is supported by the high percentage (39%) of early-stage cancers identified by performing HRCT scans annually for the regular follow-up of IPF patients reported by TOMASSETTI *et al.* [53]. Similar data were described in a Korean study where the diagnosis of early-stage lung cancer was made in 41% of IPF patients. This study also confirmed that squamous cell carcinoma and adenocarcinoma were the most represented histological patterns, with cancer mainly observed in lower lobes and lung subpleural regions close to areas of fibrosis [56, 57]. In addition, KHAN *et al.* [55] described a wide pattern of epithelial alterations within areas of honeycombing, ranging from epithelial atypia to squamous metaplasia, carcinoma *in situ* and invasive squamous cell carcinoma.

What to do

In a recent study, survival in patients with lung cancer and IPF was significantly shorter than in patients with IPF without lung cancer (median survival 38.7 *versus* 63.9 months) [49]. Survival at 1 and 3 years after IPF diagnosis was 78% and 52% in patients with lung cancer *versus* 92% and 70%, respectively, in those without lung cancer [53]. LEE *et al.* [56] have shown that the 5-year survival in surgically treated patients (37% *versus* 72.5%, p<0.001) as well as the relapse-free survival time (44.9 *versus* 66.8 months, p<0.014) was significantly reduced in patients with I-ALC compared with those with lung cancer without IPF. Interestingly, the reduced survival of I-ALC patients was not related to age, sex, pulmonary function, smoking habits, histological type or disease stage, and only partially to a lower pre-operative arterial carbon dioxide tension. In I-ALC patients, in contrast to patients who underwent to surgery for lung cancer alone, a higher incidence of respiratory deaths due to pneumonia, acute respiratory distress syndrome and acute exacerbations of IPF was observed, inducing LEE *et al.* [56] to conclude that the lower survival of I-ALC patients was mainly due to IPF. For this reason, TOMASSETTI *et al.* [53] proposed a new treatment strategy taking into consideration not only the lung cancer stage but also the degree of severity of IPF calculated using the GAP index. In general, patients with lung cancer in stage 1 and IPF in GAP stage 1 underwent surgery, whereas patients with a more advanced stage of cancer and/or more severe IPF were treated with chemotherapy, radiotherapy or supportive therapy. However, this and other studies have confirmed that the early post-operative mortality and morbidity was high in patients with I-ALC, and the risk of acute exacerbations was considered unacceptable after lobectomy, whereas in sublobar resection, the risk of complication was much lower, although a good part of these patients had a recurrence of lung cancer during follow-up [57–61]. Several studies have examined the peri-operative risk factors that may favour the occurrence of acute exacerbations. MIZUNO *et al.* [62] have described a relationship between the amount of intraoperative fluid infused and the occurrence of fatal acute exacerbations, suggesting that minimising intravenous fluid administration could be important for their prevention. Less invasive treatments, such as thermo- or cryoablation, could be a valid alternative to traditional surgery but they need to be further explored in the specific context of I-ALC. A further, different approach is represented by stereotactic body radiotherapy. This procedure is characterised by a very high local control of radiation and, therefore, has become widespread for the treatment of pulmonary lesions in specific circumstances. It is also considered safe, although adverse events such as radiation pneumonitis have been described. After a case report showing the occurrence of radiation pneumonitis in one patient with lung cancer and subclinical IPF, proper studies on a larger number of patients with lung cancer and radiological signs of lung fibrosis were performed [63]. Disappointingly, these studies demonstrated that the rate of extensive and fatal radiation pneumonitis was higher in patients with subclinical ILDs. This finding led the authors of these studies to conclude that the presence of signs of lung fibrosis in patients with lung cancer should be considered a contraindication for radiotherapy [64, 65].

Unfortunately, chemotherapy and "traditional" radiotherapy are no better therapeutic solutions, although their role for the treatment of I-ALC is still controversial. MINEGISHI et al. [66] evaluated a paclitaxel/carboplatin regimen in patients with I-ALC, observing that this treatment was as effective and well tolerated as in patients without IPF. In this study, the overall response rate was of 61% with a median progression-free survival of 5.3 months; only one (5.3%) patient experienced an acute exacerbation of IPF following treatment. Conversely, other studies reported an acute exacerbation rate of 30% or more, together with a high rate of pulmonary toxicity [66–68]. Acute exacerbations of IPF have also been reported following radiotherapy for lung cancer [69, 70]. Furthermore, ISOBE et al. [70] have shown that 24% of patients who received chemotherapy had acute respiratory deterioration that caused lethal respiratory failure in 60% of them. Respiratory deterioration was entirely ascribed to IPF progression, with typical clinical and HRCT signs of acute IPF exacerbation such as the appearance of bilateral ground-glass opacities. In these patients, any other possible cause of respiratory damage, such as pulmonary embolism, congestive heart failure or infection, was excluded. In contrast, no acute respiratory deterioration was observed in those patients who only received best supportive care [70]. TOMASSETTI et al. [53] reported similar findings in their 12 patients treated with chemotherapy, six of whom suffered of severe adverse events: heart failure, pneumothorax, empyema, pancytopenia and two acute exacerbations, one of which was fatal. This study, in agreement with previous observations, confirmed the high percentage of patients with I-ALC that died of respiratory failure due to IPF (43%), whereas 13% of them died from the progression of lung cancer. Interestingly, a consistent part of proportion of these patients (17%) died because of the complications associated with diagnostic procedures as well as surgical and medical treatments.

The relative rarity of the association between lung cancer and IPF prevents the possibility to arrange proper prospective, randomised studies analysing the different possible therapeutic approaches for I-ALC. All available data come instead from retrospective studies suggesting that treatment, and specifically surgical treatment, should be reserved for those patients with less advanced cancer and less severe IPF. In other patients, where cancer and/or IPF is more advanced, there is no clear evidence that chemotherapy or radiotherapy will prolong their survival, whereas many studies have confirmed that both chemotherapy and radiotherapy may be the cause of severe complications.

Based on its high incidence, I-ALC can be considered a true comorbidity of patients with IPF. IPF patients should be recognised as a population at high risk of lung cancer and, therefore, should undergo to a proper screening programme based on annual HRCT, which may be helpful in disclosing lung cancer at early stages. It is well known that a similar approach with low-dose CT reduced mortality by 6.7% for lung cancer in adult heavy smokers. Unfortunately, the presence of IPF, even if an early diagnosis of lung cancer is made, virtually precludes the possibility of an effective treatment for lung cancer. The lack of effective and safe therapeutic options for patients with I-ALC, and the subsequent poor prognosis that characterises this association of diseases makes the therapeutic approach to these patients extremely complicated. In a recent review dealing with the management of the comorbidities of IPF, FULTON and RYERSON [71] suggested treating patients with I-ALC on a case-by-case basis, trying to find a balance between the possibility of curing or practising palliation on one hand, and the potential complications that may be induced by diagnostic procedures and therapeutic approaches on the other hand. All that should be seen in the light of the overall dramatically poor prognosis that characterises IPF.

References

1. Chilosi M, Poletti V, Rossi A. The pathogenesis of COPD and IPF: distinct horns of the same devil? *Respir Res* 2012; 13: 3.
2. Cottin V. The impact of emphysema in pulmonary fibrosis. *Eur Respir Rev* 2013; 22: 153–157.
3. Lee JS. The role of gastroesophageal reflux and microaspiration in idiopathic pulmonary fibrosis. *Clin Pulm Med* 2014; 21: 81–85.
4. Mitchell PD, Das JP, Murphy DJ, *et al.* Idiopathic pulmonary fibrosis with emphysema: evidence of synergy among emphysema and idiopathic pulmonary fibrosis in smokers. *Respir Care* 2015; 60: 259–268.
5. Harari S, Caminati A. IPF: new insight on pathogenesis and treatment. *Allergy* 2010; 65: 537–553.
6. Tanjore H, Blackwell TS, Lawson WE. Emerging evidence for endoplasmic reticulum stress in the pathogenesis of idiopathic pulmonary fibrosis. *Am J Physiol Lung Cell Mol Physiol* 2012; 302: L721–L729.
7. Macneal K, Schwartz DA. The genetic and environmental Causes of Pulmonary Fibrosis. *Proc Am Thorac Soc* 2012; 9: 120–125.
8. Leung J, Cho Y, Lockey RF, *et al.* The role of aging in idiopathic pulmonary fibrosis. *Lung* 2015; 193: 605–610.
9. López-Otín C, Blasco MA, Partridge L, *et al.* The hallmarks of aging. *Cell* 2013; 153: 1194–1217.
10. Copley SJ, Wells AU, Hawtin KE, *et al.* Lung morphology in the elderly: comparative CT study of subjects over 75 years old *versus* those under 55 years old. *Radiology* 2009; 251: 566–573.
11. Vancheri C. Idiopathic pulmonary fibrosis and cancer: do they really look similar? *BMC Med* 2015; 13: 220.
12. Antoniou KM, Tomassetti S, Tsitoura E, *et al.* Idiopathic pulmonary fibrosis and lung cancer: a clinical and pathogenesis update. *Curr Opin Pulm Med* 2015; 21: 626–633.
13. Vancheri C, Cottin V, Kreuter M, *et al.* IPF, comorbidities and management implications. *Sarcoidosis Vasc Diffuse Lung Dis* 2015; 32: Suppl. 1, 17–23.
14. Stella GM, Inghilleri S, Pignochino Y, *et al.* Activation of oncogenic pathways in idiopathic pulmonary fibrosis. *Transl Oncol* 2014; 7: 650–655.
15. Vancheri C, Failla M, Crimi N, *et al.* Idiopathic pulmonary fibrosis: a disease with similarities and links to cancer biology. *Eur Respir J* 2010; 35: 496–504.
16. Tanjore H, Blackwell TS, Lawson WE. Emerging evidence for endoplasmic reticulum stress in the pathogenesis of idiopathic pulmonary fibrosis. *Am J Physiol Lung Cell Mol Physiol* 2012; 302: L721–L729.
17. Macneal K, Schwartz DA. The genetic and environmental causes of pulmonary fibrosis. *Proc Am Thorac Soc* 2012; 9: 120–125.
18. Kim KK, Kugler MC, Wolters PJ, *et al.* Alveolar epithelial cell mesenchymal transition develops *in vivo* during pulmonary fibrosis and is regulated by the extracellular matrix. *Proc Natl Acad Sci USA* 2006; 103: 13180–13185.
19. Li J, Yang M, Li P, *et al.* Idiopathic pulmonary fibrosis will increase the risk of lung cancer. *Chin Med J (Engl)* 2014; 127: 3142–3149.
20. Sanders YY, Kumbla P, Hagood JS. Enhanced myofibroblastic differentiation and survival in Thy-1⁻ lung fibroblasts. *Am J Respir Cell Mol Biol* 2007; 36: 226–235.
21. Sanders YY, Pardo A, Selman M, *et al.* Thy-1 promoter hypermethylation: a novel epigenetic pathogenic mechanism in pulmonary fibrosis. *Am J Respir Cell Mol Biol* 2008; 39: 610–618.
22. Hojo S, Fujita J, Yamadori I, *et al.* Heterogeneous point mutations of the p53 gene in pulmonary fibrosis. *Eur Respir J* 1998; 12: 1404–1408.
23. Uematsu K, Yoshimura A, Gemma A, *et al.* Aberrations in the fragile histidine triad (*FHIT*) gene in idiopathic pulmonary fibrosis. *Cancer Res* 2001; 61: 8527–8233.
24. Demopoulos K, Arvanitis DA, Vassilakis DA, *et al.* MYCL1, FHIT, SPARC, P16^{INK4} and TP53 genes associated to lung cancer in idiopathic pulmonary fibrosis. *J Cell Mol Med* 2002; 6: 215–222.
25. Antoniou KM, Samara KD, Lasithiotaki I, *et al.* Differential telomerase expression in idiopathic pulmonary fibrosis and non-small cell lung cancer. *Oncolog Rep* 2013; 30: 2617–2624.
26. Calado RT, Young NS. Telomere diseases. *N Engl J Med* 2009; 361: 2353–2365.
27. Vosa U, Vooder T, Kolde R, *et al.* Meta-analysis of microRNA expression in lung cancer. *Int J Cancer* 2013; 132: 2884–2893.
28. Pandit KV, Milosevic J, Kaminski N. MicroRNAs in idiopathic pulmonary fibrosis. *Transl Res* 2011; 157: 191–199.
29. Mazieres J, He B, You L, *et al.* Wnt signaling in lung cancer. *Cancer Lett* 2005; 222: 1–10.
30. Chilosi M, Poletti V, Zamò A, *et al.* Aberrant Wnt/β-catenin pathway activation in idiopathic pulmonary fibrosis. *Am J Pathol* 2003; 162: 1495–1502.

31. Caraci F, Gili E, Calafiore M, *et al.* TGF-β1 targets the GSK-3β/β-catenin pathway *via* ERK activation in the transition of human lung fibroblast into myofibroblasts. *Pharmacol Res* 2008; 57: 274–282.

32. Cantley LC. The phosphoinositide 3-kinase pathway. *Science* 2002; 296: 1655–1657.

33. Conte E, Gili E, Fruciano M, *et al.* PI3K p110g overexpression in idiopathic pulmonary fibrosis lung tissue and fibroblast cells: *in vitro* effects of its inhibition. *Lab Invest* 2013; 93: 566–576.

34. Wei X, Han J, Chen ZZ, *et al.* A phosphoinositide 3-kinase-γ inhibitor, AS605240 prevents bleomycin- induced pulmonary fibrosis in rats. *Biochem Biophys Res Commun* 2010; 397: 311–317.

35. Andrae J, Gallini R, Betsholtz C. Role of platelet-derived growth factors in physiology and medicine. *Genes Dev* 2008; 22: 1276–1312.

36. Voelkel NF, Vandivier RW, Tuder RM. Vascular endothelial growth factor in the lung. *Am J Physiol Lung Cell Mol Physiol* 2006; 290: L209–L221.

37. Dosanjh A. The fibroblast growth factor pathway and its role in the pathogenesis of lung disease. *J Interferon Cytokine Res* 2012; 32: 111–114.

38. Beyer C, Distler JH. Tyrosine kinase signaling in fibrotic disorders: translation of basic research to human disease. *Biochim Biophys Acta* 2013; 1832: 897–904.

39. Hetzel M, Bachem M, Anders D, *et al.* Different effects of growth factors on proliferation and matrix production of normal and fibrotic human lung fibroblasts. *Lung* 2005; 183: 225–237.

40. Grimminger F, Günther A, Vancheri C. The role of tyrosine kinases in the pathogenesis of idiopathic pulmonary fibrosis. *Eur Respir J* 2015; 45: 1426–1433.

41. Chaudhary NI, Roth GJ, Hilberg F, *et al.* Inhibition of PDGF, VEGF and FGF signalling attenuates fibrosis. *Eur Respir J* 2007; 29: 976–985.

42. King TEJr, Bradford WZ, Castro-Bernardini S, *et al.* A phase 3 trial of pirfenidone in patients with idiopathic pulmonary fibrosis. *N Engl J Med* 2014; 370: 2083–2092.

43. Richeldi L, du Bois RM, Raghu G, *et al.* Efficacy and safety of nintedanib in idiopathic pulmonary fibrosis. *N Engl J Med* 2014; 370: 2071–2082.

44. Li YY, Jones SJ. Drug repositioning for personalized medicine. *Genome Med* 2012; 4: 27.

45. Reck M, Kaiser R, Mellemgaard A, *et al.* Docetaxel plus nintedanib *versus* docetaxel plus placebo in patients with previously treated non-small-cell lung cancer (LUME-Lung 1): a phase 3, double-blind, randomised controlled trial. *Lancet Oncol* 2014; 15: 143–155.

46. Miura Y, Saito T, Tsunoda Y, *et al.* Clinical effect of pirfenidone on incidence of lung carcinoma in chronic interstitial pneumonia. *Eur Respir J* 2014; 44: Suppl. 58, P3497.

47. Iwata T, Yoshida S, Nagato K, *et al.* Experience with perioperative pirfenidone for lung cancer surgery in patients with idiopathic pulmonary fibrosis. *Surg Today* 2015; 45: 1263–1270.

48. Le Jeune I, Gribbin J, West J, *et al.* The incidence of cancer in patients with idiopathic pulmonary fibrosis and sarcoidosis in the UK. *Respir Med* 2007; 101: 2534–2540.

49. Matsushita H, Tanaka S, Saiki Y, *et al.* Lung cancer associated with usual interstitial pneumonia. *Pathol Int* 1995; 45: 925–932.

50. Ozawa Y, Suda T, Naito T, *et al.* Cumulative incidence of and predictive factors for lung cancer in IPF. *Respirology* 2009; 14: 723–728.

51. Usui K, Tanai C, Tanaka Y, *et al.* The prevalence of pulmonary fibrosis combined with emphysema in patients with lung cancer. *Respirology* 2011; 16: 326–331.

52. Park J, Kim DS, Shim TS, *et al.* Lung cancer in patients with idiopathic pulmonary fibrosis. *Eur Respir J* 2001; 17: 1216–1219.

53. Tomassetti S, Gurioli C, Ryu JH, *et al.* The impact of lung cancer on survival of idiopathic pulmonary fibrosis. *Chest* 2015; 147: 157–164.

54. Kishi K, Homma S, Kurosaki A, *et al.* High-resolution computed tomography findings of lung cancer associated with idiopathic pulmonary fibrosis. *J Comput Assist Tomogr* 2006; 30: 95–99.

55. Khan KA, Kennedy MP, Moore E, *et al.* Radiological characteristics, histological features and clinical outcomes of lung cancer patients with coexistent idiopathic pulmonary fibrosis. *Lung* 2015; 193: 71–77.

56. Lee T, Park JY, Lee HY, *et al.* Lung cancer in patients with idiopathic pulmonary fibrosis: clinical characteristics and impact on survival. *Respir Med* 2014; 108: 1549–1555.

57. Fujimoto T, Okazaki T, Matsukura T, *et al.* Operation for lung cancer in patients with idiopathic pulmonary fibrosis: surgical contraindication? *Ann Thorac Surg* 2003; 76: 1674–1678.

58. Kushibe K, Kawaguchi T, Takahama M, *et al.* Operative indications for lung cancer with idiopathic pulmonary fibrosis. *Thorac Cardiovasc Surg* 2007; 55: 505–508.

59. Watanabe A, Higami T, Ohori S, *et al.* Is lung cancer resection indicated in patients with idiopathic pulmonary fibrosis? *J Thorac Cardiovasc Surg* 2008; 136: 1357–1363.

60. Omori T, Tajiri M, Baba T, *et al.* Pulmonary Resection for Lung Cancer in Patients With Idiopathic Interstitial Pneumonia. *Ann Thorac Surg* 2015; 100: 954–960.

61. Kumar P, Goldstraw P, Yamada K, *et al.* Pulmonary fibrosis and lung cancer: risk and benefit analysis of pulmonary resection. *J Thorac Cardiovasc Surg* 2003; 125: 1321–1327.

62. Mizuno Y, Iwata H, Shirahashi K, *et al*. The importance of intraoperative fluid balance for the prevention of postoperative acute exacerbation of idiopathic pulmonary fibrosis after pulmonary resection for primary lung cancer. *Eur J Cardiothorac Surg* 2012; 41: e161–e165.

63. Takeda A, Enomoto T, Sanuki N, *et al*. Acute exacerbation of subclinical idiopathic pulmonary fibrosis triggered by hypofractionated stereotactic body radiotherapy in a patient with primary lung cancer and slightly focal honeycombing. *Radiat Med* 2008; 26: 504–507.

64. Yamaguchi S, Ohguri T, Ide S, *et al*. Stereotactic body radiotherapy for lung tumors in patients with subclinical interstitial lung disease: the potential risk of extensive radiation pneumonitis. *Lung Cancer* 2013; 82: 260–265.

65. Yamaguchi S, Ohguri T, Matsuki Y, *et al*. Radiotherapy for thoracic tumors: association between subclinical interstitial lung disease and fatal radiation pneumonitis. *Int J Clin Oncol* 2015; 20: 45–52.

66. Minegishi Y, Sudoh J, Kuribayasi H, *et al*. The safety and efficacy of weekly paclitaxel in combination with carboplatin for advanced non-small cell lung cancer with idiopathic interstitial pneumonias. *Lung Cancer* 2011; 71: 70–74.

67. Kenmotsu H, Naito T, Kimura M, *et al*. The risk of cytotoxic chemotherapy-related exacerbation of interstitial lung disease with lung cancer. *J Thorac Oncol* 2011; 6: 1242–1246.

68. Watanabe N, Taniguchi H, Kondoh Y, *et al*. Chemotherapy for extensive-stage small-cell lung cancer with idiopathic pulmonary fibrosis. *Int J Clin Oncol* 2014; 19: 260–265.

69. Watanabe N, Taniguchi H, Kondoh Y, *et al*. Efficacy of chemotherapy for advanced non-small cell lung cancer with idiopathic pulmonary fibrosis. *Respiration* 2013; 85: 326–331.

70. Isobe K, Hata Y, Sakamoto S, *et al*. Clinical characteristics of acute respiratory deterioration in pulmonary fibrosis associated with lung cancer following anti-cancer therapy. *Respirology* 2010; 15: 88–92.

71. Fulton BG, Ryerson CJ. Managing comorbidities in idiopathic pulmonary fibrosis. *Int J Gen Med* 2015; 8: 309–318.

Disclosures: C. Vancheri reports receiving grants and personal fees from Roche and Boehringer Ingelheim.

Chapter 13

Pulmonary hypertension

Etienne-Marie Jutant[1,2,3], Laura Price[4], S. John Wort[4], Marc Humbert[1,2,3] and David Montani[1,2,3]

IPF is often associated with PH, which principally develops due to fibrotic destruction of the vasculature and pulmonary vascular remodelling. The presence of PH worsens prognosis, especially when associated with right ventricular dysfunction. The extent of PH is not closely associated with the extent of lung fibrosis, as assessed by pulmonary lung function or radiological features, suggesting that the severity of fibrosis is not the only driving factor for PH. The term "out of proportion PH" has now been abandoned and replaced with "IPF with severe PH" in the minority of patients with a mean pulmonary artery pressure >35 mmHg. Although echocardiography is a useful indicator, right heart catheterisation remains the gold standard for PH in IPF. There is no current recommendation for PH-specific therapies in IPF, and patients should be included in clinical trials. Current treatment recommendations are optimisation of treatment of the underlying IPF, oxygen supplementation when necessary and lung transplantation, despite the increase in transplantation complications when PH is associated with IPF.

IPF is the most common of the IIPs, with prevalence in Europe between 1.25 and 23.4 cases per 100 000 population and an annual incidence between 0.22 and 7.4 per 100 000 population [1]. Pulmonary vasculature involvement in IPF leading to PH represents a major issue in the natural course of the disease. PH worsens the prognosis of IPF patients and the management of PH is extremely challenging.

Classification and definition of PH

In the recent guidelines for the diagnosis and treatment of PH [2], a revised classification of PH was adopted (table 1). Group 3 was defined as "PH due to lung diseases and/or hypoxia" and was characterised by pre-capillary PH, defined by a mean pulmonary artery pressure (P_{pa}) $\geqslant$25 mmHg and a normal pulmonary artery wedge pressure $\leqslant$15 mmHg which were assessed by right heart catheterisation (RHC). In this group, the predominant causes of PH are alveolar hypoxia associated with chronic lung diseases, impaired control of breathing or residing at high altitude. PH associated with ILD, including IPF, is included within this group.

[1]Université Paris-Sud, Faculté de Médecine, Université Paris-Saclay, Le Kremlin Bicêtre, France. [2]AP-HP, Service de Pneumologie, Hôpital Bicêtre, Le Kremlin Bicêtre, France. [3]Inserm UMR_S 999, Hôpital Marie Lannelongue, Le Plessis Robinson, France. [4]Pulmonary Hypertension Service, Royal Brompton Hospital, London, UK.

Correspondence: David Montani, Service de Pneumologie, Université Paris-Sud, Hôpital Bicêtre, 78 Rue du général Leclerc, 94270 Le Kremlin Bicêtre, France. E-mail: david.montani@aphp.fr

ERS Monogr 2016; 71: 160–174. DOI: 10.1183/2312508X.10005815

Table 1. Comprehensive classification of PH

1. Pulmonary arterial hypertension
    1.1 Idiopathic
    1.2 Heritable
        1.2.1. BMPR2 mutation
        1.2.2. Other mutations
    1.3 Drugs and toxins induced
    1.4 Associated with
        1.4.1. Connective tissue disease
        1.4.2. Human immunodeficiency virus (HIV) infection
        1.4.3. Portal hypertension
        1.4.4. Congenital heart disease
        1.4.5. Schistosomiasis
1'. Pulmonary veno-occlusive disease and/or pulmonary capillary haemangiomatosis
    1'.1 Idiopathic
    1'.2 Heritable
        1'.2.1. EIF2AK4 mutation
        1'.2.2. Other mutations
    1'.3 Drugs, toxins and radiation induced
    1'.4 Associated with:
        1'.4.1. Connective tissue disease
        1'.4.2. HIV infection
1''. Persistent pulmonary hypertension of the newborn
2. Pulmonary hypertension due to left heart disease
    2.1 Left ventricular systolic dysfunction
    2.2 Left ventricular diastolic dysfunction
    2.3 Valvular disease
    2.4 Congenital/acquired left heart inflow/outflow tract obstruction and congenital cardiomyopathies
    2.5 Congenital/acquired pulmonary vein stenosis
3. Pulmonary hypertension due to lung diseases and/or hypoxia
    3.1 Chronic obstructive pulmonary disease
    3.2 Interstitial lung disease
    3.3 Other pulmonary diseases with mixed restrictive and obstructive pattern
    3.4 Sleep-disordered breathing
    3.5 Alveolar hypoventilation disorders
    3.6 Chronic exposure to high altitude
    3.7 Developmental lung diseases
4. Chronic thromboembolic pulmonary hypertension and other pulmonary artery obstructions
    4.1 Chronic thromboembolic pulmonary hypertension
    4.2 Other pulmonary artery obstructions
        4.2.1. Angiosarcoma
        4.2.2. Other intravascular tumours
        4.2.3. Arteritis
        4.2.4. Congenital pulmonary arteries stenoses
        4.2.5. Parasites (hydatidosis)
5. Pulmonary hypertension with unclear and/or multifactorial mechanisms
    5.1 Haematological disorders: chronic haemolytic anaemia, myeloproliferative disorders, splenectomy
    5.2 Systemic disorders, sarcoidosis, pulmonary histiocytosis, lymphangioleiomyomatosis, neurofibromatosis
    5.3 Metabolic disorders: glycogen storage disease, Gaucher disease, thyroid disorders
    5.4 Others: pulmonary tumoral thrombotic microangiopathy, fibrosing mediastinitis, chronic renal failure (with/without dialysis), segmental pulmonary hypertension

Reproduced and modified from [2] with permission from the publisher.

As observed in different chronic respiratory diseases comprising Group 3 PH, the severity of PH usually correlates poorly with the severity of the underlying lung disease. In addition, a minority of patients with IPF or COPD have severe haemodynamic impairment disproportionate to their parenchymal involvement [3–6]. These patients often only have moderate lung function impairment and moderate fibrosis observed on CT scans, but they have severe PH. The term "out-of-proportion PH" has progressively been abandoned in the successive classifications, as there is no clearly defined threshold of what could be considered as a proportionate increase in mean Ppa related to the underlying parenchymal involvement. The most recent European Society of Cardiology/European Respiratory Society guidelines aimed to define a subgroup of patients with "IPF with severe PH", based on haemodynamic assessment [2]. The definition of severe PH is presented in table 2 and was defined as a mean Ppa >35 mmHg or ⩾25 mmHg in the presence of low cardiac output at rest.

Pathophysiology of IPF-PH

PH associated with ILD is included in Group 3 of the classification of PH [2]. More rarely, PH associated with ILD could be part of the other groups, in particular: pulmonary arterial hypertension (PAH) associated with connective tissue diseases (Group 1); PH due to left heart disease (Group 2) as left heart dysfunction is frequently found in patients with chronic respiratory diseases [2]; or chronic thromboembolic PH (Group 4) as patients with IPF are more likely to develop pulmonary embolism [7]. Associated comorbidities including obstructive sleep apnoea, which leads to intermittent hypoxia during sleep and is frequent in IPF [8], or concomitant emphysema may contribute to the onset of PH. Therefore, even though PH associated with IPF is usually classified in Group 3, screening for other risk factors of PAH and/or PH remains essential.

The pathophysiology of PH associated with IPF (IPF-PH) results from a combination of different mechanisms. Fibrotic destruction of the vasculature leading to vascular rarefaction appears to be the principle mechanism. Indeed, overall vessel density has been shown to be reduced with important vascular ablation, mainly in areas of honeycombing [9, 10]. As in other causes of chronic respiratory insufficiency, hypoxic pulmonary arterial vasoconstriction participates in milder degrees of IPF-PH and could be increased during exercise because of intermittent hypoxia [8] or during sleep in cases of overnight hypoxia. Vascular remodelling, microvascular injury and endothelial dysfunction may also play an important role in the development of more severe PH. In 1963, TURNER-WARWICK [11] first

---

Table 2. Haemodynamic classification of PH due to lung disease

Terminology	Haemodynamics (right heart catheterisation)
COPD/IPF/CPFE without PH	Mean Ppa <25 mmHg
COPD/IPF/CPFE with PH	Mean Ppa ⩾25 mmHg
COPD/IPF/CPFE with severe PH	Mean Ppa >35 mmHg, or mean Ppa ⩾25 mmHg in the presence of a low cardiac output (CI <2.5 L·min^{-1}·m^{-2}, not explained by other causes)

Ppa: pulmonary artery pressure; CI: cardiac index. Reproduced and modified from [2] with permission from the publisher.

described the existence of aberrant neovascularisation in IPF with the development of neovascularisation with subpleural systemic pulmonary anastomoses. Many studies since have reported abnormal and heterogenous vascular remodelling in IPF [9, 10], which could participate in the development of PH. Regarding neovascularisation, one hypothesis is that the reduction in peripheral pulmonary blood flow in relation to the hypoxic pulmonary vascular remodelling leads to a protective angiogenic response in the pulmonary capillaries, in an attempt to counteract the "pruning" of the peripheral vessels. This is supported by experiments showing that angiostatin worsens hypoxic PH [12] and that VEGF overexpression protects against hypoxic PH [13]. Moreover, it has been shown that there is an increase in the production of important pulmonary vascular mediators, including endothelin (ET)-1 [14] and VEGF [15] in fibrotic lungs. ET-1 is a potent vasoconstrictor, a pro-mitogenic protein and a promoter of smooth muscle cell growth, which also contributes to fibrosis. In a cross-sectional study, VENTETUOLO et al. [16] included 52 patients with IPF and performed RHC and measured serum ET-1. They showed that higher ET-1 levels were associated with higher mean Ppa and may be associated with higher pulmonary vascular resistance. VEGF is an important growth factor generally implicated in angiogenesis, vascular remodelling and fibrosis. However, VENTETUOLO et al. [16] also showed an absence of correlation between levels of serum VEGF and mean Ppa [16]. Finally, genetic predisposition, abnormal lymphocyte function (with autoimmune features) and variable cytokine or chemokine expression [17] are also likely to participate in the development of IPF-PH.

Prevalence of IPF-PH

The prevalence of IPF-PH has been assessed in several studies but with huge heterogeneity in the populations studied, ranging from early-stage IPF to end-stage IPF at the time of lung transplantation. This explains the large range of prevalence reported in the literature (table 3).

In mild-to-moderate IPF, the prevalence of PH is quite low, ranging from 8.1% to 14.9% [18–20]. In this population, PH is generally of moderate severity and severe PH (mean Ppa >35 mmHg) is only found in 4% of patients [20]. RAGHU et al. [21] assessed the clinical course of pulmonary haemodynamics in 117 mild-to-moderate IPF patients (excluding severe patients with a FVC <50%, extensive honeycombing on HRCT or New York Heart Association (NYHA) grade III or IV functional symptoms), from the ARTEMIS-IPF

Table 3. Prevalence of PH in principal IPF-PH studies

First author [ref.]	Study	FVC %/DLCO %	Mean Ppa mmHg	PH prevalence
HAMADA [18]	Retrospective	74/45	16±5	6/70 (8.1)
RAGHU [19]	Prospective	69/42		48/494 (9.7)
KIMURA [20]	Retrospective	70/48	19.2±6.5	15/101 (14.9)
LETTIERI [23]	Retrospective	49/31	23.4±5.1	25/79 (31.6)
SHORR [3]	Retrospective	48/no result		1163/2525 (46.1)
NATHAN [41]	Retrospective	Baseline: 49/33	Baseline: 22.6±6	Baseline: 17/44 (38.6)
			Follow-up: 32.7±9.5	Follow-up: 38/44 (86.4)
MINAI [25]	Retrospective	49/28	26.2±10	55/124 (44)

Data are presented as mean±SD or n/N (%), unless otherwise stated. Ppa: pulmonary artery pressure.

(Randomized, Placebo-Controlled Study to Evaluate Safety and Effectiveness of Ambrisentan in IPF) trial. A second RHC was performed 12 months after the first RHC, and showed that the pulmonary pressures remained stable over 1 year in most of the patients and only five out of 117 patients developed PH. The rate of increase of mean Ppa was therefore, on average, 0.4 mmHg after 48 months in this population with mild-to-moderate IPF [21]. This equates to ~0.5 mmHg·year^{-1} in COPD [22], which is above the baseline increase in Ppa of 1 mmHg per 10 years. In end-stage IPF, generally at the time of evaluation for lung transplantation, the prevalence of PH is higher (ranging from 31.6% to 46.1%) [3, 23–25] but PH remains moderate, with severe PH found in 9.1% of the patients [3]. In a retrospective study, NATHAN et al. [24] reported the evolution of mean Ppa in 44 patients with IPF between the first evaluation for transplantation and time of lung transplantation. At baseline, 38.6% (17 out of 44) of the patients had PH. The majority of the non-PH patients developed PH during the interval with a subsequent incidence of 77.8%. Finally, at the time of transplantation, 86.4% of the patients had PH. The mean Ppa change between the two RHCs was 10.1 mmHg with a monthly rate of change of 3.8±6.1 mmHg [24].

In conclusion, PH is generally mild to moderate in IPF and only a minority of patients present with severe PH, even if severe PH is more frequent than in COPD where PH is severe in only 1% of cases [5]. PH develops slowly in mild and clinically stable patients but can probably develop more rapidly in advanced stage IPF.

IPF and other comorbidities

Other comorbidities are more frequent than PH in IPF and have to be diagnosed and treated. In a Danish IPF cohort of 121 patients, the most frequently observed comorbidities were cardiovascular disease (20%), arterial hypertension (15%) and diabetes mellitus (11%) [26]. A recent review of 126 studies reported that the prevalence of other comorbidities were also frequent among IPF patients, such as obstructive sleep apnoea (6–91%), lung cancer (3–48%), COPD (6–67%), ischaemic heart disease (3–68%) and gastro-oesophageal reflux (0–94%) [27].

Pathological assessment

Lung biopsy is not part of the evaluation of PH in IPF. However, surgical lung biopsy is recommended for the diagnosis of IPF when patients present with non-diagnostic scans or the diagnosis of IPF is uncertain [28]. In cases of IPF-PH there may be remodelling of the small pulmonary arteries with wall thickening and proliferation of endothelial and smooth muscle cells, in association with histological signs of UIP (figure 1). This would suggest the presence of IPF-PH histologically, but it must be emphasised that lung biopsy is not the recommended modality to diagnose IPF-PH. This relates to the high risk of clinical deterioration, acute exacerbations of IPF [29] and adverse events related to hypoxia and bleeding due to associated PH, as well as reduced tolerance to general anaesthesia and one lung ventilation if video-assisted thoracoscopic surgery biopsy is performed.

Impact of PH on prognosis in patients with IPF

IPF has a median survival range of 2.5–3.5 years [30, 31], but when PH develops the risk of death is increased. In mild-to-moderate IPF patients, HAMADA et al. [18] found a relative risk of mortality of 2.2 at 5 years when mean Ppa is >17 mmHg. KIMURA et al. [20] showed

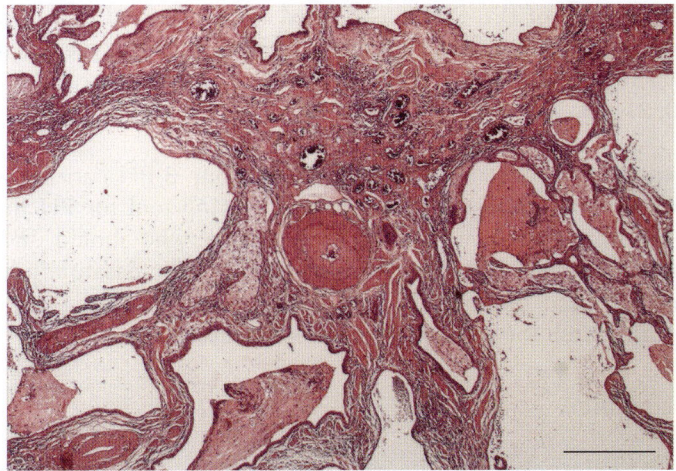

Figure 1. Pulmonary arteries from a patient with IPF and PH (haematoxylin and stain). UIP lesions associated with pulmonary arterial remodelling. Scale bar=500 µm.

that high mean P_{pa} at the initial evaluation of IPF is an independent predictor of death (HR 1.064; p=0.010). In advanced IPF, PH is also associated with a higher risk of death (OR 2.6; p=0.001) [23]. In a retrospective study, 88 IPF patients were stratified into three groups depending on systolic P_{pa} measured by echocardiography; <35 mmHg, 36–50 mmHg and >50 mmHg [32]. The median survival rates for these three groups were 4.8 years, 4.1 years and 0.7 years, respectively. Patients with a systolic P_{pa} >50 mmHg had significantly worse survival compared to other subgroups and the relative risk for death was 1.34 per 10 mmHg increase [32]. Finally, in some studies, the level of pulmonary vascular resistance and not mean P_{pa} was significantly associated with death [33].

Acute exacerbations of IPF are acute deteriorations in respiratory status of unknown aetiology and are the most severe complication of IPF leading to death in >50% of the cases [34]. A study of 55 IPF patients showed that PH at baseline was associated with a significant risk of acute exacerbations (HR 2.217, p=0.041) [35]. In addition, the development of an acute exacerbation can lead to acute PH and associated right ventricular dysfunction, most probably related to hypoxic vasoconstriction, as has been recognised and studied previously in acute exacerbations of COPD [36]. In conclusion, PH in mild-to-moderate IPF, as in advanced stages of IPF, is an adverse prognostic factor.

Screening for PH in IPF patients

There are no specific clinical signs of PH in IPF. Progressive appearance of exertional dyspnoea or worsening of pre-existing dyspnoea may suggest PH, especially if it occurs in a patient with stable interstitial disease. A prominent pulmonary component of the second heart sound may be present, with signs of right heart failure later in the disease course. Peripheral oedema may not always indicate right heart failure as it may also result from the effects of hypoxaemia and hypercapnia on the renin-angiotensin-aldosterone system [2]. Therefore, PH is difficult to recognise early in IPF and could be suspected by electrocardiogram, chest radiography or echocardiography. Interestingly, as mentioned previously, pulmonary haemodynamics do not correlate with markers of the severity of the underlying lung disease, such as FVC and TLC [3, 18, 23, 25, 32, 37].

However, the development of IPF-PH is associated with increased dyspnoea [32], increased requirement of oxygen [3, 23], lower walk distance and severe oxygen desaturation during the 6MWT [20, 21, 23, 25, 38], low partial pressure of oxygen at rest [18, 20, 25, 32], and low D_{LCO} [18, 20, 21, 23, 32].

As RHC is an invasive procedure not without risk in group 3 PH patients with high oxygen requirements, it cannot be proposed as a routine screening tool for PH in all IPF patients. Therefore, there has been extensive research to determine who should undergo RHC. As a general rule, patients presenting with symptoms or oxygen desaturations that are more severe than expected based on their PFTs should be further evaluated, in particular by echocardiography, to search for concomitant left heart dysfunction or PH [2].

Brain natriuretic peptide

In 39 patients with pulmonary fibrosis (28 with IPF), LEUCHTE *et al.* [38] reported that serum brain natriuretic peptide (BNP) concentrations correlated with haemodynamic parameters and predicted PH with a high sensitivity (100%) and specificity (89%). BNP was not associated with impairment of lung volume [38]. In a prospective study of 176 patients with chronic lung disease (including 55 with IPF), elevated BNP concentrations identified significant PH with a sensitivity of 85% and a specificity of 88% and was a risk factor of death independent of lung function impairment or hypoxaemia [39]. Thus, BNP may be an interesting tool in screening and follow-up of IPF-PH and could allow noninvasive detection of significant PH with high accuracy. However, it remains to be validated in a large IPF population and it cannot be used as a sole marker to diagnose IPF-PH.

Echocardiography

Echocardiography is an easily available, noninvasive diagnostic modality that can, in most cases, detect PH by estimating systolic P_{pa} based on the measurement of the tricuspid regurgitation jet velocity. Comparison of echocardiography and RHC measurements showed that, even if there was a correlation between systolic P_{pa} measured by echocardiography and RHC [23, 24], pressure estimations were inaccurate in 52% [40] to 60% [41], 48% of patients were misclassified as having PH and echocardiography underestimated the systolic P_{pa} in 11.6%. Estimated sensitivity, specificity and positive and negative predictive values of systolic P_{pa} for the diagnosis of PH were 85–86%, 29–55%, 39–52% and 80–87%, respectively [40, 41]. Moreover, echocardiography studies suggest that it is only possible to obtain accurate echocardiography windows in 44–55% of patients with ILD because of air distension of the lungs [40, 41], although in our experience this is not such a common problem.

Pulmonary function test

Several studies have demonstrated that lung volume impairment, including FVC and TLC which are marker of lung fibrosis destruction, are not associated with the presence of PH unlike D_{LCO} and the FVC/D_{LCO} ratio which are better markers [3, 18, 23, 25, 32, 37]. NATHAN *et al.* [42] have specifically studied the ability of FVC, D_{LCO} and the FVC/D_{LCO} ratio to predict underlying PH in a retrospective study of 118 patients with IPF-PH. There was no correlation between measurements of lung volumes and PH and there was only a modest association between D_{LCO} and PH. Thus, D_{LCO} is not sufficient to be used as a stand-alone surrogate for underlying PH [42]. It has been shown that a baseline transfer coefficient of the lung for carbon monoxide (transfer factor of the lung for carbon monoxide/alveolar volume) <50% and/or a decline in transfer coefficient of the lung for carbon monoxide >15% at 6 months predicted mortality and the development of PH onset better than the transfer factor of the lung for carbon monoxide or FVC in fibrotic IIP [43]. A composite physiological index calculated using PFT results and the extent of fibrosis on HRCT, which had been shown to be a good predictor of disease extension and mortality in IPF [44], was not associated with underlying PH [42]. The poor correlation between lung volumes and PH reinforces the hypothesis that lung destruction is not the only pathophysiological factor leading to IPF-PH.

Cardiopulmonary exercise testing

Recent guidelines reported that patients with PAH have a typical pattern on cardiopulmonary exercise testing (CPET) with a low end-tidal partial pressure of carbon dioxide, high ventilator equivalents for carbon dioxide (minute ventilation/carbon dioxide production), low oxygen pulse (oxygen uptake/heart rate) and low peak oxygen uptake [2, 45].

In a study where CPET was performed in 81 patients with IPF (57% of PH diagnosed by echocardiography), the authors reported that resting systolic Ppa correlated with CPET signs of circulatory impairment (low peak oxygen uptake, low anaerobic threshold, low peak oxygen pulse and low end-tidal partial pressure of carbon dioxide at anaerobic threshold) [46]. Although a very useful tool, even with submaximal testing, CPET may be difficult to perform in patients with severe breathlessness. CPET alone is not enough to make a diagnosis of IPF-PH but could be important in the initial evaluation for assessing prognosis and to enable follow-up of patients with IPF-PH.

CT of the chest

In 2007, Zisman et al. [4] compared CT scans from 65 patients with advanced IPF with available RHC data and found no significant correlation between mean Ppa with any of the chest CT-determined measurements including extent of fibrosis, ground-glass opacification, honeycombing and the ratio of the diameters of the main pulmonary artery and ascending aorta. This latter measurement is predictive of PH in many settings without fibrosis [47] but it is a less reliable sign in the presence of fibrotic lung disease as it can also be increased in the absence of PH [48], although it might be improved when combined with echocardiography [49]. In this last study on patients with chronic lung diseases and PH (21% with IPF), a moderate correlation between the diameter of the segmental pulmonary artery and mean Ppa was shown (R^2=0.24; p=0.001) but no correlation was shown between the diameter of the subsegmental artery and mean Ppa (R^2=0.02; p=0.3). Overall, chest CT findings alone are not useful as a screen for PH in advanced IPF [4].

Combination of parameters to detect PH

In the study by Lettieri et al. [23], the association of a need for supplemental oxygen and DLCO <40% increased the risk of PH 10-fold. Zisman et al. [37] showed that a predictor based on arterial oxygen saturation measured by pulse oximetry and FVC/DLCO has a high negative predictive value (81%) for PH in IPF. More recently Ruoco et al. [50] suggested that an algorithm including BNP, DLCO and echocardiography findings (mean Ppa, systolic Ppa and tricuspid annular plane systolic excursion) is a useful and repeatable tool to detect PH in patients with ILD and should lead to RHC when the algorithm score is >3. These results are encouraging but need to be confirmed in a larger population and validated by follow-up data.

Diagnosis of IPF-PH requires RHC

Even though several noninvasive tools are useful for screening, RHC remains the gold standard for diagnosis as a definite diagnosis of IPF-PH relies on measurements obtained during RHC [2]. IPF-PH (Group 3) is generally pre-capillary in nature (mean P_{pa} ⩾25 mmHg at rest with normal pulmonary artery wedge pressure ⩽15 mmHg) [2, 21]. In the most recent European Society of Cardiology/European Respiratory Society guidelines, the retained indications for RHC in advanced lung disease are proper diagnosis or exclusion of PH in candidates for surgical treatments like transplantation, suspected PAH or chronic thromboembolic PH, episodes of right ventricular failure and inconclusive echocardiographic findings in patients with a high level of suspicion of PH and potential therapeutic implications [51]. A new classification was recommended, depending on mean P_{pa}, and is presented in table 2 [2, 51]. As previously discussed, the severe PH group is the smallest group but should include patients suspected to have more severe vascular abnormalities. It will be interesting to identify these patients, who may share a more severe vascular phenotype, and question the potential efficacy of pulmonary vascular therapies in well-designed clinical trials.

IPF-PH: how to treat it?

In July 2015, there was an update of the international guidelines on IPF treatment, and one of the questions posed in these guidelines was whether PH should be treated in patients with IPF. The committee did not make a firm final recommendation and it was concluded that further evidence was needed to guide this clinical decision [28]. The 5th World Symposium of PH and the European Society of Cardiology/European Respiratory Society guidelines drew the same conclusion [2, 51]. It was recommended to: 1) reverse hypoxaemia by using long-term oxygen therapy in IPF-PH patients who are hypoxaemic, even if this recommendation is not supported by clinical trials; 2) control the underlying disease; and 3) include these patients in controlled trials, especially patients with milder forms of IPF and severe PH who should be referred to expert centres. Indeed, patients with suspected PAH in addition to their lung diseases may be treated according to the recommendations for PAH [2]. However, the suspicion of PAH is very difficult to confirm in IPF and assessment in an expert centre is needed. Specific PAH therapies are not recommended in Group 3 PH because although positive effects may be seen, these treatments may worsen ventilation/perfusion mismatch and hypoxaemia by disturbing hypoxic vasoconstriction. Although several studies have been performed (often with some methodological concerns), no large well-conducted studies have confirmed important outcome benefits in patients with IPF-PH where diagnosis is confirmed using RHC. Recently, three studies retrospectively reported the outcome of Group 3 PH patients treated by compassionate PH treatment despite the absence of recommendations. The first study retrospectively studied 79 Group 3 PH patients (three with IPF) and compared the outcomes of the 26 patients with severe PH treated with PH drugs to the eight patients without severe PH treated by PH drugs and the patients not treated. There was no effect of the treatment on exercise capacity but a sub-group analysis showed a benefit of survival in the severe PH treated group (HR 0.182, p=0.002) [52]. The second study compared 118 Group 3 PH patients with severe PH (eight with IPF) to 74 idiopathic PAH patients, all treated with pulmonary vasodilators. Compared to PAH patients, Group 3 PH treated patients didn't show an improvement in 6MWD or in NYHA functional class but N-terminal pro-BNP was decreased. Survival was worse in the Group 3 PH group compared to PAH patients; this was driven by the ILD sub-group which had the poorest survival [53]. Finally, a recent report which compared 151 patients with IIP and PH receiving PH treatment (113 with IPF) with 798 PAH patients from the COMPERA (Comparative, Prospective Registry of Newly Initiated Therapies for Pulmonary Hypertension) registry showed a median improvement in 6MWD of 24.5 m in patients with PH-IIP and an improvement in NYHA functional class in 29.5% of patients, but survival rates were significantly worse in PH-IIP than PAH (3-year survival 34.0% *versus* 68.6%; p<0.001) [54]. In the last two studies, there was no comparison with a non-treated group. These studies are not enough to encourage a compassionate treatment in IPF-PH and prospective long-term randomised studies are needed. The studies to date are detailed below and summarised in table 4.

Prostacyclin

Long-term studies of prostacyclin in IPF-PH are missing. In 1999, OLSCHEWSKI *et al.* [55] studied eight patients with pulmonary fibrosis (one with IPF) and compared the haemodynamic effects of intravenous and inhaled prostacyclin and inhaled nitric oxide in a randomised fashion. They found that inhaled prostacyclin caused pulmonary vasodilatation with maintenance of gas exchange and systemic arterial pressure whereas intravenous prostacyclin was not pulmonary selective, resulting in a significant drop in systemic arterial pressure and a marked increase in shunt flow [55]. Intravenous prostacyclin also increased ventilation/perfusion mismatch and caused systemic hypotension in patients with IPF-PH, although without adverse events [56]. Therefore, limited evidence can suggest physiological benefit for inhaled but not intravenous prostacyclin in IPF-PH.

Phosphodiesterase type-5 inhibitors and soluble guanylate cyclase stimulator

The phosphodiesterase type (PDE)-5 inhibitor sildenafil has also been studied in IPF-PH, although long-term large, randomised and double-blind studies are missing. In a small open-label trial of 16 patients with pulmonary fibrosis (including seven with IPF) and

Table 4. Clinical trials with a specific PH drug in IPF-PH

First author [ref.]	Drug	Patients n	Study type	Follow-up	Primary end-point	Results
OLSHEWSKI [55]	Prostacyclin	8	P/R	Acute	None	
GHOFRANI [56]	Sildenafil	16	P/C/R	Acute	↓ PVRI	Significant
COLLARD [57]	Sildenafil	14	P	12 weeks	Δ6MWD	Significant
HAN [59]	Sildenafil	119	C/R	12 weeks	Δ6MWD	Significant
HOEPER [68]	Riociguat	21	P	12 weeks	Safety	Significant
CORTE [64]	Bosentan	66	P/C/R/B	16 weeks	↓ PVRI >20%	NS
RAGHU [19]	Ambrisentan	492	P/C/R/B	35 weeks	Time to IPF progression	Stopped

P: prospective; R: randomised; C: control; B: blinded; PVRI: pulmonary vascular resistance index; NS: nonsignificant.

severe PH confirmed by RHC (mean $P_{pa} \geqslant 35$ mmHg), GHOFRANI *et al.* [56] compared the acute haemodynamic effects of sildenafil and infused prostacyclin. Oral sildenafil and intravenous prostacyclin both decreased the pulmonary resistance vascular index but only oral sildenafil (and inhaled nitric oxide) maintained ventilation/perfusion matching and systemic blood pressure [56]. A more recent open-label study demonstrated an improvement in 6MWD with sildenafil in patients with IPF-PH [57]. This was followed by STEP-IPF (Sildenafil Trial of Exercise Performance in Idiopathic Pulmonary Fibrosis), a double-blind, randomised, placebo-controlled multicentre study which compared the effects of sildenafil with placebo on 6MWD in advanced IPF (D_{LCO} <30%). This showed no difference with the main criteria at 12 weeks but some improvements in secondary end-points (dyspnoea, QoL and partial pressure of oxygen) [58]. A *post hoc* analysis of echocardiography by HAN *et al.* [59] in 119 out of 180 STEP-IPF patients (studied in a blinded retrospective manner) showed that sildenafil improved exercise capacity and QoL compared with placebo in subjects with IPF and right ventricular dysfunction, but not in those with only right ventricular hypertrophy. In an observational open-label pilot study of 10 patients with ILD and PH (including six with IPF), treatment with sildenafil or tadalafil led to an increase in the cardiac index and a significant decrease in pulmonary vascular resistance [60]. Therefore, available data suggest beneficial effects of PDE-5 inhibitors in terms of pulmonary haemodynamics, exercise tolerance and QoL, and suggest that this drug is well tolerated in IPF-PH; but the longer term effects on morbidity and mortality remain elusive.

Riociguat is the first of the new "soluble guanylyl cyclase stimulators" designed to restore cyclic guanosine monophosphate levels independently of nitric oxide [23]. In a multicentre pilot trial of 21 patients with mild ILD (59% with IPF) and PH, HOEPER *et al.* [61] studied the safety of riociguat and showed that it was well tolerated. Cardiac output and pulmonary vascular resistance, were also improved but mean P_{pa} was not [61]. A randomised, double-blind, placebo-controlled phase II trial on efficacy and safety of riociguat in patients with symptomatic PH associated with IIPs (RISE-IIP) is ongoing [62].

Endothelin receptor antagonists

In the BUILD-3 (Bosentan Use in Interstitial Lung Disease) study, the dual endothelin receptor agonist bosentan was well tolerated in patients suffering from IPF without PH, but did not change the time to worsening in IPF compared to placebo [63]. The B-PHIT (Bosentan in Pulmonary Hypertension Associated with Fibrotic Idiopathic Interstitial Pneumonia) study was a randomised, double-blind, placebo-controlled study of bosentan in 66 patients with IIP (46 IPF) and PH [64]. In this study no difference was found between patients treated with bosentan or placebo in terms of pulmonary haemodynamics, clinical parameters or lung function. There were no adverse events related to bosentan, including effects on gas exchange [64]. ARTEMIS-IPF was a phase 3 study of ambrisentan, the selective endothelin A receptor antagonist, on disease progression in patients with IPF-PH. The study excluded patients with severe IPF. Patients underwent RHC at baseline and follow-up, and were stratified on the basis of the presence of PH. The composite primary end-point (time to IPF disease progression) was not met and the study was stopped early because of the greater disease progression and increased hospitalisations for respiratory complication in the ambrisentan group [19]. This study has resulted in a strong recommendation against the use of ambrisentan in IPF, independent of the presence of PH [28].

These large well-designed studies confirm that endothelin receptor antagonists (including bosentan and ambrisentan) provide no benefit in IPF-PH, and that ambrisentan may cause harm.

Tyrosine kinase inhibitors and PH

Tyrosine kinase inhibitors are of potential interest in IPF because they inhibit IPF-relevant cell proliferation, extracellular matrix production and cytokine activity [65]. There are no studies of tyrosine kinase inhibitors in IPF-PH, and in IPF without PH there is a strong recommendation against the use of imatinib because of a lack of efficacy and concerns regarding safety and cost [28, 66]. In PAH, imatinib is not recommended because of a lack of efficacy and reports of serious adverse events, including subdural haematomas [67–69]. Moreover, dasatinib, a nonselective tyrosine kinase inhibitor used in chronic myelogenous leukaemia, is associated with causing PH [70, 71]. Therefore, there is no information on the effect of TKI on IPF-PH and one should remain vigilant about the use of TKI in this population.

Pulmonary rehabilitation

In PH guidelines, it is recommended that patients suffering from PAH (Group 1) should avoid excessive physical activity but when physically deconditioned may undertake exercise rehabilitation. They must exercise at a steady state and exercise training programmes should be implemented by centres experienced in both PAH patient care and rehabilitation of compromised patients [2]. There are no recommendations regarding rehabilitation in PH in Group 3. In IPF without PH, some studies on rehabilitation showed an improvement in walk distance, symptoms and QoL [72, 73]. Therefore, in the IPF guidelines there is a weak recommendation for the use of pulmonary rehabilitation in the majority of patients with IPF [74]. In a study of 402 patients with ILD (50% with IPF and 28% with PH) receiving pulmonary rehabilitation, patients with IPF-PH also benefited from rehabilitation [75], although to a lesser extent. Therefore, we might suggest that pulmonary rehabilitation should have positive outcomes in IPF-PH patients, but clearly prospective clinical trials are necessary.

Impact of PH in transplanted patients with IPF

Lung transplantation remains the only curative treatment for IPF. The presence of PH should alert clinicians to consider earlier referral for lung transplantation assessment. However, caution is necessary because PH could increase transplantation complications. WHELAN et al. [76] showed that PH increased 90-day mortality following lung transplantation for IPF. In a prospective, multicentre cohort study, FANG et al. [77] evaluated the relationship between pulmonary haemodynamic parameters and the incidence of primary graft dysfunction in those undergoing lung transplantation for IPF. They showed that mean Ppa was 8.9 mmHg higher in patients with primary graft dysfunction than those without. Moreover, each incremental 10-mmHg increase in mean Ppa further increased the odds of developing primary graft dysfunction by nearly 65%.

Conclusion

PH has to systematically be taken into account in the evaluation, follow-up and treatment of IPF. Indeed, PH is frequent in IPF, it negatively impacts on prognosis and confirming the diagnosis of PH in IPF may be difficult without RHC. Clinical trials are urgently needed to find new and effective treatments.

References

1. Nalysnyk L, Cid-Ruzafa J, Rotella P, *et al.* Incidence and prevalence of idiopathic pulmonary fibrosis: review of the literature. *Eur Respir Rev* 2012; 21: 355–361.
2. Galiè N, Humbert M, Vachiery JL, *et al.* 2015 ESC/ERS guidelines for the diagnosis and treatment of pulmonary hypertension. *Eur Respir J* 2015; 46: 903–975.
3. Shorr AF, Wainright JL, Cors CS, *et al.* Pulmonary hypertension in patients with pulmonary fibrosis awaiting lung transplant. *Eur Respir J* 2007; 30: 715–721.
4. Zisman DA, Karlamangla AS, Ross DJ, *et al.* High-resolution chest CT findings do not predict the presence of pulmonary hypertension in advanced idiopathic pulmonary fibrosis. *Chest* 2007; 132: 773–779.
5. Chaouat A, Bugnet A-S, Kadaoui N, *et al.* Severe pulmonary hypertension and chronic obstructive pulmonary disease. *Am J Respir Crit Care Med* 2005; 172: 189–194.
6. Thabut G, Dauriat G, Stern JB, *et al.* Pulmonary hemodynamics in advanced COPD candidates for lung volume reduction surgery or lung transplantation. *Chest* 2005; 127: 1531–1536.
7. Dalleywater W, Powell HA, Fogarty AW, *et al.* Venous thromboembolism in people with idiopathic pulmonary fibrosis: a population-based study. *Eur Respir J* 2014; 44: 1714–1715.
8. Lee RN, Kelly E, Nolan G, *et al.* Disordered breathing during sleep and exercise in idiopathic pulmonary fibrosis and the role of biomarkers. *QJM* 2015; 108: 315–323.
9. Renzoni EA, Walsh DA, Salmon M, *et al.* Interstitial vascularity in fibrosing alveolitis. *Am J Respir Crit Care Med* 2003; 167: 438–443.
10. Ebina M, Shimizukawa M, Shibata N, *et al.* Heterogeneous increase in CD34-positive alveolar capillaries in idiopathic pulmonary fibrosis. *Am J Respir Crit Care Med* 2004; 169: 1203–1208.
11. Turner-Warwick M. Precapillary systemic-pulmonary anastomoses. *Thorax* 1963; 18: 225–237.
12. Pascaud MA, Griscelli F, Raoul W, *et al.* Lung overexpression of angiostatin aggravates pulmonary hypertension in chronically hypoxic mice. *Am J Respir Cell Mol Biol* 2003; 29: 449–457.
13. Partovian C, Adnot S, Eddahibi S, *et al.* Heart and lung VEGF mRNA expression in rats with monocrotaline- or hypoxia-induced pulmonary hypertension. *Am J Physiol* 1998; 275: H1948–H1956.
14. Uguccioni M, Pulsatelli L, Grigolo B, *et al.* Endothelin-1 in idiopathic pulmonary fibrosis. *J Clin Pathol* 1995; 48: 330–334.
15. Ando M, Miyazaki E, Ito T, *et al.* Significance of serum vascular endothelial growth factor level in patients with idiopathic pulmonary fibrosis. *Lung* 2010; 188: 247–252.
16. Ventetuolo CE, Kawut SM, Lederer DJ. Plasma endothelin-1 and vascular endothelial growth factor levels and their relationship to hemodynamics in idiopathic pulmonary fibrosis. *Respiration* 2012; 84: 299–305.
17. Feghali-Bostwick CA, Tsai CG, Valentine VG, *et al.* Cellular and humoral autoreactivity in idiopathic pulmonary fibrosis. *J Immunol* 2007; 179: 2592–2599.
18. Hamada K, Nagai S, Tanaka S, *et al.* Significance of pulmonary arterial pressure and diffusion capacity of the lung as prognosticator in patients with idiopathic pulmonary fibrosis. *Chest* 2007; 131: 650–656.
19. Raghu G, Behr J, Brown KK, *et al.* Treatment of idiopathic pulmonary fibrosis with ambrisentan: a parallel, randomized trial. *Ann Intern Med* 2013; 158: 641–649.
20. Kimura M, Taniguchi H, Kondoh Y, *et al.* Pulmonary hypertension as a prognostic indicator at the initial evaluation in idiopathic pulmonary fibrosis. *Respiration* 2013; 85: 456–463.
21. Raghu G, Nathan SD, Behr J, *et al.* Pulmonary hypertension in idiopathic pulmonary fibrosis with mild-to-moderate restriction. *Eur Respir J* 2015; 46: 1370–1377.
22. Weitzenblum E, Sautegeau A, Ehrhart M, *et al.* Long-term course of pulmonary arterial pressure in chronic obstructive pulmonary disease. *Am Rev Respir Dis* 1984; 130: 993–998.
23. Lettieri CJ, Nathan SD, Barnett SD, *et al.* Prevalence and outcomes of pulmonary arterial hypertension in advanced idiopathic pulmonary fibrosis. *Chest* 2006; 129: 746–752.
24. Nathan SD, Shlobin OA, Ahmad S, *et al.* Serial development of pulmonary hypertension in patients with idiopathic pulmonary fibrosis. *Respiration* 2008; 76: 288–294.
25. Minai OA, Santacruz JF, Alster JM, *et al.* Impact of pulmonary hemodynamics on 6-min walk test in idiopathic pulmonary fibrosis. *Respir Med* 2012; 106: 1613–1621.
26. Hyldgaard C, Hilberg O, Bendstrup E. How does comorbidity influence survival in idiopathic pulmonary fibrosis? *Respir Med* 2014; 108: 647–653.
27. Raghu G, Amatto VC, Behr J, *et al.* Comorbidities in idiopathic pulmonary fibrosis patients: a systematic literature review. *Eur Respir J* 2015; 46: 1113–1130.
28. Raghu G, Rochwerg B, Zhang Y, *et al.* An Official ATS/ERS/JRS/ALAT Clinical Practice Guideline: Treatment of Idiopathic Pulmonary Fibrosis. An Update of the 2011 Clinical Practice Guideline. *Am J Respir Crit Care Med* 2015; 192: e3–19.
29. Kondoh Y, Taniguchi H, Kitaichi M, *et al.* Acute exacerbation of interstitial pneumonia following surgical lung biopsy. *Respir Med* 2006; 100: 1753–1759.

30. Martinez FJ, Safrin S, Weycker D, *et al.* The clinical course of patients with idiopathic pulmonary fibrosis. *Ann Intern Med* 2005; 142: 963–967.

31. Bjoraker JA, Ryu JH, Edwin MK, *et al.* Prognostic significance of histopathologic subsets in idiopathic pulmonary fibrosis. *Am J Respir Crit Care Med* 1998; 157: 199–203.

32. Nadrous HF, Pellikka PA, Krowka MJ, *et al.* Pulmonary hypertension in patients with idiopathic pulmonary fibrosis. *Chest* 2005; 128: 2393–2399.

33. Corte TJ, Wort SJ, Gatzoulis MA, *et al.* Pulmonary vascular resistance predicts early mortality in patients with diffuse fibrotic lung disease and suspected pulmonary hypertension. *Thorax* 2009; 64: 883–888.

34. Collard HR, Moore BB, Flaherty KR, *et al.* Acute exacerbations of idiopathic pulmonary fibrosis. *Am J Respir Crit Care Med* 2007; 176: 636–643.

35. Judge EP, Fabre A, Adamali HI, *et al.* Acute exacerbations and pulmonary hypertension in advanced idiopathic pulmonary fibrosis. *Eur Respir J* 2012; 40: 93–100.

36. Abraham AS, Cole RB, Green ID, *et al.* Factors contributing to the reversible pulmonary hypertension of patients with acute respiratory failure studies by serial observations during recovery. *Circ Res* 1969; 24: 51–60.

37. Zisman DA, Karlamangla AS, Kawut SM, *et al.* Validation of a method to screen for pulmonary hypertension in advanced idiopathic pulmonary fibrosis. *Chest* 2008; 133: 640–645.

38. Leuchte HH, Neurohr C, Baumgartner R, *et al.* Brain natriuretic peptide and exercise capacity in lung fibrosis and pulmonary hypertension. *Am J Respir Crit Care Med* 2004; 170: 360–365.

39. Leuchte HH, Baumgartner RA, Nounou ME, *et al.* Brain natriuretic peptide is a prognostic parameter in chronic lung disease. *Am J Respir Crit Care Med* 2006; 173: 744–750.

40. Arcasoy SM, Christie JD, Ferrari VA, *et al.* Echocardiographic assessment of pulmonary hypertension in patients with advanced lung disease. *Am J Respir Crit Care Med* 2003; 167: 735–740.

41. Nathan SD, Shlobin OA, Barnett SD, *et al.* Right ventricular systolic pressure by echocardiography as a predictor of pulmonary hypertension in idiopathic pulmonary fibrosis. *Respir Med* 2008; 102: 1305–1310.

42. Nathan SD, Shlobin OA, Ahmad S, *et al.* Pulmonary hypertension and pulmonary function testing in idiopathic pulmonary fibrosis. *Chest* 2007; 131: 657–663.

43. Corte TJ, Wort SJ, MacDonald PS, *et al.* Pulmonary function vascular index predicts prognosis in idiopathic interstitial pneumonia. *Respirology* 2012; 17: 674–680.

44. Wells AU, Desai SR, Rubens MB, *et al.* Idiopathic pulmonary fibrosis: a composite physiologic index derived from disease extent observed by computed tomography. *Am J Respir Crit Care Med* 2003; 167: 962–969.

45. Sun XG, Hansen JE, Oudiz RJ, *et al.* Exercise pathophysiology in patients with primary pulmonary hypertension. *Circulation* 2001; 104: 429–435.

46. Boutou AK, Pitsiou GG, Trigonis I, *et al.* Exercise capacity in idiopathic pulmonary fibrosis: the effect of pulmonary hypertension. *Respirology* 2011; 16: 451–458.

47. Ng CS, Wells AU, Padley SP. A CT sign of chronic pulmonary arterial hypertension: the ratio of main pulmonary artery to aortic diameter. *J Thorac Imaging* 1999; 14: 270–278.

48. Devaraj A, Wells AU, Meister MG, *et al.* The effect of diffuse pulmonary fibrosis on the reliability of CT signs of pulmonary hypertension. *Radiology* 2008; 249: 1042–1049.

49. Devaraj A, Wells AU, Meister MG, *et al.* Detection of pulmonary hypertension with multidetector CT and echocardiography alone and in combination. *Radiology* 2010; 254: 609–616.

50. Ruocco G, Cekorja B, Rottoli P, *et al.* Role of BNP and echo measurement for pulmonary hypertension recognition in patients with interstitial lung disease: an algorithm application model. *Respir Med* 2015; 109: 406–415.

51. Seeger W, Adir Y, Barberà JA, *et al.* Pulmonary hypertension in chronic lung diseases. *J Am Coll Cardiol* 2013; 62: 25 Suppl, D109–D116.

52. Lange TJ, Baron M, Seiler I, *et al.* Outcome of patients with severe PH due to lung disease with and without targeted therapy. *Cardiovasc Ther* 2014; 32: 202–208.

53. Brewis MJ, Church AC, Johnson MK, *et al.* Severe pulmonary hypertension in lung disease: phenotypes and response to treatment. *Eur Respir J* 2015; 46: 1378–1389.

54. Hoeper MM, Behr J, Held M, *et al.* Pulmonary hypertension in patients with chronic fibrosing idiopathic interstitial pneumonias. *PLoS One* 2015; 10: e0141911.

55. Olschewski H, Ghofrani HA, Walmrath D, *et al.* Inhaled prostacyclin and iloprost in severe pulmonary hypertension secondary to lung fibrosis. *Am J Respir Crit Care Med* 1999; 160: 600–607.

56. Ghofrani HA, Wiedemann R, Rose F, *et al.* Sildenafil for treatment of lung fibrosis and pulmonary hypertension: a randomised controlled trial. *Lancet* 2002; 360: 895–900.

57. Collard HR, Anstrom KJ, Schwarz MI, *et al.* Sildenafil improves walk distance in idiopathic pulmonary fibrosis. *Chest* 2007; 131: 897–899.

58. Idiopathic Pulmonary Fibrosis Clinical Research Network, Zisman DA, Schwarz M, *et al.* A controlled trial of sildenafil in advanced idiopathic pulmonary fibrosis. *N Engl J Med* 2010; 363: 620–628.

59. Han MK, Bach DS, Hagan PG, *et al.* Sildenafil preserves exercise capacity in patients with idiopathic pulmonary fibrosis and right-sided ventricular dysfunction. *Chest* 2013; 143: 1699–1708.

60. Zimmermann GS, von Wulffen W, Huppmann P, *et al.* Haemodynamic changes in pulmonary hypertension in patients with interstitial lung disease treated with PDE-5 inhibitors. *Respirology* 2014; 19: 700–706.
61. Hoeper MM, Halank M, Wilkens H, *et al.* Riociguat for interstitial lung disease and pulmonary hypertension: a pilot trial. *Eur Respir J* 2013; 41: 853–860.
62. Bayer. Efficacy and Safety of Riociguat in Patients With Symptomatic Pulmonary Hypertension (PH) Associated With Idiopathic Interstitial Pneumonias (IIP) (RISE-IIP). NCT02138825. https://clinicaltrials.gov/ct2/show/NCT02138825?term=riociguat+and+Idiopathic+Interstitial+Pneumonias&rank=1 Date last accessed: February 4, 2016. Date last updated: January 11, 2016.
63. King TE, Brown KK, Raghu G, *et al.* BUILD-3: a randomized, controlled trial of bosentan in idiopathic pulmonary fibrosis. *Am J Respir Crit Care Med* 2011; 184: 92–99.
64. Corte TJ, Keir GJ, Dimopoulos K, *et al.* Bosentan in pulmonary hypertension associated with fibrotic idiopathic interstitial pneumonia. *Am J Respir Crit Care Med* 2014; 190: 208–217.
65. Grimminger F, Günther A, Vancheri C. The role of tyrosine kinases in the pathogenesis of idiopathic pulmonary fibrosis. *Eur Respir J* 2015; 45: 1426–1433.
66. Daniels CE, Lasky JA, Limper AH, *et al.* Imatinib treatment for idiopathic pulmonary fibrosis: randomized placebo-controlled trial results. *Am J Respir Crit Care Med* 2010; 181: 604–610.
67. Humbert M. Impression, sunset. *Circulation* 2013; 127: 1098–1100.
68. Hoeper MM, Barst RJ, Bourge RC, *et al.* Imatinib mesylate as add-on therapy for pulmonary arterial hypertension: results of the randomized IMPRES study. *Circulation* 2013; 127: 1128–1138.
69. Frost AE, Barst RJ, Hoeper MM, *et al.* Long-term safety and efficacy of imatinib in pulmonary arterial hypertension. *J Heart Lung Transplant* 2015; 34: 1366–1375.
70. Montani D, Bergot E, Günther S, *et al.* Pulmonary arterial hypertension in patients treated by dasatinib. *Circulation* 2012; 125: 2128–2137.
71. Simonneau G, Gatzoulis MA, Adatia I, *et al.* Updated clinical classification of pulmonary hypertension. *J Am Coll Cardiol* 2013; 62: 25 Suppl, D34–D41.
72. Holland AE, Hill CJ, Conron M, *et al.* Short term improvement in exercise capacity and symptoms following exercise training in interstitial lung disease. *Thorax* 2008; 63: 549–554.
73. Nishiyama O, Kondoh Y, Kimura T, *et al.* Effects of pulmonary rehabilitation in patients with idiopathic pulmonary fibrosis. *Respirology* 2008; 13: 394–399.
74. Raghu G, Collard HR, Egan JJ, *et al.* An official ATS/ERS/JRS/ALAT statement: idiopathic pulmonary fibrosis: evidence-based guidelines for diagnosis and management. *Am J Respir Crit Care Med* 2011; 183: 788–824.
75. Huppmann P, Sczepanski B, Boensch M, *et al.* Effects of inpatient pulmonary rehabilitation in patients with interstitial lung disease. *Eur Respir J* 2013; 42: 444–453.
76. Whelan TPM, Dunitz JM, Kelly RF, *et al.* Effect of preoperative pulmonary artery pressure on early survival after lung transplantation for idiopathic pulmonary fibrosis. *J Heart Lung Transplant* 2005; 24: 1269–1274.
77. Fang A, Studer S, Kawut SM, *et al.* Elevated pulmonary artery pressure is a risk factor for primary graft dysfunction following lung transplantation for idiopathic pulmonary fibrosis. *Chest* 2011; 139: 782–787.

Disclosures: S.J. Wort reports grants and personal fees from Actelion Pharmaceuticals and Bayer, and personal fees from GSK. M. Humbert reports grants and personal fees from Actelion, Bayer and GSK, and personal fees from Novartis and Pfizer. D. Montani reports grants and personal fees from Actelion and Bayer, and personal fees from BMS, GSK, Novartis and Pfizer outside the submitted.

Acknowledgements: The authors would like to thank P. Dorfmüller and M-R. Ghigna (Service d'anatomopathologie, Centre Chirurgical Marie Lannelongue, Le Plessis-Robinson, France) for the histology image.

Chapter 14

CPFE: distinctive and non-distinctive features

Athol U. Wells[1], George A. Margaritopoulos[1], Katerina M. Antoniou[2], Hilario Nunes[3] and Ulrich Costabel[4]

Emphysema is highly prevalent in patients with IPF. However, the question of whether CPFE should be viewed as a syndrome or merely as the coincidental existence of two disease processes remains uncertain. Distinctive pathogenetic features have yet to be demonstrated in CPFE. It is unclear whether observed mortality trends and the reported high prevalence of PH are specific CPFE characteristics or merely reflect a greater reduction in pulmonary reserve due to the coexistence of two processes. No data currently exist to suggest that, in CPFE, pulmonary fibrosis is more progressive or that the presence of PH results from a unique microvascular phenotype. Thus, CPFE syndrome designation is not, at this stage, justified by proven pathogenetic insights or prognostic utility. The strongest current argument for a CPFE syndrome relates to the definition of disease progression in treatment trials and clinical practice, with emerging data suggesting that CPFE has an important confounding effect on serial FVC trends.

In clinical series of patients with IPF, concurrent smoking-related emphysema is present on HRCT in up to 40% of cases. The association was first recognised in the medical literature in 1990 [1], but it was not until well after the millennium that it was first suggested that CPFE should be viewed as a discrete syndrome [2]. The purpose of this chapter is to review the clinical and pathogenetic implications of the entity of CPFE, with particular regard to its validity as a discrete syndrome, and to explore current uncertainties in its definition and evaluation.

Historical perspective

IPF is generally viewed as a classic restrictive disorder, characterised by reductions in TLC and FVC, a lesser reduction in FEV1 and an increased FEV1/FVC ratio. Quantified as percentages of predicted normal values, D_{LCO} levels tend to be 10–25% lower than measures of lung volume, including FVC. Carbon monoxide uptake per unit alveolar volume, quantified as the transfer coefficient of the lung for carbon monoxide (K_{CO}, synonymous

[1]Interstitial Lung Disease Unit, Royal Brompton Hospital, London, London, UK. [2]Dept of Thoracic Medicine, Medical School, University of Crete, Heraklion, Greece. [3]Service de Pneumologie, Hôpital Avicenne, Bobigny, France. [4]Ruhrlandklinik, Westdeutsches Lungenzentrum, am Universitätsklinikum, Essen, Germany.

Correspondence: Athol U. Wells, Interstitial Lung Disease Unit, Royal Brompton Hospital, Sydney St, London, SW3 6NP, UK.
E-mail: RBHILD@rbht.nhs.uk

with D_{LCO}/alveolar volume) is usually low, in the normal range or slightly reduced in IPF, in the absence of concurrent emphysema or pulmonary vasculopathy.

In 1990, WIGGINS *et al.* [1] reported a small series of IPF patients characterised by concurrent smoking-related emphysema and a unique pulmonary function phenotype, consisting of a misleading preservation of lung volumes (median FVC 98.7%, range 68–131%) in association with a devastating reduction in gas transfer (median D_{LCO} 32%, range 9–35%). In this early series, outcome was not reported. The severe D_{LCO} reduction was ascribed to the combined impact of the two disease processes although the spurious preservation of lung volumes was not, at first, well understood.

In 1993, STRICKLAND *et al.* [3] evaluated the well-recognised phenomenon in IPF of false positive diagnoses of pulmonary embolism due to the presence, on ventilation–perfusion scintigraphy, of prominent areas with normal ventilation but absent perfusion. HRCT scanning, performed concurrently with scintigraphy, showed conclusively that the pulmonary embolism-like scintigraphic abnormalities were due to areas of honeycombing or, less frequently, areas of bullous emphysematous change that were ventilated normally (unlike emphysematous abnormalities in patients with COPD). These findings can be explained by traction on small airways due to interstitial fibrosis, preventing the typical small airway collapse characteristic of smoking-related emphysema and resulting in preserved ventilation of areas of bullous destruction (and a corresponding overall increase in measured lung volumes).

In 1997, in a comparison between 54 IPF patients and 14 patients with CPFE, the separate pulmonary function consequences of ILD and emphysema were quantified [4]. After adjustment for the extent of ILD (scored using a reproducible HRCT scoring system), the presence of emphysema was associated with preservation of lung volumes (a 5–10% increase, on average) and a greater reduction in D_{LCO} and K_{CO}, by 15% and 35%, respectively. The K_{CO} effect was especially striking, with concurrent emphysema much more influential than the extent of IPF as a determinant of the reduction in K_{CO}. Importantly, on multivariate analysis, after the extent of IPF in HRCT and the presence of emphysema had been taken into account, the smoking history had no independent effect on pulmonary function impairment.

The study discussed above led directly to the development, in 2003, of a composite physiological index (CPI) in a prospective evaluation of 212 consecutive IPF patients (including 89 with concurrent emphysema) [5]. The CPI, derived in 112 patients and tested in 112 patients, was found to correlate more strongly with the extent of IPF on HRCT and to predict survival more accurately than individual pulmonary function variables. The CPI formula $(91.0-(0.65 \times D_{LCO} \text{ % pred})-(0.53 \times FVC \text{ % pred})+(0.34 \times FEV_1 \text{ % pred}))$ expressed the combination of pulmonary function variables that captured the functional impact of IPF while excluding the functional consequences of emphysema. Reverse weighting of FEV_1 played a crucial role in this regard. Lower D_{LCO} and FVC levels resulted in higher CPI values. However, with FVC included in the equation, lower FEV_1 levels (resulting in lower CPI scores) were indicative of a less restrictive FEV_1/FVC ratio, in keeping with the additional loss of D_{LCO} due to concurrent emphysema. Thus, the CPI can be viewed as an adjusted D_{LCO} level, quantifying the reduction in D_{LCO} due to IPF while excluding the reduction in D_{LCO} due to emphysema. This conclusion was confirmed in a sub-analysis of patients without concurrent emphysema: CPI and D_{LCO} levels were strikingly similar both in correlating with the extent of IPF on HRCT and in predicting survival.

Findings in the CPI study did not change when the analysis was confined to patients meeting American Thoracic Society (ATS)/European Respiratory Society (ERS) diagnostic criteria for IPF, following the 2002 reclassification of the IIPs [6], suggesting that the CPFE pulmonary function phenotype applies equally to IPF and to other idiopathic fibrotic disorders (such as fibrotic NSIP). Another important observation was that despite the inclusion of some patients with moderately extensive emphysema, overt airflow obstruction was not present in any case in the CPI cohort. It appears that unless emphysema is clearly the predominant disease process, FEV1/FVC ratios associated with the presence of emphysema tend to be normal or less restrictive than in isolated pulmonary fibrosis, but are not generally reduced. Thus, the exclusion criteria applied in most recent IPF treatment trials (*e.g.* an FEV1/FVC ratio <70%) do not exclude a significant sub-group of IPF patients with extensive emphysema on HRCT.

Up to this point in time, CPFE had been viewed as the coincidental coexistence of IPF and emphysema, with a common pathogenetic linkage to smoking. In 2005, in a mouse model of tumour necrosis factor-α overexpression, Lundblad *et al.* [7] reported morphological abnormalities consistent with both pulmonary fibrosis and emphysema, in association with generalised lung inflammation. The authors concluded that their findings did not model any single human disease but this prompted immediate disagreement from Cottin and Cordier [8], who argued that the experimental model reinforced the recognition of CPFE as an "under-recognised syndrome". Earlier in 2005, Cottin *et al.* [2] had reported a retrospective analysis of 61 patients with emphysema, predominantly in the upper zones, and fibrotic ILD, predominantly in the lower zones. The characteristic pulmonary function phenotype described previously was confirmed in this series as a defining feature of CPFE and, in addition, PH was diagnosed at presentation in 54% of patients and was a malignant prognostic determinant. The authors concluded that the characteristic functional profile, taken together with their observation of a high prevalence of PH, provided support for "the individualisation of… (CPFE as a discrete entity)… apart from both idiopathic pulmonary fibrosis and pulmonary emphysema" [2]. Cottin and Cordier [9] subsequently nuanced their views in an eloquent 2009 editorial, arguing that "The syndrome of combined pulmonary fibrosis and emphysema (CPFE) is not just a distinct phenotype of IPF. It deserves the terminology of syndrome as a result of the association of symptoms and clinical manifestations, each with a probability of being present increased by the presence of the other".

In the intervening period, Mura *et al.* [10] provided further confirmation, in 2006, of the characteristic functional profile of CPFE. In a study of 21 patients with IPF and emphysema, compared with 21 patients with IPF but no emphysema, the presence of emphysema had a significant independent effect on lung volumes, measures of gas transfer, 6MWT data and the severity of exertional dyspnoea. The CPI was closely related to the extent of IPF on HRCT and also to the dyspnoea score.

Some of the many subsequent series in which patients with CPFE are included, cited later in this chapter, provide arguments for and against the designation of CPFE as a discrete syndrome. Given that syndrome status was first proposed for the entity of CPFE more than 10 years ago, it is perhaps surprising that in a recent European-wide IPF meeting no overall consensus on this question could be reached, based on audience voting, with the "uncertain" response easily the most popular option. In order to address this issue, it is necessary to first consider the larger question of the level of evidence required to justify syndrome designation.

Justification for the designation of a clinical entity as a syndrome

A syndrome, as classically defined, consists of a disease or disorder that involves a particular group of signs and symptoms. However, the acceptance of a syndrome requires a greater provenance than the mere recognition of an association, be it between clinical variables or underlying disease processes. Patients with lung cancer are most commonly smokers and a large proportion have concurrent smoking-related emphysema: however, there is no current support for a lung cancer and emphysema syndrome. IPF and emphysema are both linked to smoking and it is inevitable that clinicians should frequently encounter patients with both diseases. In ILD, the complex diagnostic terminology is a major problem for patients and less experienced doctors: the addition of yet another acronym (CPFE) to this field requires the justification of added value. To gain acceptance, it is generally accepted that a proposed syndrome must provide either clinical utility (*i.e.* serve as an aid to diagnosis, prognostic evaluation or management) or pathogenetic insights (*i.e.* underlying pathogenetic mechanisms unique to the syndrome are present), providing an avenue for the development of new therapies.

Issues in the diagnosis and quantification of disease

The term "CPFE" can be applied to a large number of individual ILDs in which emphysema coexists with fibrosis, but in idiopathic disease it applies to patients with fibrotic IIP. However, this group of diseases includes patients with IPF, fibrotic NSIP and unclassifiable disease. This complicates the evaluation of the prognostic significance of CPFE: based on well-established differences in outcome, it can be expected that survival will be better in NSIP–CPFE patients than in IPF–CPFE patients. Thus, it is likely that prognostic distinctions between IPF and CPFE, examined in a number of studies, will be influenced by the proportion of patients with NSIP in the CPFE group, going some way to explain the discrepancies in outcome findings discussed later in this chapter. While NSIP is less prevalent than IPF, and the majority of patients with NSIP are nonsmokers [11], CPFE is frequent in current or former smokers with NSIP (14 out of 18 smokers with NSIP in one series [12]).

In some series, an attempt is made to examine CPFE specifically in patients with IPF. However, this goal is complicated by the lack of histological confirmation of UIP in most CPFE patients with suspected IPF: surgical biopsies are seldom performed in this patient group due to the greater reduction in gas transfer than in IPF patients with emphysema and the high prevalence of PH. The diagnosis of IPF is mostly based upon HRCT appearance, but herein lies a difficulty unique to CPFE: the discrimination between true honeycomb changes (required for an HRCT diagnosis of IPF) and the admixture of emphysema and pulmonary fibrosis, in which "pseudo-honeycomb change" is observed, is a major difficulty. In a recent study of inter-observer variation between 112 observers using the current ATS/ERS/Japanese Respiratory Society/Latin American Thoracic Association criteria for a diagnosis of UIP, agreement was only moderate on the overall HRCT pattern and also on the presence and absence of both emphysema and honeycombing [13]. Thus, it appears inevitable that even in series of IPF patients with CPFE, some diagnostic contamination is unavoidable.

Exactly the same constraint applies to the quantification of emphysema. In patients with CPFE, emphysema often merges imperceptibly with pulmonary fibrosis in the mid zones and the quantification of emphysema, as opposed to honeycombing, is not straightforward.

In many series, little or no attempt is made to quantify emphysema: cardinal analyses are based on the presence, rather than the extent, of emphysema. The current consensus is that density masking, often advocated for emphysema quantification, is poorly suited for use in CPFE. Density masking cannot discriminate between low density areas due to emphysema and areas of similarly low density doe to honeycomb cysts or traction bronchiectasis. In over 40 published manuscripts exploring the entity of CPFE, density masking has been attempted in only five series [14–18], mostly in an effort to examination functional–morphological correlations.

Definitive prognostic evaluation of CPFE, with particular reference to comparisons between CPFE and isolated pulmonary fibrosis, requires quantification of both pulmonary fibrosis and emphysema. It cannot be assumed that pulmonary fibrosis will be similarly extensive in both patient groups. Even within the entity of CPFE, significant extent differences exist: CPFE patients with IPF have been observed to have more extensive fibrosis than CPFE patients with other forms of UIP (mostly rheumatoid arthritis, systemic sclerosis and asbestosis) [19]. In another series, patients with CPFE had significantly less extensive pulmonary fibrosis than IPF patients without emphysema [20]. This finding appears logical as patients present when symptoms become significant. For example, when pulmonary reserve is impaired due to pre-existing emphysema, exercise limitation will be associated with less extensive fibrosis than in patients with isolated pulmonary fibrosis. However, an important caveat exists in the interpretation of this series: CPFE was diagnosed only when the extent of emphysema on HRCT was greater than 10% of the lung volume. The application of the 10% threshold, with the designation of patients with less extensive emphysema as non-CPFE patients, was wholly arbitrary and is not generally accepted (although agreement on what constitutes "trivial emphysema" may appear desirable). The use of this threshold may explain the discrepancy with a recent series, in which the extent of fibrosis did not differ significantly between patients with CPFE and those with isolated pulmonary fibrosis [16].

Prognostic significance of CPFE

As discussed earlier, CPFE was initially reported to have a poor prognosis (which was worse than in most historical series of pulmonary fibrosis) [2]. This observation was confirmed in some subsequent series, with CPFE sub-groups mostly or wholly made up of IPF patients [16, 18, 21–23]. However, in other series, mortality was reported to be similar in CPFE and in isolated pulmonary fibrosis [20, 24] or was lower in patients with CPFE [25–27]. These differences are difficult to rationalise, but possible explanations include diagnostic contamination (with a higher proportion of NSIP cases in CPFE populations with better survival) and differences in the selection of patients with CPFE. It is not clear whether, in series with better CPFE outcomes, patients with more extensive emphysema than fibrosis, including those with trivial fibrosis, are overrepresented. It is also possible that variations in the baseline severity of pulmonary function impairment may be influential in survival analyses, although the characteristic pulmonary function profile of CPFE described in early series, consisting of relative preservation of lung volumes and greater reduction in D_{LCO} levels, have been repeatedly confirmed [14, 17, 20, 22, 23–28].

Given the discordance between outcomes discussed above, it is difficult to argue that a proposed CPFE syndrome is strongly supported by mortality analyses. The difficulty lies in the failure, in most series, to adjust survival models for baseline D_{LCO} levels (capturing the combined functional impact of emphysema, fibrosis and PH and, in this way, quantifying and excluding excess mortality due to greater loss of pulmonary reserve). The unresolved question is whether IPF progresses more rapidly when there is concurrent emphysema, or whether progression is similar in IPF and in IPF–CPFE, with mortality primarily linked to baseline severity. What data exists in this regard seems to suggest that ILD progression differs little between the two sub-groups. In IPF cohorts of 110 and 249 patients, respectively, survival was not influenced by the presence of emphysema, after adjusting for the severity of ILD as judged by pulmonary function variables and the presence of PH [23] or as judged by pulmonary function variables and HRCT scoring of disease extent [29]. Conflicting information exists on serial changes in FVC and D_{LCO}. In one cohort, the 3-year change in both variables did not differ between IPF and IPF–CPFE [30], but in another series, patients with IPF–CPFE were characterised by less decline in FVC and D_{LCO} than that observed in IPF patients without emphysema [31]. In one recent series, the intriguing observation was made, using quantitative HRCT imaging, that in CPFE serial HRCT change mostly results from an increase in emphysema (as quantified by automated scoring of areas of low lung density) [15]. However, it is uncertain whether this finding represents increasing emphysema due to fibrotic traction, worsening honeycombing (with honeycomb cysts scored as "emphysema" using density thresholds) or, as seems likely, a combination of both.

At the time of writing, less rapid FVC decline has been reported in abstract form in CPFE–IPF patients, compared with IPF patients without emphysema, in two pharmaceutical cohorts. Although critical scrutiny of these data must await peer-reviewed publication, the possibility that serial changes in FVC, now the favoured primary end-point in IPF treatment trials, may be confounded by concurrent emphysema has major implications for future IPF trial design. The inclusion criteria in the ASCEND (Assessment of pirfenidone to confirm efficacy and safety in idiopathic pulmonary fibrosis) trial of pirfenidone in IPF [32] were designed to exclude patients with a significant functional impact from concurrent emphysema (*i.e.* an overtly restrictive FEV1/FVC ratio was required). Confirmation that CPFE is characterised by less rapid FVC decline would also have important implications for the routine monitoring of IPF, both in the identification of disease progression and in prognostic evaluation. In IPF cohorts, containing patients with and without emphysema, serial FVC trends have consistently predicted mortality. However, in IPF–CPFE patients with moderate-to-severe emphysema on HRCT, significant declines in FEV1 (>10%) over 12 months were the only pulmonary function trends predictive of mortality in one series [33].

CPFE and concurrent disease processes

PH was a highly prevalent association with CPFE in an early report [2], as discussed earlier, and this finding was examined in greater detail in two well characterised cohorts. In the series of MEJIA *et al.* [23], emphysema was present in 31 (28%) out of 110 IPF patients. Severe PH (pulmonary artery systolic pressure >75 mmHg) was present in 21 (72%) out of 29 CPFE patients undergoing echocardiography, compared with only eight (12%) out of 68 IPF patients without emphysema and was a malignant prognostic determinant, which, taken together with the greater pulmonary impairment in CPFE patients, accounted for the higher mortality associated with CPFE in this series. In a subsequent evaluation of 40 patients with IPF–CPFE and PH proven at right heart catheterisation, the outcome was poor with a mortality of 40% at 1 year: higher pulmonary vascular resistance, higher heart rate, lower cardiac index and lower D_{LCO} levels were associated with shorter survival [34].

Recent data from a retrospective case-matched evaluation have indicated that the risk of lung cancer is higher in patients with CPFE than in those with emphysema (although the lung cancer risk did not differ significantly between CPFE and IPF without associated emphysema) [35]. In keeping with this finding is the observation that in lung cancer patients, CPFE was significantly more frequent than pulmonary fibrosis in isolation (8.9% *versus* 1.3%), although emphysema without coexisting pulmonary fibrosis was much more prevalent (35.3%) [36]. The association between lung cancer and CPFE is important clinically because it impacts on cancer management. In a series of 47 CPFE patients with lung cancer, standard of care cancer treatment (as recommended in international guidelines) could not be instituted in 20 cases, including eight cases in which limitations in treatment were directly related to the presence of CPFE [37]. There is conflicting information about the prognostic significance of CPFE in patients receiving therapy for lung cancer. In 365 patients undergoing resection of nonsmall cell lung cancer, the presence of CPFE was found to be an independent predictor of worse survival [38]. However, in an evaluation of the whole range of cancer therapies in 1536 patients with lung cancer of all types, the presence of CPFE was not an independent prognostic factor [39].

CPFE in connective tissue diseases

CPFE was first reported in connective tissue disease in 34 patients with rheumatoid arthritis (n=18), systemic sclerosis (n=10) or other disorders (n=6) [40]. Morphological and pulmonary function abnormalities were similar to those documented in idiopathic CPFE. In all cases, there was emphysema in the upper zones and pulmonary fibrosis in the lower zones on HRCT. Patients with CPFE had relatively preserved lung volumes and lower measures of gas transfer compared with patients with pulmonary fibrosis in isolation. Four patients were lifelong nonsmokers a fact that was not emphasised in this manuscript, but was highly relevant to the findings in a subsequent large cohort of 333 patients with systemic sclerosis-related ILD [41]. Emphysema was present in 41 cases (12.3%), including in 26 (19.7%) out of 132 current or former smokers and 15 (7.5%) out of 201 lifelong nonsmokers. After adjustment for the extent of fibrosis on HRCT, emphysema was associated with an average additional reduction of 24.1% from baseline DLCO levels and an increase of 34.8% in the FVC/DLCO ratio, but there was no overall significant effect on FVC levels. These effects did not differ between smokers and nonsmokers, and on multivariate analysis PFTs were not influenced by either smoking status or the total pack-year smoking dose, after adjustment for the extent of pulmonary fibrosis or the presence of emphysema. Emphysema was generally limited in extent, with half of the patients having trivial disease (*i.e.* <5% of the total lung volume on HRCT). However, measures of gas transfer were significantly more impaired, even in patients with trivial emphysema, than in systemic sclerosis patients with pulmonary fibrosis in isolation. These findings were especially relevant to the recently proposed DETECT algorithm [42], in which an elevated FVC/DLCO ratio is one of several criteria proceeding echocardiography in screening for PH. In the study by Antoniou *et al.* [41], the FVC/DLCO ratio was confounded by the presence of emphysema and was not a reliable marker for echocardiographic features of PH.

The sporadic presence of emphysema in lifelong nonsmokers with systemic sclerosis-associated ILD (prevalence 7.5%, 95% CI 4–12% [41]) must be interpreted with caution in the absence of a control cohort of healthy nonsmoking adults. However, in a study of 12 368 lifelong nonsmokers, the prevalence of emphysema on CT was <2% [43], suggesting an increased predilection for emphysema in systemic sclerosis. Similarly, there is a surprisingly high prevalence of emphysema in current or former smokers with rheumatoid lung [44]. Taken together with the low pack-year smoking histories associated with CPFE in smokers with both rheumatoid arthritis and systemic sclerosis, the observations in these studies raise the possibility of an autoimmune contribution to emphysema pathogenesis.

Pathogenetic considerations

Thus far, no primary pathogenetic pathways unique to CPFE have been identified. A number of pathways common to pulmonary fibrosis and emphysema have been identified, including oxidative stress, protein citrullination and matrix metalloproteinase imbalance. Emphysema on HRCT was found to be approximately five-fold more prevalent than expected, after adjustment for age, gender and pack-year smoking history, in IPF and rheumatoid lung, compared with smokers without pulmonary fibrosis [44]. In both diseases and in systemic sclerosis-associated ILD, the pack-year smoking history associated with the presence of emphysema was lower than reported in a large cohort of smokers [41, 44]. Thus, it appears that all three fibrosing diseases cluster with the presence of emphysema, raising the possibility of a shared predilection triggered by smoking in a subset of patients with ILD. Also in favour of linked pathogenesis is the observation that short telomeres lower the threshold of cigarette smoke-induced damage in a model of telomerase null mice, and may contribute to age-related onset of emphysema in humans [45]. In the same paper the authors identified a family with a deletion in the Box H domain of TERC, including the proband affected with emphysema, her father with IPF and her sister with CPFE. A family has been reported with both fibrotic IIPs and/or emphysema, including one case with pathologically proven NSIP, one with CPFE and one with isolated emphysema [46]. Similarly, CPFE has been described in familial surfactant protein C mutation [47].

However, if a pathogenetic CPFE syndrome exists, it is questionable whether it will be applicable to all patients with CPFE. Inevitably, despite the phenomenon of clustering of emphysema with pulmonary fibrosis, the two diseases will coexist in some patients simply as coincidental smoking-related processes. The definition of a patient group with a unique pathogenetic pathway is likely to require careful morphological evaluation of histopathological and HRCT features. In a recent autopsy study, thick-walled cystic lesions (with emphysematous destruction and surrounding dense wall fibrosis) were present histologically in over 70% of patients with CPFE, but were never observed in patients with either isolated pulmonary fibrosis or isolated emphysema [48]. Patterns of emphysema on HRCT in CPFE have been classified into three broad groups: 1) progressive transition with diffuse emphysema and a zone of transition between bullae and honeycombing; 2) paraseptal emphysema with predominant subpleural bullae (enlarging in size at the bases); and 3) separate processes with discrete areas of fibrosis and emphysema [49]. Much work remains to be done to define CPFE morphological sub-types, but without this the identification of signature pathogenetic pathways may be difficult to achieve.

Is a discrete CPFE syndrome justified?

Currently, the proposed CPFE syndrome cannot be defended on pathogenetic grounds, although the authors strongly suspect that key pathogenetic pathways will emerge, based on the high prevalence of emphysema in smokers with IPF and rheumatoid lung. However, currently, the acceptance of a CPFE syndrome is dependent on its perceived clinical utility. It is difficult to argue that the syndrome is justified based on its mortality, given the conflicting outcomes found in comparisons with isolated IPF in a number of series.

It can be argued that the high prevalence of PH justifies a syndrome designation, if the practical consequence is the earlier identification of this lethal complication. However, this view would carry more weight if an effective PH treatment existed, shown to prolong life expectancy in ILD. Furthermore, no evidence exists indicating that ILD in IPF–CPFE patients should be managed differently from IPF patients without emphysema: both patient subsets were included in the recent successful antifibrotic treatment trials.

The strongest argument for a syndrome may relate to monitoring of disease progression in patients with CPFE, given the recent advent of antifibrotic agents and the need to identify progressive disease accurately in individual cases. Serial FVC trends, which are generally viewed as the cardinal monitoring measure in IPF, may be less reliable in IPF–CPFE, with a lower prognostic significance than in the remaining IPF patients. If endorsed at peer review, emerging information based on analyses of pharmaceutical cohorts may lead to the use of different primary end-points in future trials of CPFE patients.

Taken in their entirety, the considerations summarised above suggest that CPFE is, at the very least, a "nearly syndrome". The authors believe that it is possible, based on either clinical utility or pathogenetic considerations, that justification for a syndrome will emerge, perhaps in the near future if a treatment effect is proven in PH in IPF and a designated CPFE syndrome facilitates earlier recognition of PH and, thus, earlier intervention. However, it is important that syndrome designation should be endorsed by expert groups, based on force of argument rather than strength of conviction.

References

1. Wiggins J, Strickland B, Turner-Warwick M. Combined cryptogenic fibrosing alveolitis and emphysema: the value of high resolution computed tomography in assessment. *Respir Med* 1990; 84: 365–369.
2. Cottin V, Nunes H, Brillet PY, *et al.* Combined pulmonary fibrosis and emphysema: a distinct underrecognised entity. *Eur Respir J* 2005; 26: 586–593.
3. Strickland NH, Hughes JM, Hart DA, *et al.* Cause of regional ventilation-perfusion mismatching in patients with idiopathic pulmonary fibrosis: a combined CT and scintigraphic study. *AJR Am J Roentgenol* 1993; 161: 719–725.
4. Wells AU, King AD, Rubens MB, *et al.* Lone cryptogenic fibrosing alveolitis: a functional-morphologic correlation based on extent of disease on thin-section computed tomography. *Am J Respir Crit Care Med* 1997; 155: 1367–1375.
5. Wells AU, Desai SR, Rubens MB, *et al.* Idiopathic pulmonary fibrosis: a composite physiologic index derived from disease extent observed by computed tomography. *Am J Respir Crit Care Med* 2003; 167: 962–969.
6. American Thoracic Society, European Respiratory Society. American Thoracic Society/European Respiratory Society international multidisciplinary consensus classification of the idiopathic interstitial pneumonias. *Am J Respir Crit Care Med* 2002; 165: 277–304.
7. Lundblad LK, Thompson-Figueroa J, Leclair T, *et al.* Tumor necrosis factor-α overexpression in lung disease: a single cause behind a complex phenotype. *Am J Respir Crit Care Med* 2005; 171: 1363–1370.
8. Cottin V, Cordier JF. Combined pulmonary fibrosis and emphysema: an experimental and clinically relevant phenotype. *Am J Respir Crit Care Med* 2005; 172: 1605–1606.
9. Cottin V, Cordier JF. The syndrome of combined pulmonary fibrosis and emphysema. *Chest* 2009; 136: 1–2.
10. Mura M, Zompatori M, Pacilli AM, *et al.* The presence of emphysema further impairs physiologic function in patients with idiopathic pulmonary fibrosis. *Respir Care* 2006; 51: 257–265.
11. Travis WD, Hunninghake G, King TE Jr, *et al.* Idiopathic nonspecific interstitial pneumonia: report of an American Thoracic Society project. *Am J Respir Crit Care Med* 2008; 177: 1338–1347.
12. Marten K, Milne D, Antoniou KM, *et al.* Non-specific interstitial pneumonia in cigarette smokers: a CT study. *Eur Radiol* 2009; 19: 1679–1685.

13. Walsh SL, Calandriello L, Sverzellati N, *et al.* Interobserver agreement for the ATS/ERS/JRS/ALAT criteria for a UIP pattern on CT. *Thorax* 2016; 71: 45–51.

14. Matsuoka S, Yamashiro T, Matsushita S, *et al.* Quantitative CT evaluation in patients with combined pulmonary fibrosis and emphysema: correlation with pulmonary function. *Acad Radiol* 2015; 22: 626–631.

15. Matsuoka S, Yamashiro T, Matsushita S, *et al.* Morphological disease progression of combined pulmonary fibrosis and emphysema: comparison with emphysema alone and pulmonary fibrosis alone. *J Comput Assist Tomogr* 2015; 39: 153–159.

16. Choi SH, Lee HY, Lee KS, *et al.* The value of CT for disease detection and prognosis determination in combined pulmonary fibrosis and emphysema (CPFE). *PLoS One* 2014; 9: e107476.

17. Ando K, Sekiya M, Tobino K, *et al.* Relationship between quantitative CT metrics and pulmonary function in combined pulmonary fibrosis and emphysema. *Lung* 2013; 191: 585–591.

18. Lee CH, Kim HJ, Park CM, *et al.* The impact of combined pulmonary fibrosis and emphysema on mortality. *Int J Tuberc Lung Dis* 2011; 15: 1111–1116.

19. Mitchell PD, Das JP, Murphy DJ, *et al.* Idiopathic pulmonary fibrosis with emphysema: evidence of synergy among emphysema and idiopathic pulmonary fibrosis in smokers. *Respir Care* 2015; 60: 259–268.

20. Ryerson CJ, Hartman T, Elicker BM, *et al.* Clinical features and outcomes in combined pulmonary fibrosis and emphysema in idiopathic pulmonary fibrosis. *Chest* 2013; 144: 234–240.

21. Sugino K, Ishida F, Kikuchi N, *et al.* Comparison of clinical characteristics and prognostic factors of combined pulmonary fibrosis and emphysema *versus* idiopathic pulmonary fibrosis alone. *Respirology* 2014; 19: 239–245.

22. Ye Q, Huang K, Ding Y, *et al.* Cigarette smoking contributes to idiopathic pulmonary fibrosis associated with emphysema. *Chin Med J (Engl)* 2014; 127: 469–474.

23. Mejia M, Carrillo G, Rojas-Serrano J, *et al.* Idiopathic pulmonary fibrosis and emphysema: decreased survival associated with severe pulmonary arterial hypertension. *Chest* 2009; 136: 10–15.

24. Jankowich MD, Rounds S. Combined pulmonary fibrosis and emphysema alters physiology but has similar mortality to pulmonary fibrosis without emphysema. *Lung* 2010; 188: 365–373.

25. Bodlet A, Maury G, Jamart J, *et al.* Influence of radiological emphysema on lung function test in idiopathic pulmonary fibrosis. *Respir Med* 2013; 107: 1781–1788.

26. Kurashima K, Takayanagi N, Tsuchiya N, *et al.* The effect of emphysema on lung function and survival in patients with idiopathic pulmonary fibrosis. *Respirology* 2010; 15: 843–848.

27. Todd NW, Jeudy J, Lavania S, *et al.* Centrilobular emphysema combined with pulmonary fibrosis results in improved survival. *Fibrogenesis Tissue Repair* 2011; 4: 6.

28. Tasaka S, Mizoguchi K, Funatsu Y, *et al.* Cytokine profile of bronchoalveolar lavage fluid in patients with combined pulmonary fibrosis and emphysema. *Respirology* 2012; 17: 814–820.

29. Antoniou KM, Hansell DM, Rubens MB, *et al.* Idiopathic pulmonary fibrosis: outcome in relation to smoking status. *Am J Respir Crit Care Med* 2008; 177: 190–194.

30. Kim YJ, Shin SH, Park JW, *et al.* Annual change in pulmonary function and clinical characteristics of combined pulmonary fibrosis and emphysema and idiopathic pulmonary fibrosis: over a 3-year follow-up. *Tuberc Respir Dis (Seoul)* 2014; 77: 18–23.

31. Akagi T, Matsumoto T, Harada T, *et al.* Coexistent emphysema delays the decrease of vital capacity in idiopathic pulmonary fibrosis. *Respir Med* 2009; 103: 1209–1215.

32. King TE Jr, Bradford WZ, Castro-Bernardini S, *et al.* A phase 3 trial of pirfenidone in patients with idiopathic pulmonary fibrosis. *N Engl J Med* 2014; 370: 2083–2092.

33. Schmidt SL, Nambiar AM, Tayob N, *et al.* Pulmonary function measures predict mortality differently in IPF *versus* combined pulmonary fibrosis and emphysema. *Eur Respir J* 2011; 38: 176–183.

34. Cottin V, Le Pavec J, Prévot G, *et al.* Pulmonary hypertension in patients with combined pulmonary fibrosis and emphysema syndrome. *Eur Respir J* 2010; 35: 105–111.

35. Kwak N, Park CM, Lee J, *et al.* Lung cancer risk among patients with combined pulmonary fibrosis and emphysema. *Respir Med* 2014; 108: 524–530.

36. Usui K, Tanai C, Tanaka Y, *et al.* The prevalence of pulmonary fibrosis combined with emphysema in patients with lung cancer. *Respirology* 2011; 16: 326–331.

37. Girard N, Marchand-Adam S, Naccache JM, *et al.* Lung cancer in combined pulmonary fibrosis and emphysema: a series of 47 Western patients. *J Thorac Oncol* 2014; 9: 1162–1170.

38. Kumagai S, Marumo S, Yamanashi K, *et al.* Prognostic significance of combined pulmonary fibrosis and emphysema in patients with resected non-small-cell lung cancer: a retrospective cohort study. *Eur J Cardiothorac Surg* 2014; 46: e113–e119.

39. Minegishi Y, Kokuho N, Miura Y, *et al.* Clinical features, anti-cancer treatments and outcomes of lung cancer patients with combined pulmonary fibrosis and emphysema. *Lung Cancer* 2014; 85: 258–263.

40. Cottin V, Nunes H, Mouthon L, *et al.* Combined pulmonary fibrosis and emphysema syndrome in connective tissue disease. *Arthritis Rheum* 2011; 63: 295–304.

41. Antoniou KM, Margaritopoulos GA, Goh NS, *et al.* Combined pulmonary fibrosis and emphysema in scleroderma lung disease has a major confounding effect on lung physiology and screening for pulmonary hypertension. *Arthritis Rheumatol* 2015 [in press; DOI: 10.1002/art.39528].

42. Coghlan JG, Denton CP, Grünig E, *et al.* Evidence-based detection of pulmonary arterial hypertension in systemic sclerosis: the DETECT study. *Ann Rheum Dis* 2013; 73: 1340–1349.

43. Henschke CI, Yip R, Boffetta P, *et al.* CT screening for lung cancer: importance of emphysema for never smokers and smokers. *Lung Cancer* 2015; 88: 42–47.

44. Antoniou KM, Walsh SL, Hansell DM, *et al.* Smoking-related emphysema is associated with idiopathic pulmonary fibrosis and rheumatoid lung. *Respirology* 2013; 18: 1191–1196.

45. Alder JK, Guo N, Kembou F, *et al.* Telomere length is a determinant of emphysema susceptibility. *Am J Respir Crit Care Med* 2011; 184: 904–912.

46. Nunes H, Monnet I, Kannengiesser C, *et al.* Is telomeropathy the explanation for combined pulmonary fibrosis and emphysema syndrome?: report of a family with TERT mutation). *Am J Respir Crit Care Med* 2014; 189: 753–754.

47. Cottin V, Reix P, Khouatra C, *et al.* Combined pulmonary fibrosis and emphysema syndrome associated with familial SFTPC mutation. *Thorax* 2011; 66: 918–919.

48. Inomata M, Ikushima S, Awano N, *et al.* An autopsy study of combined pulmonary fibrosis and emphysema: correlations among clinical, radiological, and pathological features. *BMC Pulm Med* 2014; 14: 104.

49. Brillet PY, Cottin V, Letoumelin P, *et al.* Combined apical emphysema and basal fibrosis syndrome (emphysema/fibrosis syndrome): CT imaging features and pulmonary function tests. *J Radiol* 2009; 90: 43–51.

Disclosures: A.U. Wells reports consultancy and/or lecturing fees from Boehringer Ingelheim, Intermune/Roche, Bayer, Gilead, Fibrogen and Cheisi, all outside the submitted work. U. Costabel reports consultancy and/or lecturing fees from Boehringer Ingelheim, Intermune, Roche, Bayer, Gilead, GSK, Centocor, UCB Celltech and Biogen, all outside the submitted work. H. Nunes reports acting as an investigator in clinical trials for Intermune, Roche, Boehringer Ingelheim and Sanofi in areas relevant to the submitted work, and for Centocor outside the submitted work.

Chapter 15

Other comorbidities

Michael Kreuter[1,2], Eva Brunnemer[1], Svenja Ehlers-Tenenbaum[1], Nicolas Kahn[1,2], Jacques Bruhwyler[3] and Martin Kolb[4]

IPF is a chronic, progressive disease that has a significant impact on QoL. It is also associated with poor survival. Several comorbidities have been reported to be more common in IPF than in the general population; these may additionally worsen QoL and prognosis. Important comorbidities include cardiovascular and thromboembolic diseases, depression, sleep disorders, and diabetes. For some of these (*e.g.* GERD), a possible association between the comorbid condition and IPF may exist and specific treatment of the comorbidity might influence the course of IPF. In GERD, retrospective data suggested a possible positive effect of antacid therapy (AAT) leading to a conditional recommendation for AAT in the current IPF guidelines; for several reasons this is highly debatable and demonstrates that prospective trials are needed to determine the interactions of treatments for comorbidities and IPF. Currently, patients with IPF should be actively screened for comorbidities; these comorbidities should then be treated as in non-IPF patients.

Patients with IPF are generally elderly and, as is typical of an ageing population, they have substantial comorbidities [1–3]. While death in IPF patients is mainly attributed to IPF itself or to infections of the respiratory system, nonrespiratory disorders, such as cardiovascular diseases and cancer, are also frequent causes of death [4]. Further, comorbidities might worsen QoL and symptoms in IPF.

The relationship between IPF and its comorbidities may be in part due to common risk factors, such as cigarette smoking, which is associated with IPF, emphysema, lung cancer, and cardiovascular disease. Another association is the process of ageing. During ageing, the telomeres at the ends of all chromosomes shorten; defects in these telomeres and/or their repair can result in various diseases. Several groups reported that telomerase mutations occur in up to 15% of patients with familial IPF [5–7]. Mutations in telomerase reverse transcriptase or telomerase RNA component, which cause telomere shortening, increase susceptibility to the subsequent onset of IPF [6]. At the same time, there is substantial evidence that telomere attrition is associated with, and possibly causative of, cancer [8] and emphysema [9]. This makes the hypothesis that IPF and some of its comorbidities share a possible pathogenic cause, being diseases of ageing, quite plausible. With regard to lung cancer, other possible common pathogenetic pathways with IPF may exist [10]. Diabetes

[1]Centre for Interstitial and Rare Lung Diseases, Pneumology and Respiratory Critical Care Medicine, Thoraxklinik, University of Heidelberg, Heidelberg, Germany. [2]Translational Lung Research Center, Heidelberg, Germany. [3]Dept of Biostatistics, ECSOR, Gembloux, Belgium. [4]Dept of Respiratory Medicine, Pathology and Molecular Medicine, McMaster University, Hamilton, ON, Canada.

Correspondence: Michael Kreuter, Centre for Interstitial and Rare Lung Diseases, Pneumology and Respiratory Critical Care Medicine, Thoraxklinik, University of Heidelberg, Röntgenstr. 1, D-69126 Heidelberg, Germany. E-mail: kreuter@uni-heidelberg.de

Copyright ©ERS 2016. Print ISBN: 978-1-84984-067-5. Online ISBN: 978-1-84984-068-2. Print ISSN: 2312-508X. Online ISSN: 2312-5098.

could influence the progression or initiation of IPF by hyperglycaemia-associated pulmonary inflammation. With regard to GERD, repetitive microaspiration may lead to chronic inflammation causing fibrotic proliferation [11–13]. Further, increased procoagulant activities in the lungs may lead to the initiation of a fibrotic stimulus [14, 15].

Only a few reports have been published on the prevalence of comorbidities in IPF patients and the source of data for these investigations may explain the variability of reported prevalence. In a recently published prospective German IPF registry [2], the most common comorbidity was arterial hypertension (54%) followed by coronary heart disease (CHD) (25%), diabetes mellitus (DM) (21%), PH (17%), and emphysema (10%). A single-centre retrospective evaluation of a tertiary referral centre for ILDs [1] reported cardiovascular disease (27%) as the main comorbidity followed by PH and depression (21% each), arterial hypertension and ischaemic heart disease (18% each), and DM (17%). Similar prevalence has been found in our own tertiary referral centre for ILDs in a retrospective analysis (M. Kreuter, unpublished data).

General approaches to the management of comorbidities in IPF

General approaches include lifestyle modifications, with weight reduction in case of obesity and sleep apnoea, smoking cessation (CHD, lung cancer, and IPF), a reduction in cardiovascular risks, and long-term oxygen therapy [16, 17]. The latter may in addition have a positive influence on the development and progression of PH. Pulmonary rehabilitation has also been shown to improve the course of IPF [18, 19] and may positively influence depression and cardiovascular diseases.

GERD in IPF

GERD is a common disease in developed countries with a population prevalence of about 10%. Initially, reflux was thought to be a solely gastro-oesophageal problem, but recent research has provided more insights into the different aspects of GERD. Different pulmonary disorders and symptoms are thought to be related to reflux and microaspiration, *e.g.* chronic cough. Furthermore, several reports demonstrated a potential association of reflux with other pulmonary diseases, such as severe asthma, COPD, IPF, and other fibrotic ILDs [20].

Depending on the study design, the reported incidence of GERD in IPF ranges between 8% (single-centre retrospective study) [1] and 29.5% (multicentre prospective registry) [2], and up to 87% in pH-monitored patients [21]. Gastro-oesophageal reflux appears to be more common in IPF than in the general population [22]. As early as 1976, MAYS *et al.* [23] proposed a relationship between reflux and pulmonary fibrosis. In a prospective analysis, TOBIN *et al.* [24] were the first to describe a higher prevalence of acid reflux in IPF patients compared to controls. This initiated discussions on a potential causative role of reflux for IPF and also other ILDs [11, 12, 22, 25, 26]. Some observations, including data from animal experiments, suggested that (micro)aspiration of acid refluxate caused parenchymal injuries, leading to pneumonitis, increased epithelial permeability, and stimulated fibrotic proliferation; this is comparable to the aspiration of gastroduodenal contents, which can trigger pulmonary injury leading to bronchiolitis obliterans syndrome after lung transplantation ([27] and reviewed in [28]). Another hypothesis is that IPF might develop only in patients with reflux whose gastric juice contains *Helicobacter pylori*. *H. pylori* produces cytotoxins that can cause mucosal damage; this might result in inflammatory changes of the interstitium, potentially influencing the development of pulmonary fibrosis [29, 30]. In a recent study by BENNETT *et al.* [31], *H. pylori* seroprevalence was associated with more advanced disease and reduced lung function in patients with IPF. However, KREUTER *et al.* [32] did not detect *H. pylori* DNA in the lung tissue of IPF patients. While a direct involvement of *H. pylori* is questioned by the latter study, a systemic immune response initiated by *H. pylori* should be investigated further.

Some authors hypothesised that microaspiration could be a cause for acute exacerbation of IPF; therefore, withholding microaspiration may have an important role in IPF management [33–35]. Further data supported these observations leading to frequent medical treatment with either proton pump inhibitors (PPIs) or H_2 blockers in IPF patients with, at least symptomatic, GERD in clinical routine [36].

Yet, the optimal management strategy for GERD in IPF is still unclear. In a study of patients with severe IPF listed for lung transplantation, LINDEN *et al.* [27] described the outcome of laparoscopic fundoplication in IPF patients diagnosed with reflux disease by pH-monitoring. Surprisingly, perioperatively no deaths were observed in these severely compromised patients. Compared to IPF patients without reflux surgery, those who had received fundoplication showed a stabilisation of functional parameters. A recent retrospective analysis by LEE *et al.* [37] reported that GERD-specific therapy, especially antacid drug treatment (PPIs, H_2 blockers) was associated with less radiographic fibrosis and was an independent predictor of longer survival in IPF patients. The authors concluded that these findings support the hypothesis that GERD and consecutive chronic microaspiration may play an important role in the pathobiology of IPF. Further work by the same group [38] reported the outcome of IPF patients from the placebo arms of three randomised controlled trials of the IPFNet, a clinical research network sponsored by the US National Heart, Lung, and Blood Institute. Of 242 IPF patients, 51% were treated with PPIs or H_2 blockers. After adjusting for sex und pulmonary function, patients on AAT showed significantly less deterioration of FVC than patients not receiving AAT. There were also fewer acute exacerbations in patients receiving AAT. However, no differences were observed for all-cause mortality or all-cause hospitalisation.

On the basis of these reports, the current IPF guidelines suggest a conditional recommendation for the treatment of asymptomatic gastro-oesophageal reflux in patients with IPF. Yet, according to an editorial statement [39], many conflicted members of this task force, who were prohibited from discussing, formulating, grading, and voting on the recommendations, would have preferred making no recommendation. Furthermore, according to unpublished data presented at the 2015 ERS meeting (M. Kreuter, unpublished data), (G. Raghu, University of Washington Medical Center, Seattle, WA, USA; personal communication) the effects of AAT are currently under discussion and potentially several more side-effects, including pulmonary infection, should be taken into account [40].

Still, several limitations on a potential association between reflux and ILDs have to be considered. First, while intriguing and in some way intuitive, no study to date has proved a pathogenetic mechanism that would explain and prove this association. Moreover, pulmonary fibrosis may also influence the function of the lower oesophageal sphincters through traction or abnormal intrathoracic pressures during coughing, potentially leading to or increasing symptomatic reflux. Also, medical treatment strategies only have an antacid effect and do not influence reflux *per se*; the kind of drug (PPI *versus* H_2 blockers) used, treatment duration, and the optimal treatment of weak or non-acid reflux are not established. Despite being a common part of the toolkit for the management of IPF, the effect of AAT on IPF needs to be confirmed in prospective randomised controlled trials.

Cardiovascular diseases in IPF

Multiple studies have shown an increased prevalence of cardiovascular diseases among patients with IPF [41–43]. They are at least twice as likely to have coronary artery disease (CAD) compared to control populations, even after adjusting for potential coronary risk factors [41]. This increased risk of vascular disease in IPF patients is most evident for acute coronary syndrome after the diagnosis of IPF has been made [42]. A study performed by NATHAN et al. [44] compared the prevalence and impact of CAD in patients with IPF to COPD patients in transplant candidates whose work-up included left heart catheterisation. The incidence of CAD was higher in IPF patients (65.8%) compared to the matched group of patients with COPD (46.1%). The authors concluded that this increased association was independent of common coronary artery risk factors. In addition, survival of IPF patients with significant CAD was worse than those with no or nonsignificant disease [44] underscoring the importance of evaluating patients with IPF for cardiovascular diseases and treating patients appropriately to minimise cardiovascular risks. The same group also reported on the value of CT scanning for the detection of CAD. They were able to demonstrate that coronary calcification, as assessed by HRCTs for the underlying ILD, was a significant predictor for CAD in IPF patient [45]. Hence, the interpretation of HRCT in IPF patients may also drive further investigations for the diagnosis, and potentially treatment, of CHD. In addition, a study by KIM et al. [41] revealed that the incidence of newly diagnosed cardiovascular disease was higher in patients with IPF (6.8%) compared to controls (2.8%). Thus far, the pathophysiology behind this increased risk of cardiovascular diseases in fibrotic lung disease is not well understood. Common risk factors, such as cigarette smoking, may contribute, but cannot explain it alone. For example, IZBICKI et al. [46] reported CAD in 28.6% of patients with fibrotic lung disease compared to 9.8% of patients with emphysema, despite the fact that 98% of those with emphysema and only 31% of patients with lung fibrosis were heavy smokers. The authors developed an interesting hypothesis by proposing that pulmonary fibrosis may not only promote fibrogenesis, but also atherosclerosis, perhaps through the release of cytokines and growth factors leading to hypercoagulability and chronic inflammation (reviewed in [47]). In contrast, in a large epidemiological study of 3211 IPF patients and 12 307 controls, DALLEYWATER et al. [43] found that several risk factors for cardiovascular diseases were more prevalent in IPF than in controls. In their study, patients with IPF were also more likely to have cardiovascular and ischaemic heart disease, arterial hypertension, and DM compared with controls. These results are in line with earlier hypothesis that certain risk factors for CAD, such as DM, are more prevalent in patients with IPF [48–50]. Data by REED et al. [50] demonstrated a higher prevalence of hyperlipidaemia, hypertension, and a higher body mass index among patients with IPF compared to those with COPD. Still, the prevalence of cardiovascular risk factors in patients with IPF has yet to be explored in large epidemiological studies, while optimised treatment strategies are yet to be established.

Venous thromboembolism

Patients with IPF are more likely to have a prothrombotic state than the general population. Recently, NAVARATNAM et al. [15] described a four-fold risk for a prothrombotic state in IPF patients. In this study, patients with a prothrombotic state were also likely to have more severe disease (*i.e.* FVC <70% predicted) and had a three-fold mortality risk. While decreased mobility in dyspnoeic patients causing venous stasis may explain this in part, another possible reason is the more direct involvement of the coagulation cascade in IPF pathogenesis. More than 20 years ago, KOTANI *et al.* [51] described increased procoagulant and antifibrinolytic activities in the lungs of IPF patients. GÜNTHER *et al.* [52] confirmed that patients with ILD have enhanced tissue factor pathway activity and fibrin turnover in the alveolar compartment. The net enhancement of fibrin turnover seems to be correlated with the decrease in lung compliance [52]. Therefore, an uncontrolled activation of the coagulation cascade after lung injury may contribute to the development of lung inflammation and fibrosis [53]. In addition to their procoagulant functions, many of the coagulation proteases can exhibit cellular and humoral effects that may contribute to fibrotic processes in the lung. One of many recent examples is the protease-activated receptor 2/tissue factor/factor VIIa axis, which seems to profoundly influence the development of pulmonary fibrosis [54]. Also, increased local expression of coagulation factor X can contribute to the fibrotic response in human and murine lung injury [55]. Therefore, anticoagulation was considered to be of benefit for IPF patients. While a first small study reported that anticoagulant therapy with vitamin K antagonists may have beneficial effects on survival in patients with IPF [56], a recent placebo-controlled clinical trial by the IPFNet did not confirm these data [57]. In contrast to KUBO *et al.* [56], treatment with warfarin was even associated with an increased risk of mortality in an IPF population who lacked other indications for anticoagulation. A negative effect may even exist for patients who are on anticoagulation therapy, mainly vitamin K antagonists, for medical reasons other than IPF (*e.g.* atrial fibrillation) [1, 58]. This may be explained by the fact that vitamin K antagonists may adversely influence the coagulation cascade [59] and that the simultaneous inhibition of vitamin K-dependent pro-coagulative factors and protein C could adversely affect inflammation and remodelling [53, 60]. Therefore, other treatments for IPF targeting the coagulation cascade, such as inhaled heparin [61] or direct thrombin inhibition [62], are currently being discussed and should be explored in future in clinical trials.

Depression in IPF

The increased prevalence of psychiatric diseases in chronically ill patients, especially those with chronic lung diseases, is well known [63]. Patients who experience dyspnoea or fatigue due to lung diseases frequently develop anxiety or depression. Data from a small IPF cohort showed that about 25% of patients had depression and that breathlessness correlated significantly with depressive symptoms. Moreover, there was a strong association between depression and dyspnoea, pain, sleep quality, and FVC [63]. AKHTAR *et al.* [64] reported an even higher incidence of 49.2% of IPF patients with significant depressive symptoms. However, disease severity, age, duration since diagnosis, and the number of comorbidities were not correlated with depression in this study. Not surprisingly, depressive symptoms in IPF patients diminish QoL [65, 66]. Furthermore, depression is a risk factor for nonadherence to medical treatment in patients with chronic disease [67]. Possible confounding roles of ILD treatment, particularly higher dose steroids, in precipitating or causing depressive symptoms have to be taken into account. Pulmonary rehabilitation can have beneficial effects not only on the typical symptoms related to IPF but also on the severity of depression [68]. Given the high prevalence and its impact on symptoms, some authors recommend that all patients with ILD should be screened routinely and treated for depression [47, 63, 66].

Sleep disorders

Sleep disturbances, including OSA are common in IPF patients, and hypoventilation during sleep can aggravate hypoxaemia and worsen coexisting PH [69–71]. Therefore, sleep disturbances play a role in overall QoL as well as in morbidity and mortality. The assessment of OSA is complicated by subjective complaints, such as daytime fatigue, that are common in both IPF and OSA patients. MERMIGKIS et al. [70] were first in reporting on the importance of OSA in IPF. Obesity and the extent of pulmonary function impairment were recognised as predictive factors for OSA. The lower lung volumes of fibrotic lungs can reduce upper airway stability and increase resistance due to decreased traction on the upper airway. This led to the interesting hypothesis of upper airway collapse occurring in IPF patients, especially during REM sleep when functional residual capacity is further reduced due to the inactivity of the intercostal muscle (reviewed in [72]). In the first prospective study of OSA in IPF [69], OSA was diagnosed in 88% of participants, but no relationship between FVC and the apnoea/hypopnoea index was demonstrated. The authors speculated that the lack of correlation might be due to performing pulmonary function testing in the standing rather than the supine position. The study was further limited by many patients receiving corticosteroids, which may increase OSA as a result of fat deposition in the neck area. Later reports from MERMIGKIS et al. [73] and PIHTILI et al. [74] confirmed that OSA is a common comorbidity in IPF. However, OSA and IPF are both diseases of the elderly, which may partly explain the high incidence [72]. With regard to therapy, a recent study that used CPAP therapy in 12 patients with IPF and moderate-to-severe OSA reported improved QoL as measured by the Functional Outcomes in Sleep Questionnaire [75]. While this is the first study demonstrating improved QoL in patients with IPF and OSA who use CPAP, the impact of CPAP on mortality is yet unclear.

Besides OSA, nocturnal desaturation, which is potentially related to underlying OSA, is common in IPF patients; it is associated with PH and carries an elevated mortality risk. Therefore, regular screening for nocturnal desaturation for all IPF (ILD) patients followed by screening and treatment for OSA, or in case of non-OSA nocturnal oxygen supplementation, should be recommended [76].

Diabetes

Endocrine disorders, especially DM are frequent comorbidities in IPF and might contribute to the pathophysiology of this disease. A report from the ILD database of the University of Chicago found that 31% of enrolled patients had DM, compared to a prevalence of about 8% in the general population [77]. A case-control study of IPF patients in Japan attained a similar result (32.7% of IPF patients had DM versus 11.4% of controls) [78]. This is a possible pathogenetic interrelation of IPF with DM through hyperglycaemia-mediated lung damage. Using a mouse model, HUNT et al. [79] demonstrated that hyperglycaemia impedes lung bacterial clearance in cystic fibrosis-related diabetes; a comparable condition may exist for diabetes in IPF patients. Increased advanced glycation end product/receptor for advanced glycation end product interaction might play a significant role in the pathogenesis of IPF [80]. However, the relationship between DM and IPF might also be attributed to the still frequent use of corticosteroids in IPF patients causing iatrogenic DM. Further studies on this important observation are still missing and the effects of DM prevention and therapy on the course of IPF have not been studied so far.

Future perspectives

Early identification and treatment of significant comorbidities in patients with IPF can translate into improved QoL, and perhaps even better survival. We have recently proposed an "IPF comorbidome", which is analogous to the COPD comorbidome (M. Kreuter, unpublished data) [81]. This describes the prevalence of comorbidities and their strength of association with outcomes in patients with IPF. Once validated, it may be used as a predictor for mortality risk in IPF. Furthermore, potential treatment of IPF and respective comorbidities by one combined therapeutic approach should be discussed; one such approach may be early palliative care [82]. Another example of a combined therapeutic approach is to target the coagulation cascade with thrombin inhibitors as a potential treatment option for IPF and for concomitant thromboembolic disease, as discussed earlier. While treatment with warfarin negatively affected outcome [1, 39, 57, 58] other anticoagulants may qualify as antifibrotic approaches, e.g. thrombomodulin. A recent study reported that the use of thrombomodulin in acute exacerbated IPF was associated with a better survival for thrombomodulin-treated, acute exacerbated IPF patients [83].

Conclusion

As stated in the recently updated ATS/ERS/ALAT/JRS guidelines, patients with IPF can have subclinical or overt comorbidities; these affect symptoms, physiology, QoL, and prognosis [3, 39]. From the data available so far, it is clear that patients with IPF should be actively screened for comorbidities and they should consequently be treated along the lines of non-IPF patients. However, some treatments may negatively affect the course of IPF, such as cancer drugs or anticoagulants; these have to be thoroughly monitored, perhaps even more so in IPF patients. Future studies and prospective trials are needed to determine the possible interaction of treatments for comorbid conditions, the course of IPF and IPF-specific therapies, and whether treatment of significant comorbidities affects long-term outcome and survival in IPF.

References

1. Hyldgaard C, Hilberg O, Bendstrup E. How does comorbidity influence survival in idiopathic pulmonary fibrosis? *Respir Med* 2014; 108: 647–653.
2. Behr J, Kreuter M, Hoeper MM, *et al.* Management of patients with idiopathic pulmonary fibrosis in clinical practice: the INSIGHTS-IPF registry. *Eur Respir J* 2015; 46: 186–196.
3. Raghu G, Collard HR, Egan JJ, *et al.* An official ATS/ERS/JRS/ALAT statement: idiopathic pulmonary fibrosis: evidence-based guidelines for diagnosis and management. *Am J Respir Crit Care Med* 2011; 183: 788–824.
4. Ley B, Collard HR, King TE Jr. Clinical course and prediction of survival in idiopathic pulmonary fibrosis. *Am J Respir Crit Care Med* 2011; 183: 431–440.
5. Armanios MY, Chen JJ, Cogan JD, *et al.* Telomerase mutations in families with idiopathic pulmonary fibrosis. *N Engl J Med* 2007; 356: 1317–1326.
6. Tsakiri KD, Cronkhite JT, Kuan PJ, *et al.* Adult-onset pulmonary fibrosis caused by mutations in telomerase. *Proc Natl Acad Sci U S A* 2007; 104: 7552–7557.
7. Mushiroda T, Wattanapokayakit S, Takahashi A, *et al.* A genome-wide association study identifies an association of a common variant in TERT with susceptibility to idiopathic pulmonary fibrosis. *J Med Genet* 2008; 45: 654–656.
8. Calado R, Young N. Telomeres in disease. *F1000 Med Rep* 2012; 4: 8.
9. Alder JK, Guo N, Kembou F, *et al.* Telomere length is a determinant of emphysema susceptibility. *Am J Respir Crit Care Med* 2011; 184: 904–912.
10. Vancheri C. Common pathways in idiopathic pulmonary fibrosis and cancer. *Eur Respir Rev* 2013; 22: 265–272.
11. Greenfield LJ, Singleton RP, McCaffree DR, *et al.* Pulmonary effects of experimental graded aspiration of hydrochloric acid. *Ann Surg* 1969; 170: 74–86.

12. Mitsuhashi T, Shimazaki M, Chanoki Y, *et al.* Experimental pulmonary fibrosis induced by trisodium citrate and acid-citrate-dextrose. *Exp Mol Pathol* 1985; 42: 261–270.

13. Mertens V, Blondeau K, Vanaudenaerde B, *et al.* Gastric juice from patients "on" acid suppressive therapy can still provoke a significant inflammatory reaction by human bronchial epithelial cells. *J Clin Gastroenterol* 2010; 44: e230–e235.

14. Kotani I, Sato A, Hayakawa H, *et al.* Increased procoagulant and antifibrinolytic activities in the lungs with idiopathic pulmonary fibrosis. *Thromb Res* 1995; 77: 493–504.

15. Navaratnam V, Fogarty AW, McKeever T, *et al.* Presence of a prothrombotic state in people with idiopathic pulmonary fibrosis: a population-based case-control study. *Thorax* 2014; 69: 207–215.

16. O'Keefe JH, Gheewala NM, O'Keefe JO. Dietary strategies for improving post-prandial glucose, lipids, inflammation, and cardiovascular health. *J Am Coll Cardiol* 2008; 51: 249–255.

17. Festi D, Scaioli E, Baldi F, *et al.* Body weight, lifestyle, dietary habits and gastroesophageal reflux disease. *World J Gastroenterol* 2009; 15: 1690–1701.

18. Dowman L, Hill CJ, Holland AE. Pulmonary rehabilitation for interstitial lung disease. *Cochrane Database Syst Rev* 2014; 10: CD006322.

19. Huppmann P, Sczepanski B, Boensch M, *et al.* Effects of inpatient pulmonary rehabilitation in patients with interstitial lung disease. *Eur Respir J* 2013; 42: 444–453.

20. Hu X, Lee JS, Pianosi PT, *et al.* Aspiration-related pulmonary syndromes. *Chest* 2015; 147: 815–823.

21. Raghu G, Freudenberger TD, Yang S, *et al.* High prevalence of abnormal acid gastro-oesophageal reflux in idiopathic pulmonary fibrosis. *Eur Respir J* 2006; 27: 136–142.

22. Savarino E, Carbone R, Marabotto E, *et al.* Gastro-oesophageal reflux and gastric aspiration in idiopathic pulmonary fibrosis patients. *Eur Respir J* 2013; 42: 1322–1331.

23. Mays EE, Dubois JJ, Hamilton GB. Pulmonary fibrosis associated with tracheobronchial aspiration. A study of the frequency of hiatal hernia and gastroesophageal reflux in interstitial pulmonary fibrosis of obscure etiology. *Chest* 1976; 69: 512–515.

24. Tobin RW, Pope CE 2nd, Pellegrini CA, *et al.* Increased prevalence of gastroesophageal reflux in patients with idiopathic pulmonary fibrosis. *Am J Respir Crit Care Med* 1998; 158: 1804–1808.

25. Ghebremariam YT, Cooke JP, Gerhart W, *et al.* Pleiotropic effect of the proton pump inhibitor esomeprazole leading to suppression of lung inflammation and fibrosis. *J Transl Med* 2015; 13: 249.

26. Lozo Vukovac E, Lozo M, Mise K, *et al.* Bronchoalveolar pH and inflammatory biomarkers in newly diagnosed IPF and GERD patients: a case-control study. *Med Sci Monit* 2014; 20: 255–261.

27. Linden PA, Gilbert RJ, Yeap BY, *et al.* Laparoscopic fundoplication in patients with end-stage lung disease awaiting transplantation. *J Thorac Cardiovasc Surg* 2006; 131: 438–446.

28. Allaix ME, Fisichella PM, Noth I, *et al.* The Pulmonary Side of Reflux Disease: from Heartburn to Lung Fibrosis. *J Gastrointest Surg* 2013; 17: 1526–1535.

29. Ibrahim WH. *Helicobacter pylori* eradication in the management of idiopathic pulmonary fibrosis. *Eur Respir J* 2007; 30: 395–396.

30. Adriani A, Repici A, Hickman I, *et al.* *Helicobacter pylori* infection and respiratory diseases: actual data and directions for future studies. *Minerva Med* 2014; 105: 1–8.

31. Bennett D, Bargagli E, Refini RM, *et al.* *Helicobacter pylori* seroprevalence in patients with idiopathic pulmonary fibrosis. *Eur Respir J* 2014; 43: 635–638.

32. Kreuter M, Kirsten D, Bahmer T, *et al.* Screening for *Helicobacter pylori* in idiopathic pulmonary fibrosis lung biopsies. *Respiration* 2016; 91: 3–8.

33. Lee JS, Song JW, Wolters PJ, *et al.* Bronchoalveolar lavage pepsin in acute exacerbation of idiopathic pulmonary fibrosis. *Eur Respir J* 2012; 39: 352–358.

34. Tcherakian C, Cottin V, Brillet PY, *et al.* Progression of idiopathic pulmonary fibrosis: lessons from asymmetrical disease. *Thorax* 2011; 66: 226–231.

35. Lee JS, Collard HR, Raghu G, *et al.* Does chronic microaspiration cause idiopathic pulmonary fibrosis? *Am J Med* 2010; 123: 304–311.

36. Pacheco-Galván A, Hart SP, Morice AH. Relationship between gastro-oesophageal reflux and airway diseases: the airway reflux paradigm. *Arch Bronconeumol* 2011; 47: 195–203.

37. Lee JS, Ryu JH, Elicker BM, *et al.* Gastroesophageal reflux therapy is associated with longer survival in patients with idiopathic pulmonary fibrosis. *Am J Respir Crit Care Med* 2011; 184: 1390–1394.

38. Lee JS, Collard HR, Anstrom KJ, *et al.* Anti-acid treatment and disease progression in idiopathic pulmonary fibrosis: an analysis of data from three randomised controlled trials. *Lancet Respir Med* 2013; 1: 369–376.

39. Raghu G, Rochwerg B, Zhang Y, *et al.* An official ATS/ERS/JRS/ALAT clinical practice guideline: treatment of idiopathic pulmonary fibrosis. An update of the 2011 clinical practice guideline. *Am J Respir Crit Care Med* 2015; 192: e3–e19.

40. Myles PR, Hubbard RB, Gibson JE, *et al.* The impact of statins, ACE inhibitors and gastric acid suppressants on pneumonia mortality in a UK general practice population cohort. *Pharmacoepidemiol Drug Saf* 2009; 18: 697–703.

41. Kim WY, Mok Y, Kim GW, *et al.* Association between idiopathic pulmonary fibrosis and coronary artery disease: a case-control study and cohort analysis. *Sarcoidosis Vasc Diffuse Lung Dis* 2015; 31: 289–296.

42. Hubbard RB, Smith C, Le Jeune I, *et al.* The association between idiopathic pulmonary fibrosis and vascular disease: a population-based study. *Am J Respir Crit Care Med* 2008; 178: 1257–1261.

43. Dalleywater W, Powell HA, Hubbard RB, *et al.* Risk factors for cardiovascular disease in people with idiopathic pulmonary fibrosis: a population-based study. *Chest* 2015; 147: 150–156.

44. Nathan SD, Basavaraj A, Reichner C, *et al.* Prevalence and impact of coronary artery disease in idiopathic pulmonary fibrosis. *Respir Med* 2010; 104: 1035–1041.

45. Nathan SD, Weir N, Shlobin OA, *et al.* The value of computed tomography scanning for the detection of coronary artery disease in patients with idiopathic pulmonary fibrosis. *Respirology* 2011; 16: 481–486.

46. Izbicki G, Ben-Dor I, Shitrit D, *et al.* The prevalence of coronary artery disease in end-stage pulmonary disease: is pulmonary fibrosis a risk factor? *Respir Med* 2009; 103: 1346–1349.

47. King C, Nathan SD. Identification and treatment of comorbidities in idiopathic pulmonary fibrosis and other fibrotic lung diseases. *Curr Opin Pulm Med* 2013; 19: 466–473.

48. Gribbin J, Hubbard R, Smith C. Role of diabetes mellitus and gastro-oesophageal reflux in the aetiology of idiopathic pulmonary fibrosis. *Respir Med* 2009; 103: 927–931.

49. Enomoto T, Usuki J, Azuma A, *et al.* Diabetes mellitus may increase risk for idiopathic pulmonary fibrosis. *Chest* 2003; 123: 2007–2011.

50. Reed RM, Eberlein M, Girgis RE, *et al.* Coronary artery disease is under-diagnosed and under-treated in advanced lung disease. *Am J Med* 2012; 125: 1228.e13–1228.e22.

51. Kotani I, Sato A, Hayakawa H, *et al.* Increased procoagulant and antifibrinolytic activities in the lungs with idiopathic pulmonary fibrosis. *Thromb Res* 1995; 77: 493–504.

52. Günther A, Mosavi P, Ruppert C, *et al.* Enhanced tissue factor pathway activity and fibrin turnover in the alveolar compartment of patients with interstitial lung disease. *Thromb Haemost* 2000; 83: 853–860.

53. Chambers RC. Procoagulant signalling mechanisms in lung inflammation and fibrosis: novel opportunities for pharmacological intervention? *Br J Pharmacol* 2008; 153: Suppl. 1, 367–378.

54. Wygrecka M, Kwapiszewska G, Jablonska E, *et al.* Role of protease-activated receptor-2 in idiopathic pulmonary fibrosis. *Am J Respir Crit Care Med* 2011; 183: 1703–1714.

55. Scotton CJ, Krupiczojc MA, Königshoff M, *et al.* Increased local expression of coagulation factor X contributes to the fibrotic response in human and murine lung injury. *J Clin Invest* 2009; 119: 2550–2563.

56. Kubo H, Nakayama K, Yanai M, *et al.* Anticoagulant therapy for idiopathic pulmonary fibrosis. *Chest* 2005; 128: 1475–1482.

57. Noth I, Anstrom KJ, Calvert SB, *et al.* A placebo-controlled randomized trial of warfarin in idiopathic pulmonary fibrosis. *Am J Respir Crit Care Med* 2012; 186: 88–95.

58. Kreuter M, Wijsenbeek MS, Vasakova M, *et al.* Unfavourable effects of medically indicated oral anticoagulation on survival in IPF. *Eur Respir J* 2016 [in press; DOI: 10.1183/13993003.02087-2015].

59. José RJ, Williams AE, Chambers RC. Proteinase-activated receptors in fibroproliferative lung disease. *Thorax* 2014; 69: 190–192.

60. Coughlin SR, Camerer E. PARticipation in inflammation. *J Clin Invest* 2003; 111: 25–27.

61. Markart P, Nass R, Ruppert C, *et al.* Safety and tolerability of inhaled heparin in idiopathic pulmonary fibrosis. *J Aerosol Med Pulm Drug Deliv* 2010; 23: 161–172.

62. Bogatkevich GS, Ludwicka-Bradley A, Silver RM. Dabigatran, a direct thrombin inhibitor, demonstrates antifibrotic effects on lung fibroblasts. *Arthritis Rheum* 2009; 60: 3455–3464.

63. Ryerson CJ, Arean PA, Berkeley J, *et al.* Depression is a common and chronic comorbidity in patients with interstitial lung disease. *Respirology* 2012; 17: 525–532.

64. Akhtar AA, Ali MA, Smith RP. Depression in patients with idiopathic pulmonary fibrosis. *Chron Respir Dis* 2013; 10: 127–133.

65. De Vries J, Kessels BL, Drent M. Quality of life of idiopathic pulmonary fibrosis patients. *Eur Respir J* 2001; 17: 954–961.

66. Elfferich MD, De Vries J, Drent M. Type D or 'distressed' personality in sarcoidosis and idiopathic pulmonary fibrosis. *Sarcoidosis Vasc Diffuse Lung Dis* 2011; 28: 65–71.

67. DiMatteo MR, Lepper HS, Croghan TW. Depression is a risk factor for noncompliance with medical treatment: meta-analysis of the effects of anxiety and depression on patient adherence. *Arch Intern Med* 2000; 160: 2101–2107.

68. Ferreira A, Garvey C, Connors GL, *et al.* Pulmonary rehabilitation in interstitial lung disease: benefits and predictors of response. *Chest* 2009; 135: 442–447.

69. Lancaster LH, Mason WR, Parnell JA, *et al.* Obstructive sleep apnea is common in idiopathic pulmonary fibrosis. *Chest* 2009; 136: 772–778.

70. Mermigkis C, Chapman J, Golish J, *et al.* Sleep-related breathing disorders in patients with idiopathic pulmonary fibrosis. *Lung* 2007; 185: 173–178.

71. Mermigkis C, Stagaki E, Amfilochiou A, *et al.* Sleep quality and associated daytime consequences in patients with idiopathic pulmonary fibrosis. *Med Princ Pract* 2009; 18: 10–15.

72. Schiza S, Mermigkis C, Margaritopoulos GA, *et al.* Idiopathic pulmonary fibrosis and sleep disorders: no longer strangers in the night. *Eur Respir Rev* 2015; 24: 327–339.

73. Mermigkis C, Stagaki E, Tryfon S, *et al.* How common is sleep-disordered breathing in patients with idiopathic pulmonary fibrosis? *Sleep Breath* 2010; 14: 387–390.

74. Pihtili A, Bingol Z, Kiyan E, *et al.* Obstructive sleep apnea is common in patients with interstitial lung disease. *Sleep Breath* 2013; 17: 1281–1288.

75. Mermigkis C, Bouloukaki I, Antoniou KM, *et al.* CPAP therapy in patients with idiopathic pulmonary fibrosis and obstructive sleep apnea: does it offer a better quality of life and sleep? *Sleep Breath* 2013; 17: 1137–1143.

76. Corte TJ, Wort SJ, Talbot S, *et al.* Elevated nocturnal desaturation index predicts mortality in interstitial lung disease. *Sarcoidosis Vasc Diffuse Lung Dis* 2012; 29: 41–50.

77. Patel S, Takahashi S, Demchuk C, *et al.* Gastro-oesophageal reflux disease in patients with idiopathic pulmonary fibrosis. *Am J Respir Crit Care Med* 2009; 179: A4063.

78. Enomoto T, Usuki J, Azuma A, *et al.* Diabetes mellitus may increase risk for idiopathic pulmonary fibrosis. *Chest* 2003; 123: 2007–2011.

79. Hunt WR, Zughaier SM, Guentert DE, *et al.* Hyperglycemia impedes lung bacterial clearance in a murine model of cystic fibrosis-related diabetes. *Am J Physiol Lung Cell Mol Physiol* 2014; 306: L43–L49.

80. Kyung SY, Byun KH, Yoon JY, *et al.* Advanced glycation end-products and receptor for advanced glycation end-products expression in patients with idiopathic pulmonary fibrosis and NSIP. *Int J Clin Exp Pathol* 2013; 7: 221–228.

81. Divo MJ, Cote C, de Torres JP, *et al.* Comorbidities and risk of mortality in patients with chronic obstructive pulmonary disease. *Am J Respir Crit Care Med* 2012; 186: 155–161.

82. Kreuter M, Herth FJ. Supportive and palliative care of advanced nonmalignant lung disease. *Respiration* 2011; 82: 307–316.

83. Kataoka K, Taniguchi H, Kondoh Y, *et al.* Recombinant human thrombomodulin in acute exacerbation of idiopathic pulmonary fibrosis. *Chest* 2015; 148: 436–443.

Disclosures: M. Kreuter and his institution have received grants from InterMune/Roche and Boehringer Ingelheim as well fees for consulting. E. Brunnemer has received fees for consulting from Roche and Boehringer Ingelheim. M. Kolb reports receiving the following outside the submitted work: grants and personal fees from Roche and Boehringer Ingelheim; personal fees from GSK, Gilead, Prometic, Genoa and AstraZeneca; and grants from Actelion and Respivert. J. Bruhwyler reports receiving personal fees from Thoraxklinik (University Heidelberg, Heidelberg, Germany) during the conduct of the study.

Chapter 16

Pharmacological management

Vincent Cottin[1] and Claudia Valenzuela[2]

Recently, two drugs have been approved in a number of countries for the treatment of IPF. Pirfenidone and nintedanib, the first antifibrotic pharmacological drugs to treat IPF, target downstream pathways of the fibrogenesis process. Randomised controlled trials have demonstrated that treatment of IPF patients with pirfenidone reduces lung function decline and improves progression-free survival. Pooled data demonstrate that pirfenidone significantly reduces the risk of all-cause mortality at 1 year. Randomised controlled trials have demonstrated that treatment of IPF patients with nintedanib reduces disease progression. Nintedanib reduces the risk of adjudicated confirmed or suspected acute exacerbations. Both pirfenidone and nintedanib have a manageable safety and tolerability profile in patients with IPF, and have a consistent effect across a variety of baseline characteristics in subgroup analysis. The primary treatment-related adverse events associated with pirfenidone therapy are gastrointestinal upset, rash and photosensitivity, and that of nintedanib is diarrhoea. Management of adverse events through treatment interruption, dose reduction, symptomatic treatment and patient education is critical to help patients remain on treatment over the long term. Pirfenidone, nintedanib and antiacid therapy are recommended (conditional recommendation) for the treatment of IPF in the 2015 update of international clinical practice guidelines.

IPF is a chronic, irreversible, progressively destructive, chronic lung disease that culminates in respiratory failure and death [1, 2]. It is associated with a radiological and/ or histopathological pattern of UIP [1], and a poor prognosis with a median survival of 2–4 years from diagnosis [2]. IPF is therefore more lethal than many common malignancies [3]. IPF rarely occurs before the age of 50 years, and the incidence is increased in smokers and ex-smokers, in individuals who have been exposed to wood or metal dust [4], and in subjects with a family history of IPF or carrying certain genetic polymorphisms or gene mutations [5]. Although IPF is a rare disease [6, 7], its incidence, prevalence and specific mortality are continuously rising [8].

The natural history of IPF is highly heterogeneous, therefore raising a number of questions regarding management. There seems to be a number of asymptomatic patients with subclinical, undiagnosed disease, especially among the elderly [9, 10]. Some patients remain relatively stable for a prolonged period of time, while others progress rapidly [2] and some experience acute exacerbations of IPF, e.g. acute respiratory worsening [11] of unidentified cause [12] that causes non-elective hospitalisation and frequently death [13]. IPF has a broad and profound impact on patients' health-related QoL [14, 15].

[1]Dept of Respiratory Medicine, National Reference Center for Rare Pulmonary Diseases, Louis Pradel Hospital, Hospices Civils de Lyon, and University of Lyon, University Claude Bernard Lyon 1, Lyon, France. [2]Hospital Universitario de la Princesa, Madrid, Spain.

Correspondence: Vincent Cottin, Hôpital Louis Pradel – Batiment Aile A4 pneumologie, Service de Pneumologie, 28 Avenue Doyen Lepine, 69677 Lyon Cedex, France. E-mail: vincent.cottin@chu-lyon.fr

Copyright ©ERS 2016. Print ISBN: 978-1-84984-067-5. Online ISBN: 978-1-84984-068-2. Print ISSN: 2312-508X. Online ISSN: 2312-5098.

IPF is believed to be initiated by persistent, multifocal, subclinical injury to the alveolar epithelial cells, followed by aberrant wound healing, and ultimately, destruction of the alveolar–capillary basement membrane and of the lung architecture [16–18]. Loss of epithelial integrity facilitated by some gene variants and/or gene expression in the ageing lung results in the failure of the alveoli to correctly respond to lung injury and to mechanical stretch. Aberrant activation of and miscommunication between epithelial cells and fibroblasts result in fibroblast proliferation, migration and differentiation of fibroblasts into myofibroblasts, and in the exaggerated production and accumulation of extracellular matrix, ultimately with structural remodelling leading to loss of alveolar function [19].

Recently, two drugs have been approved in a number of countries for the treatment of IPF. Pirfenidone and nintedanib, the first antifibrotic pharmacological drugs to treat IPF, target downstream pathways of the fibrogenesis process (*e.g.* myofibroblast migration and fibroblast synthesis of collagen). Pirfenidone has some further anti-inflammatory and antioxidant effects. Nintedanib also downregulates inflammation, autophagy and angiogenesis. This chapter will summarise the evidence and experience with antifibrotic drugs, including a discussion of safety and tolerability data drawn from long-term clinical trial observations and published real-world experience, put in the perspective of the current international guidelines for the management of IPF.

Pirfenidone

Drug development and pharmacology

Pirfenidone was approved by Japan in 2008, then by the European Medicines Agency in March 2011. It was the first licensed therapy for IPF in Europe (European Union, Iceland and Norway) and was approved in Canada in 2012. In October 2014, pirfenidone was approved by the Food and Drug Administration as a treatment for IPF in the USA, simultaneously with nintedanib.

Pirfenidone, or 5-methyl-1-phenyl-2-(1H)-pyridone, is a small, orally available chemical molecule, which has antifibrotic activity by attenuating the expression, synthesis and/or accumulation of collagen [20], and inhibition of the recruitment and/or expression of extracellular matrix-producing cells (*i.e.* fibroblasts) [21]. In addition, pirfenidone has some anti-inflammatory effects and protects against oxidative stress [22]. It reduces experimentally induced pulmonary fibrosis across multiple *in vitro* and *in vivo* animal models [23] in a dose-related manner, in part through modulation of cytokines and growth factors including TGF-β [24–26], basic fibroblast growth factor [25] and tumour necrosis factor-α [27–29]. Comparable antifibrotic properties were observed across multiple organ systems in *in vivo* animal models, in both prophylactic and therapeutic dosing regimens, and at clinically relevant doses, with supportive results from cell-based studies [23]. Pirfenidone also reduced transplant-related pulmonary fibrosis in a model of post-transplant obliterative bronchiolitis [24].

Clinical trials

Pilot trial
The first clinical use of pirfenidone in pulmonary fibrosis was published in 1999 (17 years after the first demonstration of an antifibrotic effect in animals), when Raghu *et al.* [30]

pioneered an open-label, compassionate, prospective, phase II trial in 54 consecutive, terminally ill patients with advanced IPF. The mean age was 62 years, mean duration of symptoms was 4.6 years and time since lung biopsy was 3.2 years. 1- and 2-year survival was 78% (95% CI 66–89%) and 63% (95% CI 50–76%), respectively [30]. Patients whose lung functions had deteriorated prior to enrolment appeared to stabilise after beginning treatment. Adverse effects were relatively minor. Although interpretation of these findings was limited by the design, this study showed that pirfenidone had the potential to stabilise lung function, warranting further clinical studies. The efficacy and safety of pirfenidone for the treatment of IPF has been extensively evaluated in randomised clinical trials in the past 10 years [31–34].

Japanese trials

Pirfenidone was investigated in a randomised, double-blind, placebo-controlled trial in 107 Japanese patients with IPF [31]. The study was prematurely stopped following a planned interim analysis at 24 weeks, which showed an increased incidence of acute exacerbations among patients randomised to the placebo arm. The decline in vital capacity (VC) at 36 weeks was significantly reduced in patients treated with pirfenidone, as compared with placebo [31]. In another randomised, double-blind, placebo-controlled, phase III trial in 275 Japanese patients with IPF, treatment with pirfenidone (1800 mg·day^{-1}) was associated with a significant reduction in the decline in VC at week 52 (p=0.042) and improved progression-free survival (p=0.028) [32].

The CAPACITY programme

Pirfenidone was further evaluated in two large, multinational, randomised, double-blind, placebo-controlled, pivotal, phase III trials (PIPF004/CAPACITY 2 (NCT00287716, clinicaltrials.gov), n=435; and PIPF006/CAPACITY 1 (NCT00287729, clinicaltrials.gov), n=344) [33] (table 1). Although nearly identical, these studies had different results. In both studies, patients were eligible if they had mild-to-moderate IPF, as defined by FVC $\geqslant$50% predicted and DLCO $\geqslant$35% of predicted, and the primary end-point was the absolute change in % predicted FVC at week 72. In study PIPF004, patients were randomised to pirfenidone 2403 mg·day^{-1}, pirfenidone 1197 mg·day^{-1} or placebo in a 2:1:2 ratio, while in study PIPF006, patients were assigned to pirfenidone 2403 mg·day^{-1} or placebo in a 1:1 ratio. In study PIPF004, the primary end-point was met (35% relative reduction; −8.0% reduction in FVC versus −12.4% in the pirfenidone 2403 mg·day^{-1} and placebo groups, respectively; p=0.001) and progression-free survival time (defined as time to confirmed $\geqslant$10% decline in % predicted FVC, $\geqslant$15% decline in % predicted DLCO or death) was improved (hazard ratio (HR) 0.64, 95% CI 0.44–0.95; p=0.023). In study PIPF006, the primary end-point was not met (−9.0% versus −9.6% in the pirfenidone and placebo groups, respectively; p=0.501), although a significant pirfenidone treatment effect was observed at study time-points prior to week 72. A pooled analysis of the pirfenidone 2403 mg·day^{-1} arms of both studies showed a significant pirfenidone treatment effect in the primary end-point (8.5% mean change in predicted FVC versus −11.0%, respectively (p=0.005); 2.5% absolute reduction, 22.8% relative reduction). In the pooled analysis, a significant difference was also found between groups for categorical change of $\geqslant$10% FVC decline (21% versus 31%, respectively; p=0.003), mean change in 6MWD (−52.8 m versus −76.8 m, respectively (p<0.001); 24 m absolute difference, 31% relative difference) and progression-free survival time (HR 0.74, 95% CI 0.57–0.96; p=0.025) [33]. The magnitude of treatment effect was clinically meaningful overall for change in FVC, 6MWD and progression-free survival time [35–37]. No significant difference was observed in overall survival but the trials were not powered to assess mortality.

Table 1. Overview of recent published phase II and phase III trials using pirfenidone or nintedanib in patients with IPF

Drug	Mode of action	Study description	Patients n	Doses studied	Primary end-point	Outcome	First author [ref.]
Pirfenidone	Oral, synthetic pyridine compound Antifibrotic (downregulation of TGF-β) Anti-inflammatory Antioxidant	Shionogi phase II (Japan) Double blind Randomised Placebo controlled Planned 12-month treatment period	107	Pirfenidone 1800 mg·day^{-1} versus placebo	Change from baseline in the lowest oxygen saturation during a 6MWT	Prematurely stopped after 9 months of treatment; acute exacerbations had occurred in 14% of placebo and 0% of pirfenidone patients, respectively (p=0.0031). Pirfenidone had a favourable effect on VC change from baseline (p=0.0366)	AZUMA [31]
		Shionogi phase III (Japan) Double blind Randomised Placebo controlled	275	Pirfenidone 1800 mg·day^{-1} or 1200 mg·day^{-1}, or placebo (ratio 2:1:2)	Change in VC at week 52	Treatment with pirfenidone (1800 mg·day^{-1}) decreased the rate of decline in VC at 52 weeks (p=0.042) Secondary end-point: increase in progression free survival time at 52 weeks (p=0.028)	TANIGUCHI [32]
		CAPACITY 2 (PIPF 004) Multinational Double blind Randomised Placebo controlled Phase III	435	Pirfenidone 2403 mg·day^{-1} or 1197 mg·day^{-1}, or placebo (ratio 2:1:2)	Absolute change in % predicted FVC at week 72	Mean FVC change at week 72 was −8.0% in the pirfenidone 2403 mg·day^{-1} group and −12.4% in the placebo group; pirfenidone reduced decline in FVC (p=0.001)[#,¶,+]	NOBLE [33]

Continued

199

Table 1. Continued

Drug	Mode of action	Study description	Patients n	Doses studied	Primary end-point	Outcome	First author [ref.]
Pirfenidone (cont.)		CAPACITY 1 (PIPF 006) Multinational Double blind Randomised Placebo-controlled Phase III	344	Pirfenidone 2403 mg·day^{-1} or placebo (ratio 1:1)	Absolute change in % predicted FVC at week 72	FVC change at week 72 was −9.0% in the pirfenidone group and −9.6% in the placebo group. (p=0.501) However, a significant pirfenidone effect was observed until week 48 (p=0.005) and in an analysis of all study time-points (p=0.007)#¶+	NOBLE [33]
		ASCEND (PIPF 016) Multinational Double blind Randomised Placebo controlled Phase III Requested by the FDA	555	Pirfenidone 2403 mg·day^{-1} or placebo	Change in FVC or death at week 52	A relative reduction of 47.9% in the proportion of patients who had an absolute decline of ⩾10 %-points in % predicted FVC or who died in the pirfenidone group compared with placebo. There was also a relative increase of 132.5% in the proportion of patients with no decline in FVC (p<0.001)¶+	KING [34]

Continued

Table 1. Continued

Drug	Mode of action	Study description	Patients n	Doses studied	Primary end-point	Outcome	First author [ref.]
Nintedanib	Intracellular inhibitor of multiple tyrosine kinases, including the VEGF, FGF, and PDGF receptors Interferes with fibroblast proliferation, migration and differentiation to myofibroblasts	TOMORROW Double blind Randomised Placebo controlled Phase II Dose finding	432	Nintedanib 50 mg once daily, 50 mg twice daily, 100 mg twice daily or 150 mg twice daily, or placebo	Annual rate of decline in FVC at 12 months	The annual rate of decline in FVC was 0.06 L·year^{-1} with nintedanib 150 mg twice daily versus 0.19 L·year^{-1} with placebo (p=0.01)	RICHELDI [65]
		INPULSIS Two replicates Randomised Parallel group Phase III	1066	Nintedanib 150 mg twice daily versus placebo (ratio 3:2)	Rate of decline in FVC at 52 weeks	In both trials, the annual rate of decline in FVC was significantly lower in the nintedanib group than in the placebo group Analysis of pooled data showed a difference versus placebo of 109.9 L·year^{-1} (95% CI 75.9–144.0 L·year^{-1}, p<0.001)	RICHELDI [67]

FGF: fibroblast growth factor; PDGF: platelet-derived growth factor; FDA: Food and Drug Administration; VC: vital capacity. #: a pooled analysis of the PIPF 004 and PIPF 006 pirfenidone 2403 mg·day^{-1} arms in both studies showed a significant difference in the primary end-point; ¶: in a pooled analysis of the three multinational trials for the pre-specified end-points, with 1247 patients included, at 1 year, pirfenidone reduced the proportion of patients with >10% decline in % predicted FVC or death by 43.8% (95% CI 29.3–55.4%). +: a pre-specified pooled analysis incorporating results from the CAPACITY trials demonstrated that treatment with pirfenidone for 1 year resulted in a significant reduction in the risk of death from any cause (p=0.01) and from IPF (p=0.006).

An independent Cochrane Collaboration meta-analysis [38] including studies PIPF004, PIPF006 and the Japanese phase III study (n=1046) [32, 33] showed that pirfenidone significantly improved progression-free survival time (HR 0.70, 95% CI 0.56–0.88; p=0.002) [38], with a magnitude of progression-free survival comparable to that observed in nonsmall cell lung cancer trials [35].

The ASCEND study

Pirfenidone has subsequently been investigated in another multinational, placebo-controlled, randomised trial, ASCEND (n=555), which was specifically requested by the Food and Drug Administration [34]. This trial was conducted with similar pre-specified design as PIPF004 and PIPF006, which enabled pooling of data to generate precise estimates of the magnitude of treatment effect. In the ASCEND trial, 555 patients with IPF were randomly assigned to receive either oral pirfenidone (2403 mg per day) or placebo for 52 weeks. The primary end-point was the change in FVC or death at week 52. Secondary end-points were the 6MWD, progression-free survival, dyspnoea, and death from any cause or from IPF. Compared to the PIPF004 and PIPF006 trials, eligibility criteria were slightly modified, with an upper limit of FEV_1/FVC of 0.80 (likely excluding most patients with significant emphysema), and the use of a centralised review of spirometry, chest HRCT, surgical lung biopsy data and an adjudication committee for death events. Notably, 95% of the patients had a pattern of "definite" UIP at chest HRCT, and approximatively 30% of patients had a lung biopsy by video-assisted thoracic surgery demonstrating a pattern of UIP, ensuring high confidence in the diagnosis of IPF according to international guidelines. Altogether, it is likely that this modification of eligibility criteria as compared to the CAPACITY studies enabled enrichment of the study cohort for patients at risk of disease progression and resulted in a more homogeneous study population [39].

A relative reduction of 47.9% was observed in the proportion of patients who had an absolute decline of 10 %-points or more in predicted FVC or who died in the pirfenidone group, as compared with the placebo group. In addition, with pirfenidone, there was a relative increase of 132.5% in the proportion of patients with no decline in FVC (p<0.001), a reduction in the decline in the 6MWD (p=0.04) and an improvement in progression-free survival (p<0.001). There was no significant between-group difference in rates of death. Sensitivity analysis confirmed the robustness of the statistical finding on the primary end-point of change in FVC and corroborated the estimated magnitude of the pirfenidone treatment effect in patients with IPF [40].

Data on outcomes at 1 year from the multinational trials were then pooled for the pre-specified end-points, with a total of 1247 patients included in the analysis. At 1 year, pirfenidone reduced the proportion of patients with a ⩾10% decline in % predicted FVC or death by 43.8% (95% CI 29.3–55.4%) and increased the proportion of patients with no decline by 59.3% (95% CI 29.0–96.8%). A treatment benefit was also observed for progression-free survival, 6MWD and dyspnoea [41]. Furthermore, a pre-specified pooled analysis incorporating results from the CAPACITY trials demonstrated that treatment with pirfenidone for 1 year resulted in a significant reduction in the risk of death from any cause (p=0.01) and from IPF (p=0.006). Pirfenidone reduced the risk of death at 1 year by 48% compared to placebo (HR 0.52, 95% CI 0.31–0.87; p=0.01) [34]. Adverse events were in line with previous studies, with gastrointestinal and skin-related adverse events more common than in the placebo group but rarely leading to treatment discontinuation. A sensitivity analysis confirmed the robustness of the data [41].

Other clinical studies

Data from the phase III trials were further supported by several "real-life" retrospective studies from academic centres. In a small, retrospective study in 18 Japanese patients, pirfenidone therapy was associated with a decrease in the rate of FVC decline in patients with advanced-stage IPF and progressive disease, defined as patients experiencing $\geqslant$10% relative decline in FVC within the 6$\pm$2 months preceding enrolment [42]. In a retrospective study on 38 patients treated with pirfenidone and 40 age-matched controls, a higher proportion of patients treated with pirfenidone *versus* placebo had stable disease based on PFTs and changes on CT, and the changes in CT correlated with the change in VC [43]. In a retrospective analysis of two independent IPF cohorts from Italy and Germany, the annual slope of decline in FVC decreased under pirfenidone therapy as compared to the period of time before treatment, while it did not change in a control cohort of patients, in line with controlled trials [44]. Results were strikingly heterogeneous at the level of a single patient and the benefit of therapy apparently was most pronounced in those patients with the greatest decline in FVC evident before treatment [44]. Similarly, a retrospective Italian study of 128 patients diagnosed with IPF suggested that pirfenidone treatment was associated with a slower decline in FVC with no change in the decline in D_{LCO} in comparison to the pre-treatment period [45]. The change in the FVC slope with treatment was more pronounced in patients with the most severe disease. Other studies similarly suggested comparable results [46–48].

The long-term treatment of pirfenidone is being further evaluated in the RECAP study (PIPF012, NCT00662038), an open-label extension study in patients with IPF who completed the CAPACITY trials [49]. Although the design of the RECAP study is more appropriate for the evaluation of treatment tolerance than efficacy, it is reassuring to observe that the proportion of patients experiencing $\geqslant$10% FVC decline at week 60 was 16.6%, compared with 16.8% and 24.8% in the pirfenidone and placebo arms of the pooled CAPACITY trials, respectively [49].

Safety and tolerance

The tolerance of pirfenidone has been evaluated in individual studies as well as in pooled data from randomised studies. In a comprehensive analysis of safety across four clinical trials evaluating pirfenidone in patients with IPF [50], 789 patients were exposed to pirfenidone for a median duration of 2.6 years and a cumulative total exposure of 2059 person exposure years. Gastrointestinal and skin-related events were the most commonly reported adverse events, were almost always mild to moderate in severity and rarely led to treatment discontinuation. Elevations (more than three times the upper limit of normal) in alanine aminotransferase (ALT) or aspartate aminotransferase (AST) occurred in 2.7% patients, with an adjusted incidence of AST/ALT elevations of 1.7 per 100 person exposure years. In a meta-analysis of six randomised controlled trials and a total of 1073 patients treated [51], the number of individuals who discontinued pirfenidone therapy was significantly higher than patients receiving placebo. The study confirmed a higher rate of gastrointestinal (nausea, dyspepsia, diarrhoea and anorexia), neurological (dizziness and fatigue) and dermatological (photosensitivity and rash) adverse events in patients receiving placebo. In a prospective, multicentre, observational study of 502 patients in Germany [52], 44.2% of these received pirfenidone (as monotherapy in two thirds of them), with no unidentified emergent adverse event.

Overall, the long-term experience with pirfenidone confirmed results of large phase III randomised studies regarding the safety and tolerability of the drug, with a treatment discontinuation rate of about 15% due to gastrointestinal and skin-related adverse events. Recommendations drawn from clinical experience for managing drug-related reactions greatly facilitate treatment adherence and tolerability [53].

Clinical use

Pirfenidone has been approved for the treatment of IPF in Japan, Europe, Canada and the USA. The recommended dose is 2403 mg per day (*e.g.* three capsules of 267 mg three times daily) administered with food. Temporary treatment interruption, dose reduction or symptomatic treatments (prokinetic agents or antiemetic therapy) are recommended for the management of adverse events, especially nausea and gastric discomfort. Liver enzymes should be monitored before and periodically during pirfenidone treatment, and liver enzyme elevations managed through treatment interruption or dose reduction. Patients should be instructed to avoid sun exposure, to wear protective clothing and to use sun screen (protecting against both ultraviolet (UV)A and UVB) on areas of skin exposed to the sun [53].

Nintedanib

Drug development and molecular targets

Nintedanib, previously known as molecule BIBF 1120, is an intracellular inhibitor of several tyrosine kinases that has recently been approved for the treatment of IPF in the USA and Europe [54]. It should be noted that nintedanib was identified as part of a process to develop small-molecule inhibitors of angiogenesis as an anticancer drug. It has been developed in oncology especially in lung, ovarian and colorectal cancer, renal cell carcinoma, and hepatocellular carcinoma [55]. As in oncology, combination therapy or the use of pleiotropic drugs is an important part of drug development in IPF, on the basis of pathogenetic considerations and by analogy with other chronic respiratory diseases (COPD, asthma and pulmonary artery hypertension) [56]. Indeed, as in cancer, monotherapies specific to individual pathways seem intrinsically unlikely to prove efficacious in IPF, due to biological redundancy [56].

As a result of the drug development, nintedanib potently blocks at least 12 tyrosine kinases, including platelet-derived growth factor receptors α and β, VEGF receptors 1–3 and fibroblast growth factor (FGF) receptors 1–3, as well as FMS-like tyrosine kinase 3, and the nonreceptor tyrosine kinases Src, Lyn and Lck [57], which are involved in lung fibrosis [58]. This contrasts with imatinib, which inhibits platelet-derived growth factor receptor, and failed to show clinical benefit in a clinical trial [59]. Overall, nintedanib has some effects on multiple signalling pathways that play a key role in the development and progression of fibrosis [54], with potential redundancy. As the effects of TGF-β, a key player in the pathogenesis of lung fibrosis, are mediated in part by FGF-2 release, and upregulation of FGF receptor 1 and 2 expression [60], it is likely that nintedanib has indirect effects on the TGF-β pathway. Indeed, *in vitro* studies using fibroblasts from patients with IPF have demonstrated that nintedanib interferes with fibroblast proliferation, migration and differentiation to myofibroblasts, and the secretion of extracellular matrix [60–63]. Nintedanib also inhibited TGF-β-induced fibroblast to myofibroblast transformation of primary human lung fibroblasts from IPF patients, as well as TGF-β-stimulated collagen secretion and deposition by primary human lung fibroblasts [60, 62]. In animal models of bleomycin- and silica-induced lung fibrosis, preventive and therapeutic treatment with nintedanib inhibits mRNA expression of

TGF-β [60], and has antifibrotic and anti-inflammatory effects [62]. In addition, recent experimental data support the notion that nintedanib has further broader effects that may mediate antifibrotic activity, including downregulation of extracellular matrix production (fibronectin and collagen 1a1) independent of TGF-β signalling, induction of non-canonical autophagy in IPF fibroblasts (an adaptive stress response impaired in IPF), and, most importantly, inhibition of TGF-β signalling [64].

Pharmacokinetics

Nintedanib has a half-life of 9.5 h and steady-state plasma concentrations are achieved within 1 week [54]. Maximum plasma concentrations are achieved ~2-4 h after oral administration with food. The absolute bioavailability of nintedanib 100 mg is 4.7% [54]. It is metabolised mainly by hydrolytic cleavage by esterases followed by glucuronidation, while biotransformation by cytochrome P450 (CYP), primarily CYP 3A4, plays a minor role. The major route of elimination of nintedanib is faecal/biliary excretion (>90% of dose), with renal excretion contributing to <1% of total clearance. Co-administration with ketoconazole or rifampicin increases (by 60%) or decreases (by 50%) exposure to nintedanib, respectively. Concomitant use of nintedanib and P-glycoprotein and CYP3A4 inducers should therefore be avoided.

Clinical trials

The TOMORROW trial

In the phase II, dose-finding TOMORROW trial, 432 patients with IPF were randomised to receive nintedanib 50 mg once daily, 50 mg twice daily, 100 mg twice daily or 150 mg twice daily, or placebo for 12 months [65]. The primary end-point was the annual rate of decline in FVC, which was 0.06 L·year^{-1} with nintedanib 150 mg twice daily *versus* 0.19 L·year^{-1} with placebo. In the primary analysis, in which a closed testing procedure was used to correct for multiplicity, the primary end-point approached statistical significance for nintedanib 150 mg twice daily *versus* placebo (p=0.06). Using a pre-specified hierarchical test, without correction for multiplicity, the difference in the annual rate of decline in FVC was significantly superior for nintedanib 150 mg twice daily *versus* placebo (p=0.01) [65]. As there were no significant differences between the lower doses of nintedanib and placebo in the annual rate of decline in FVC, the dose of 150 mg twice daily was selected for subsequent studies of nintedanib in pulmonary fibrosis.

The TOMORROW study further provided promising results regarding secondary end-points. Nintedanib 150 mg twice daily reduced the proportion of patients with a decrease in FVC >10% or >200 mL compared with placebo (23.8% *versus* 44.0%, p=0.004). Nintedanib 150 mg twice daily preserved health-related QoL compared with placebo, as measured by change in the St George's Respiratory Questionnaire (SGRQ) score (−0.66 *versus* +5.46 points; p=0.007), and significantly reduced the incidence of investigator-reported acute exacerbations compared with placebo (2.4 *versus* 15.7 per 100 patient-years; p=0.02). The number of deaths from respiratory causes was numerically lower in patients receiving nintedanib than placebo, but with a small number of events overall (two *versus* eight; p=0.06) [65]. Adverse events related to nintedanib were predominantly gastrointestinal in nature and dose dependent, including diarrhoea, nausea and vomiting, and leading to more treatment discontinuations than with placebo. Elevations in liver transaminases were also more frequently reported in patients treated with nintedanib 150 mg twice daily than placebo [65].

The INPULSIS trials

The INPULSIS trials were two replicate, randomised, parallel-group, phase III trials of nintedanib 150 mg twice daily *versus* placebo [66, 67]. A total of 1066 patients were randomised 3:2 to receive nintedanib or placebo for 52 weeks. The protocol of the study included practical recommendations for the management of adverse events, especially temporary interruption of treatment, dose reduction to 100 mg twice daily and the use of symptomatic therapies for the relief of diarrhoea. Concomitant therapy with stable dose of prednisone $\leqslant$15 mg·day^{-1} or equivalent was permitted. Although concomitant use of pirfenidone or other antifibrotic therapy was not permitted during the study, patients were permitted to receive azathioprine, cyclophosphamide, cyclosporin A, NAC or prednisone >15 mg·day^{-1} or equivalent after 6 months, if deemed appropriate by the investigator. Treatment was left to the discretion of the investigator in cases of acute exacerbation.

To be eligible for inclusion in the INPULSIS trials, patients were required to have an FVC of $\geqslant$50% predicted and a DLCO of 30–79% predicted. The chest HRCT scan performed within 12 months before screening was centrally reviewed by a single radiologist, to ensure presence of honeycombing and/or a combination of reticular abnormality and traction bronchiectasis, without nodules or consolidation or features suggestive of alternative causes. Notably, a significant proportion of patients enrolled in the INPULSIS trials met criteria for the possible UIP pattern at HRCT (without honeycombing features) and did not have a lung biopsy, and therefore had a diagnosis of possible/probable IPF that cannot be ascertained according to international guidelines [1], yet does correspond to a significant proportion of patients seen in the routine ILD clinic. Similarly, surgical lung biopsy specimens, if available, were reviewed by a single pathologist. The study population in the INPULSIS trials had a baseline FVC of ~80% of predicted value and a DLCO of 47% of predicted, with a wide range of lung function, including patients with relatively preserved FVC, as well as patients with moderate impairment of lung function.

In addition, to be eligible, patients had to have a FEV1/FVC ratio of $\geqslant$0.7 but patients with an HRCT scan showing emphysema were not excluded. Indeed, emphysema, which is a common comorbidity in patients with IPF [68] and associated with smaller changes in lung function over time [69], was present in 40% of patients in the INPULSIS trials [54]. Patients at increased risk of bleeding (*e.g.* those receiving full-dose anticoagulation, high-dose platelet therapy or fibrinolysis) were excluded from the trials. Patients with myocardial infarction within 6 months or unstable angina within 1 month of randomisation were not eligible [66].

The primary end-point in the INPULSIS trials was the annual rate of decline in FVC [66]. In both trials, the annual rate of decline in FVC was significantly lower in the nintedanib group than in the placebo group. Analysis of pooled data showed an annual rate of decline in FVC of −113.6 mL·year^{-1} in the nintedanib group *versus* −223.5 mL·year^{-1} in the placebo group (difference *versus* placebo 109.9 L·year^{-1}, 95% CI 75.9–144.0 L·year^{-1}; p<0.001) [67].

The effects of nintedanib on pre-specified secondary lung function end-points were consistent with the primary analysis. The absolute mean changes in FVC % predicted at week 52 were −2.9% in the nintedanib group and −6.1% in the placebo group (difference *versus* placebo 3.2%, 95% CI 2.4–4.0%; p<0.001) [27]. An absolute decline in FVC % predicted of $\geqslant$5% over 6–12 months is associated with increased mortality in patients with IPF [36, 70, 71]. A significantly higher proportion of patients in the nintedanib group than in the placebo group had an FVC response at week 52, defined as no absolute decline in

FVC >5% predicted (53.0% *versus* 38.8%; OR 1.8, 95% CI 1.4–2.4) or >10% predicted (70.1% *versus* 60.5%; OR 1.6, 95% CI 1.2–2.1) [67]. In a *post hoc* analysis, disease progression was defined as absolute and relative declines in FVC >5% or >10% predicted at week 52. Nintedanib significantly reduced the proportions of patients with absolute and relative declines in FVC >10% predicted compared with placebo (29.9% *versus* 39.5% and 35.6% *versus* 48.7%, respectively) and with absolute and relative declines in FVC >5% predicted (47.0% *versus* 61.2% and 51.1% *versus* 64.5%, respectively) [54]. Assessing the decline in FVC % predicted as a relative change may maximise the chance of identifying a ⩾10% decline in FVC % predicted without sacrificing prognostic accuracy [70].

Key secondary end-points were the time to first investigator-reported acute exacerbation and change from baseline in SGRQ total score, both assessed over 52 weeks with pre-specified pooled analyses of data [66], for which the results of the two INPULSIS trials were discordant. Using a predefined definition for acute exacerbations, no significant difference was found in INPULSIS-1 between the nintedanib and placebo groups in time to first investigator-reported acute exacerbation (HR 1.15, 95% CI 0.54–2.42; p=0.67); however, a significant benefit of nintedanib *versus* placebo was found in INPULSIS-2 (HR 0.38, 95% CI 0.19–0.77; p=0.005). In the pooled analysis, there was no significant difference in the time to first investigator-reported acute exacerbation between the nintedanib and placebo groups (HR 0.64, 95% CI 0.39–1.05; p=0.08) [65]. The majority of acute exacerbations occurred in patients with FVC ⩽70% predicted at baseline, suggesting that patients with more advanced disease may be more at risk of acute exacerbation and that the effect of nintedanib might be more pronounced in this subgroup[54]. In contrast, the discrepancy between the trials was not explained by imbalances in the races or geographical distribution of the study populations. All investigator-reported events of acute exacerbations were then reviewed by an adjudication committee of three experts in IPF based on medical documentation, and classified as a confirmed acute exacerbation, suspected acute exacerbation or not an acute exacerbation. Suspected (not confirmed) acute exacerbations events were generally those with incomplete data sets, including cases with insufficient documentation to definitely rule out possible causes of acute respiratory worsening (pulmonary embolism, infection, *etc.*). A significant difference in favour of nintedanib was found on time to first adjudicated confirmed or suspected acute exacerbation compared with placebo (HR 0.32, 95% CI 0.16–0.65; p=0.001) [67]. The differences in results observed for investigator-reported exacerbations and adjudicated confirmed/suspected exacerbations has been hypothesised to be related to the phenomenon of treatment effect dilution, *i.e.* the random inclusion of "false" acute exacerbations in the analysis, leading to decreased statistical power [72].

Regarding the other key secondary end-point, no difference in mean change from baseline in SGRQ total score was observed between the nintedanib and placebo groups in INPULSIS-1, but a significantly smaller increase (indicating benefit) in SGRQ total score occurred in the nintedanib group in INPULSIS-2 [67], with no significant difference in the pooled analysis.

Although the INPULSIS trials were not powered to show a reduction in mortality with nintedanib *versus* placebo, analysis of pooled data showed a trend towards a reduction in mortality in patients receiving nintedanib compared with placebo (all-cause mortality 5.5% *versus* 7.8% (HR 0.70, 95% CI 0.43–1.12; p=0.14); death from respiratory causes 3.8% *versus* 5.0% (HR 0.74, 95% CI 0.41–1.34; p=0.34)) [67].

Several pre-specified subgroup analyses of pooled data from the INPULSIS trials were performed [73]. There was no statistically significant difference in the effect of nintedanib for the primary end-point, or the key secondary end-points of change from baseline in SGRQ total score or time to first acute exacerbation in any subgroup. The effect of nintedanib was consistent across a range of pre-specified subgroups by patients' sex, age (<65 or ≥65 years), race (white or Asian), baseline SGRQ total score (≤40 or >40), smoking status (never or ex/current), systemic corticosteroid use (yes or no) and bronchodilator use (yes or no). Treatment effects for the key secondary end-points seemed more pronounced in subjects with baseline FVC ≤70% predicted, because the majority of acute exacerbations and a greater deterioration in SGRQ total score occurred in placebo-treated subjects in this subgroup [73]. Similarly, a comparable effect of treatment was found in patients with honeycombing at HRCT and/or confirmation of a UIP pattern by biopsy *versus* those with features of possible UIP pattern on HRCT and no biopsy. A *post hoc* analysis showed that the treatment effect of nintedanib was independent of the presence of emphysema at baseline [54]. A further *post hoc* analysis demonstrated that nintedanib reduced the annual rate of decline in FVC in patients with an FEV_1/FVC ratio >0.8 (difference *versus* placebo 126.1 mL·year^{-1}, 95% CI 81.6–170.6 mL·year^{-1}) and in patients with an FEV_1/FVC ratio ≤0.8 (difference *versus* placebo 95.5 mL·year^{-1}, 95% CI 41.9–149.1 mL·year^{-1}) with a significant treatment-by-subgroup interaction (p=0.0124) [54].

Furthermore, an analysis of pooled data from the TOMORROW and INPULSIS trials was conducted. The HR for all-cause mortality was 0.70 (95% CI 0.46–1.08, p=0.0954) and the HR for mortality from respiratory causes was 0.62 (95% CI 0.37–1.06, p=0.0779) [54]. In a further analysis of deaths that occurred between randomisation and the end of the follow-up period of both studies, a 43% reduction in risk was found favouring nintedanib (HR 0.57, 95% CI 0.34–0.97; p=0.0274) [54].

Similar to the TOMORROW study, the side-effect profile of nintedanib in the INPULSIS trials was manageable for most patients, with the most frequently reported adverse events being gastrointestinal, especially diarrhoea (62.4% of patients receiving nintedanib *versus* 18.4% of those receiving placebo), vomiting, nausea and decreased appetite [67]. Most adverse events were mild or moderate in intensity, and these led to permanent treatment discontinuation in 19.3% of patients in the nintedanib group *versus* 13.0% of patients treated with placebo. Despite the high frequency of diarrhoea, permanent treatment discontinuation was required in only 4.4% of patients, suggesting that management of diarrhoea through treatment interruption, dose reduction and the use of antidiarrhoeal therapies were successful in enabling patients to remain on treatment. Elevations in liver enzymes occurred in 5.0% of patients in the nintedanib group and 0.7% of patients in the placebo group.

The TOMORROW and INPULSIS trials were continued by ongoing open-label extension trials (NCT01170065 and INPULSIS-ON/NCT01619085, respectively). Preliminary analysis reported in international meetings suggests similar long-term safety and tolerability of nintedanib, as compared to phase II and III trials.

Clinical use

Nintedanib has been approved for the treatment of IPF in the USA and Europe. The recommended dose is 150 mg twice daily, with the two doses administered approximately 12 h apart with food. Temporary treatment interruption, dose reduction to 100 mg twice daily or symptomatic treatments (anti-diarrhoeal therapy, antiemetics and adequate hydration) are recommended for the management of adverse events especially diarrhoea. Liver enzymes should be monitored before and periodically during nintedanib treatment and liver enzyme elevations managed through treatment interruption or dose reduction. As inhibition of VEGF receptor by nintedanib may potentially increase the risk of bleeding or gastrointestinal perforation, patients at known risk for these events should be treated with nintedanib only if the anticipated benefit outweighs the risk. Nintedanib may be used as first-line therapy in patients with IPF or in patients who have previously been treated with pirfenidone.

International guidelines for the management of IPF

Methodology

Given rapidly evolving evidence for the drug management of IPF, the official American Thoracic Society/European Respiratory Society/Japanese Respiratory Society/Latin American Thoracic Society clinical practice guidelines for the treatment of IPF were updated (table 2), with the reappraisal of previously assessed treatment options and new recommendations for novel agents. Guidelines were developed by a multidisciplinary committee consisting of pulmonologists, a general internist, a radiologist, a pathologist, an information scientist, methodologists and a patient with IPF [74]. Committee members had to disclose all potential conflicts of interest, and pulmonologists with expertise in IPF who had conflicts of interest participated in the discussion of the evidence but had to abstain from formulating, grading and voting recommendations. Disease progression was defined in 2011 [1] as increasing respiratory symptoms, worsening pulmonary function test results, progression of fibrosis on HRCT scan, acute respiratory decline or death. Changes over time in FVC or D_{LCO} were considered indirect measures of disease progression for the purpose of this update of the guidelines [74]. Recommendations were developed according to GRADE (Grading of Recommendations Assessment, Development and Evaluation) and were either "strong" or "conditional" (synonymous with weak recommendation in the 2011 document [1]). A strong recommendation means for clinicians that "most individuals should receive the intervention, and that adherence to this recommendation could be used as a quality criterion or

Table 2. Summary of the official American Thoracic Society (ATS)/European Respiratory Society (ERS)/Japanese Respiratory Society (JRS)/Latin American Thoracic Society (ALAT) clinical practice guidelines for the treatment of IPF (update of the 2011 clinical practice guideline)

Strong recommendation against	Conditional recommendation against	Conditional recommendation in favour	Strong recommendation in favour
Anticoagulation (warfarin) Triple therapy (combination of prednisone +azathioprine+NAC Selective endothelin receptor antagonist (ambrisentan) Imatinib, a tyrosine kinase inhibitor with one target	Dual endothelin receptor antagonist (macitentan, bosentan) Phosphodiesterase-5 inhibitor (sildenafil) NAC monotherapy Anti-PH therapy for IPF-associated PH	Nintedanib, a tyrosine kinase inhibitor with multiple targets Pirfenidone Antacid therapy	None

performance indicator; the recommendation can be adopted as policy in most situations" [74]. A conditional recommendation means for clinicians "to recognise that different choices will be appropriate for individual patients, and that they must help each patient arrive at a management decision consistent with his or her values and preferences. Decision aids may be useful in helping individuals to make decisions consistent with their values and preferences. Policy making will require substantial debate and involvement of various stakeholders" [74].

Summary of treatment recommendations

A summary of recommendations for specific treatment questions can be found in table 2. Three drug therapies are conditionally recommended for the treatment of IPF, *i.e.* nintedanib, pirfenidone and antacid therapy. Other drug therapies had either a strong recommendation against their use based on studies that proved them to be harmful in IPF [59, 75–77] or a conditional recommendation against their use based on insufficient evidence or on studies demonstrating lack of benefit [78–86]. Negative studies not yet included in the guidelines have also been recently published using co-trimoxazole [87] and CC-chemokine ligand 2 [88].

N-acetylcysteine

Oxidative stress may contribute to the epithelial cell damage involved in the pathogenesis of IPF. A deficiency of glutathione, a major antioxidant, was observed in lungs of IPF patients [89]. NAC is a precursor of glutathione and was proposed as antioxidant therapy in IPF. Two randomised controlled trials with inhaled NAC have been performed. One compared 30 IPF patients who received aerosolised NAC *versus* control (bromhexine hydrochloride) at 12 months [83]. NAC did not influence pulmonary function, but showed a significant reduction of ground-glass score on HRCT [83]. The other study assessed the efficacy of NAC in 76 patients with early disease; the primary end-point, *i.e.* the change in FVC at 48 weeks, was not met, but FVC was stable in a subset of patients [84].

The IFIGENIA trial assessed the efficacy of high dose of oral NAC (600 mg three times a day) in combination with prednisone and azathioprine. This "triple therapy" reduced the decline in lung function at 1 year compared with prednisone and azathioprine alone [90]. The lack of a true placebo arm lead to a subsequent evaluation of the efficacy of NAC in the IPFnet-sponsored PANTHER trial, a placebo-controlled, randomised, three-arm trial [76]. The triple therapy prednisone, azathioprine and NAC (600 mg three times a day) was compared with NAC alone or placebo. A pre-specified interim analysis planned at approximately 50% of data collection found that the triple combination therapy was associated with a significant increase in all-cause mortality, hospitalisations and serious adverse events. This arm was discontinued and the PANTHER study continued with two groups, NAC *versus* placebo [85]. However, NAC monotherapy did not demonstrate significant benefit of preserving FVC in IPF patients over 60 weeks [85]. One recent study showed that the polymorphisms within the *TOLLIP* gene may influence the response profile to NAC monotherapy [91]. Specifically, a minority of patients carrying the s3750920 (*TOLLIP*) TT genotype may benefit from NAC therapy. However, results from this retrospective study should be reproduced prospectively and are not yet transposable to clinical practice.

Sildenafil

Sildenafil has been studied in two randomised controlled trials in patients with IPF [81, 82]. In the phase III STEP-IPF (Sildenafil Trial of Exercise Performance in IPF) trial, 180 patients with D_{LCO} <35% predicted were randomised to receive either sildenafil 20 mg three times daily or placebo for 12 week, followed by a 12-week open-label extension phase. No benefit was observed for the primary outcome, which was the proportion of patients who had more than 20% improvement in 6MWD at 12 weeks. However, significant differences were observed in favour of sildenafil for secondary and exploratory end-points, including improvement in shortness of breath, QoL measure, DLCO and arterial oxygen saturation [82]. A subgroup analysis suggested that patients with right ventricular systolic dysfunction at echocardiography might benefit from sildenafil, with a significant improvement in 6MWD [92]. In another, smaller study [81], no significant benefit in was observed in 6MWD with sildenafil as compared to placebo, but patients with PH or right ventricular dysfunction were excluded from the study. Pooled analysis of both studies [74] showed improvement in SGRQ but no benefit in other end-points. Overall, the use of sildenafil is not recommended in patients with IPF [74]. Further studies are needed to assess its potential role in patients with IPF and documented pre-capillary PH.

Antacid therapy

Because gastro-oesophageal reflux is highly prevalent in patients with IPF and aspiration or microaspiration is hypothesised to worsen IPF, antacid treatments have been proposed in IPF to decrease microaspiration-associated epithelial alveolar injury. In one analysis of pooled data from placebo arms of three randomised trials, patients who received proton pump inhibitors or histamine-2 blocker receptor antagonists experienced small decline in FVC during the study period than those not receiving antacid treatment and had no episode of acute exacerbation of IPF, with no difference in overall mortality [93]. In another retrospective study, a survival advantage was found in IPF patients receiving antacid therapy [94]. In light of the low cost of antacid therapy and very limited risk of treatment (possible small increase in the risk of pneumonia), it was suggested that clinicians use regular antacid treatment for patients with IPF (conditional recommendation, very low confidence in the estimates of effect). Of note, the same level of recommendation was given to antacid therapy (regardless of the presence or absence of symptomatic reflux) as well as to pirfenidone and nintedanib, for which a much greater quality of evidence is available, with well-conducted, phase III randomised controlled trials [95]. This largely reflects the methodology of the guidelines and that only non-conflicted members could vote. Further studies are needed to evaluate whether antacid therapy is beneficial in IPF and whether the benefit would be different in symptomatic *versus* nonsymptomatic patients with reflux. Omeprazole interacts with pirfenidone and should be avoided in patients receiving this drug, whereas other proton pump inhibitors can be prescribed.

Pirfenidone

Based on the evidence demonstrating efficacy of pirfenidone in IPF (see ealier), including new evidence that has become available since the 2011 guideline [1], it is suggested that "clinicians use pirfenidone in patients with IPF (conditional recommendation, moderate confidence in estimates of effect) [...]. This recommendation places a high value on the potential benefit of pirfenidone on patient-important outcomes such as disease progression as measured by rates of FVC decline and mortality and a lower value on potentially significant adverse effects and the cost of treatment" [74]. It is important that patients be educated on all potential adverse effects and on how to prevent them. Patients should share the decision of treatment. Additional data are needed in patients with more severe functional impairment or significant comorbidities including airflow obstruction and/or comorbid emphysema, although data from academic centres and subgroup analysis of randomised trials presented in meetings suggest that the treatment effect is comparable across patients subgroups. The proper duration of treatment is not known. As IPF is a progressive, irreversible disease despite treatment, the treatment goal is to slow progression of disease, which should be explained to the patient, the family, and to healthcare providers.

Nintedanib

As mentioned earlier in this chapter, there is accumulated evidence that nintedanib reduces disease progression in patients with IPF. In the 2015 update of the clinical practice guidelines on IPF, it is suggested that "clinicians use nintedanib in patients with IPF (conditional recommendation, moderate confidence in estimates of effect). […] This recommendation places a high value on the potential benefit of nintedanib on patient-important outcomes such as disease progression measured by rate of FVC decline and mortality and a lower value on potentially significant adverse effects and the expected cost of treatment" [74]. Patients must be informed of commonly reported adverse effects, especially diarrhoea, although relatively few patients discontinue the drug secondary to adverse effects. Additional data are needed in patients with more severe functional impairment or other comorbidities. The population enrolled in the nintedanib trials included patients with a HRCT scan pattern suggestive of possible or probable UIP pattern, without confirmation of UIP on surgical lung biopsy (probable IPF) (e.g. patients with a "working diagnosis" of IPF) [96]. The proper duration of treatment is not known. As for pirfenidone, the treatment goal is to slow progression of disease.

Unresolved issues and future perspectives

Treatment of IPF with mild-to-moderate functional impairment

One issue that remains to be explored relates to the optimal time to initiate antifibrotic therapy. Although no study specifically included patients with mild functional impairment or patients with no or few clinical manifestations (so-called subclinical disease), subgroup analysis of both pirfenidone and nintedanib randomised trials suggest that the drugs are equally effective across disease severity subgroups with regards to the primary end-point (FVC) [48, 97]. This observation is in favour of early initiation of therapy, if possible within local regulations (in the UK, the National Institute for Health and Care Excellence (NICE) requires that FVC be between 50% and 80% predicted for pirfenidone to be initiated). Furthermore, given interindividual differences in lung function, a patient with a baseline FVC value of 85% of predicted at the time of IPF diagnosis may in fact already have declined from 120% of predicted to 85%, a significant decline. Among factors that may limit early initiation of treatment, asymptomatic IPF patients may be less inclined to tolerate moderate severity side-effects from antifibrotic therapy than those with more severe impairment in their daily life activities. In addition, early treatment initiation implies confident diagnosis of IPF, which in early disease, may frequently require a surgical lung biopsy [98]. Overall, the patient's preference needs to be taken into account, as some will favour long-term improvement of survival with treatment, whereas others may prefer to abstain from any treatment to avoid any side-effects.

Similarly, data from randomised trials do not inform the clinicians about when to discontinue antifibrotic therapy or possibly switch drug. In the UK, NICE arbitrarily stated that pirfenidone should be discontinued if FVC decreased by $\geqslant$10%. This, however, does not take into account the inherent variability in the course of IPF progression and variability of lung function measurement. Whereas a decline in FVC is predictive of subsequent mortality, it is not an indicator of individual treatment response, and "decliners" may or may not continue to decline [99, 100]. Data from prospective registries [52] may provide useful information about discontinuation and switch of antifibrotic therapy.

Again, the patient's preference must be considered, as the benefit/tolerance ratio may vary with the progression of disease, and increased impairment of exercise capacity and QoL. Strict stopping rules may be difficult to apply in any case.

Choice of first-line therapy

Because no head-to-head trials of nintedanib and pirfenidone have been conducted, a direct comparison of drugs is not possible. Indirect comparison of nintedanib *versus* pirfenidone by network analysis (using placebo groups as a common denominator) has showed no significant difference [101]. Such analysis should be interpreted with great caution in the light of the various differences between the studies especially the patient population and the primary endpoint.

International guidelines [74] do not provide recommendations for one treatment over another, nor do they provide suggestions for or against combination regimen or sequential therapy, with the exception of a strong recommendation against the use of the triple combination therapy. The duration of treatment benefit beyond 1 year is unknown. However, long-term data from extension-phase studies suggest that both pirfenidone and nintedanib may have acceptable tolerability and safety for several years. There is uncertainty regarding the condition of possible UIP on HRCT when a diagnostic surgical lung biopsy has not been performed; it is suggested to use the terminology of "working diagnosis of IPF" on the basis of a multidisciplinary evaluation and to manage patients as those with definite UIP/IPF.

Combination therapy

Demonstration of the efficacy of pirfenidone and nintedanib in reducing the progression of IPF has created momentum for the possible use of both drugs in combination. However, data are still scarce and do not support combination of these drugs outside of clinical trials. Barriers to co-administration of drugs include shared gastrointestinal side-effects, pharmacokinetic interaction, cost, limited rationale regarding pathophysiology (both drugs are effective at least partly through inhibition of the TGF-β pathway), and lack of data regarding safety and tolerability. In a study in 50 Japanese patients with IPF, co-administration of nintedanib and pirfenidone reduced exposure to nintedanib, possibly reflecting reduced absorption but had no effect on the pharmacokinetics of pirfenidone [102]. More patients reported nausea and vomiting when nintedanib was added to pirfenidone than when it was given alone. However, no definite conclusions on the safety and tolerability of a combination of nintedanib and pirfenidone can be drawn due to the low number of patients and the short treatment duration in this study. At present, there are therefore no data to support the use of combination therapy with nintedanib and pirfenidone in patients with IPF.

Because the future of IPF treatment probably involves combination therapy [56], current and future clinical trials will largely comprise add-on trials, in which a new drug is combined with nintedanib or pirfenidone. A number of compounds are currently under evaluation for the treatment of lung fibrosis. The co-administration of monoclonal antibodies with pirfenidone or nintedanib might appropriately target multiple distinct pathways and might ultimately prove valuable to treat IPF, with presumably an acceptable tolerability and safety profile. Development of drugs used in combination will need to overcome significant challenges in study design and patient recruitment, however [39, 103]. Specifically, the background use of effective therapies by patients enrolled in clinical trials will slow disease progression, reduce event rates and increase dropout rates, thereby reducing study power or require to increase the sample size to maintain adequate statistical power [39].

Conclusion

Given the many challenges, there is a tremendous unmet need to identify biomarkers in IPF, and to personalise therapy to individuals based on biomarkers and/or genetic polymorphism. There is a number of drugs currently evaluated for IPF [56]. Recent data regarding polymorphism in the *TOLLIP* gene (coding for negative inhibitor of Toll-like receptors (TLRs), including TLR2 and TLR4, that are active in the lung, with anti-inflammatory activity) associated with a distinct safety and efficacy profile to NAC therapy [91] suggests that personalised medicine, as it developed in recent years in oncology, may also be attainable in IPF. This further highlights the importance of pharmacogenetics in IPF, which in the future, may bring us to a new era of research and individualised drug therapy in IPF.

References

1. Raghu G, Collard HR, Egan JJ, *et al.* An official ATS/ERS/JRS/ALAT statement: idiopathic pulmonary fibrosis: evidence-based guidelines for diagnosis and management. *Am J Respir Crit Care Med* 2011; 183: 788–824.
2. Ley B, Collard HR, King TE Jr. Clinical course and prediction of survival in idiopathic pulmonary fibrosis. *Am J Respir Crit Care Med* 2011; 183: 431–440.
3. Vancheri C. Common pathways in idiopathic pulmonary fibrosis and cancer. *Eur Respir Rev* 2013; 22: 265–272.
4. Ley B, Collard HR. Epidemiology of idiopathic pulmonary fibrosis. *Clin Epidemiol* 2013; 5: 483–492.
5. Kropski JA, Blackwell TS, Loyd JE. The genetic basis of idiopathic pulmonary fibrosis. *Eur Respir J* 2015; 45: 1717–1727.
6. Spagnolo P, du Bois RM, Cottin V. Rare lung disease and orphan drug development. *Lancet Respir Med* 2013; 1: 479–487.
7. Nalysnyk L, Cid-Ruzafa J, Rotella P, *et al.* Incidence and prevalence of idiopathic pulmonary fibrosis: review of the literature. *Eur Respir Rev* 2012; 21: 355–361.
8. Navaratnam V, Fleming KM, West J, *et al.* The rising incidence of idiopathic pulmonary fibrosis in the U.K. *Thorax* 2011; 66: 462–467.
9. Copley SJ, Wells AU, Hawtin KE, *et al.* Lung morphology in the elderly: comparative CT study of subjects over 75 years old *versus* those under 55 years old. *Radiology* 2009; 251: 566–573.
10. Washko GR, Hunninghake GM, Fernandez IE, *et al.* Lung volumes and emphysema in smokers with interstitial lung abnormalities. *N Engl J Med* 2011; 364: 897–906.
11. Ryerson CJ, Cottin V, Brown KK, *et al.* Acute exacerbation of idiopathic pulmonary fibrosis: shifting the paradigm. *Eur Respir J* 2015; 46: 512–520.
12. Collard HR, Moore BB, Flaherty KR, *et al.* Acute exacerbations of idiopathic pulmonary fibrosis. *Am J Respir Crit Care Med* 2007; 176: 636–643.
13. Martinez FJ, Safrin S, Weycker D, *et al.* The clinical course of patients with idiopathic pulmonary fibrosis. *Ann Intern Med* 2005; 142: 963–967.
14. Swigris JJ, Gould MK, Wilson SR. Health-related quality of life among patients with idiopathic pulmonary fibrosis. *Chest* 2005; 127: 284–294.
15. Swigris JJ, Stewart AL, Gould MK, *et al.* Patients' perspectives on how idiopathic pulmonary fibrosis affects the quality of their lives. *Health Qual Life Outcomes* 2005; 3: 61.
16. Noble PW, Barkauskas CE, Jiang D. Pulmonary fibrosis: patterns and perpetrators. *J Clin Invest* 2012; 122: 2756–2762.
17. Fernandez IE, Eickelberg O. New cellular and molecular mechanisms of lung injury and fibrosis in idiopathic pulmonary fibrosis. *Lancet* 2012; 380: 680–688.
18. Wolters PJ, Collard HR, Jones KD. Pathogenesis of idiopathic pulmonary fibrosis. *Ann Rev Pathol* 2014; 9: 157–179.

19. Selman M, Pardo A. Revealing the pathogenic and aging-related mechanisms of the enigmatic idiopathic pulmonary fibrosis. An integral model. *Am J Respir Crit Care Med* 2014; 189: 1161–1172.

20. Iyer SN, Gurujeyalakshmi G, Giri SN. Effects of pirfenidone on procollagen gene expression at the transcriptional level in bleomycin hamster model of lung fibrosis. *J Pharmacol Exp Ther* 1999; 289: 211–218.

21. Kakugawa T, Mukae H, Hayashi T, *et al.* Pirfenidone attenuates expression of HSP47 in murine bleomycin-induced pulmonary fibrosis. *Eur Respir J* 2004; 24: 57–65.

22. Carter NJ. Pirfenidone: in idiopathic pulmonary fibrosis. *Drugs* 2011; 71: 1721–1732.

23. Schaefer CJ, Ruhrmund DW, Pan L, *et al.* Antifibrotic activities of pirfenidone in animal models. *Eur Respir Rev* 2011; 20: 85–97.

24. Liu H, Drew P, Gaugler AC, *et al.* Pirfenidone inhibits lung allograft fibrosis through L-arginine-arginase pathway. *Am J Transplant* 2005; 5: 1256–1263.

25. Oku H, Shimizu T, Kawabata T, *et al.* Antifibrotic action of pirfenidone and prednisolone: different effects on pulmonary cytokines and growth factors in bleomycin-induced murine pulmonary fibrosis. *Eur J Pharmacol* 2008; 590: 400–408.

26. Zhou H, Latham CW, Zander DS, *et al.* Pirfenidone inhibits obliterative airway disease in mouse tracheal allografts. *J Heart Lung Transplant* 2005; 24: 1577–1585.

27. Iyer SN, Hyde DM, Giri SN. Anti-inflammatory effect of pirfenidone in the bleomycin-hamster model of lung inflammation. *Inflammation* 2000; 24: 477–491.

28. Nakazato H, Oku H, Yamane S, *et al.* A novel anti-fibrotic agent pirfenidone suppresses tumor necrosis factor-alpha at the translational level. *Eur J Pharmacol* 2002; 446: 177–185.

29. Oku H, Nakazato H, Horikawa T, *et al.* Pirfenidone suppresses tumor necrosis factor-alpha, enhances interleukin-10 and protects mice from endotoxin shock. *Eur J Pharmacol* 2002; 446: 167–176.

30. Raghu G, Johnson WC, Lockhart D, *et al.* Treatment of idiopathic pulmonary fibrosis with a new antifibrotic agent, pirfenidone: results of a prospective, open-label Phase II study. *Am J Respir Crit Care Med* 1999; 159: 1061–1069.

31. Azuma A, Nukiwa T, Tsuboi E, *et al.* Double-blind, placebo-controlled trial of pirfenidone in patients with idiopathic pulmonary fibrosis. *Am J Respir Crit Care Med* 2005; 171: 1040–1047.

32. Taniguchi H, Ebina M, Kondoh Y, *et al.* Pirfenidone in idiopathic pulmonary fibrosis. *Eur Respir J* 2010; 35: 821–829.

33. Noble PW, Albera C, Bradford WZ, *et al.* Pirfenidone in patients with idiopathic pulmonary fibrosis (CAPACITY): two randomised trials. *Lancet* 2011; 377: 1760–1769.

34. King TE Jr, Bradford WZ, Castro-Bernardini S, *et al.* A phase 3 trial of pirfenidone in patients with idiopathic pulmonary fibrosis. *N Engl J Med* 2014; 370: 2083–2092.

35. Vancheri C, du Bois RM. A progression-free end-point for idiopathic pulmonary fibrosis trials: lessons from cancer. *Eur Respir J* 2013; 41: 262–269.

36. du Bois RM, Weycker D, Albera C, *et al.* Forced vital capacity in patients with idiopathic pulmonary fibrosis: test properties and minimal clinically important difference. *Am J Respir Crit Care Med* 2011; 184: 1382–1389.

37. du Bois RM, Weycker D, Albera C, *et al.* Six-minute-walk test in idiopathic pulmonary fibrosis: test validation and minimal clinically important difference. *Am J Respir Crit Care Med* 2011; 183: 1231–1237.

38. Spagnolo P, Del Giovane C, Luppi F, *et al.* Non-steroid agents for idiopathic pulmonary fibrosis. *Cochrane Database Syst Rev* 2010; 9: CD003134.

39. Collard HR, Bradford WZ, Cottin V, *et al.* A new era in idiopathic pulmonary fibrosis: considerations for future clinical trials. *Eur Respir J* 2015; 46: 243–249.

40. Lederer DJ, Bradford WZ, Fagan EA, *et al.* Sensitivity analyses of the change in FVC in a phase 3 trial of pirfenidone for idiopathic pulmonary fibrosis. *Chest* 2015; 148: 196–201.

41. Noble PW, Albera C, Bradford WZ, *et al.* Pirfenidone for idiopathic pulmonary fibrosis: analysis of pooled data from three multinational phase 3 trials. *Eur Respir J* 2016; 47: 243–253.

42. Sugino K, Ishida F, Kikuchi N, *et al.* Comparison of clinical characteristics and prognostic factors of combined pulmonary fibrosis and emphysema *versus* idiopathic pulmonary fibrosis alone. *Respirology* 2014; 19: 239–245.

43. Iwasawa T, Ogura T, Sakai F, *et al.* CT analysis of the effect of pirfenidone in patients with idiopathic pulmonary fibrosis. *Eur J Radiol* 2014; 83: 32–38.

44. Loeh B, Drakopanagiotakis F, Bandelli GP, *et al.* Intraindividual response to treatment with pirfenidone in idiopathic pulmonary fibrosis. *Am J Respir Crit Care Med* 2015; 191: 110–113.

45. Harari S, Caminati A, Albera C, *et al.* Efficacy of pirfenidone for idiopathic pulmonary fibrosis: An Italian real life study. *Respir Med* 2015; 109: 904–913.

46. Oltmanns U, Kahn N, Palmowski K, *et al.* Pirfenidone in idiopathic pulmonary fibrosis: real-life experience from a German tertiary referral center for interstitial lung diseases. *Respiration* 2014; 88: 199–207.

47. Cottin V, Maher T. Long-term clinical and real-world experience with pirfenidone in the treatment of idiopathic pulmonary fibrosis. *Eur Respir Rev* 2015; 24: 58–64.

48. Kreuter M. Pirfenidone: an update on clinical trial data and insights from everyday practice. *Eur Respir Rev* 2014; 23: 111–117.

49. Costabel U, Albera C, Bradford WZ, *et al.* Analysis of lung function and survival in RECAP: An open-label extension study of pirfenidone in patients with idiopathic pulmonary fibrosis. *Sarcoidosis Vasc Diffuse Lung Dis* 2014; 31: 198–205.

50. Valeyre D, Albera C, Bradford WZ, *et al.* Comprehensive assessment of the long-term safety of pirfenidone in patients with idiopathic pulmonary fibrosis. *Respirology* 2014; 19: 740–747.

51. Jiang C, Huang H, Liu J, *et al.* Adverse events of pirfenidone for the treatment of pulmonary fibrosis: a meta-analysis of randomized controlled trials. *PLoS One* 2012; 7: e47024.

52. Behr J, Kreuter M, Hoeper MM, *et al.* Management of patients with idiopathic pulmonary fibrosis in clinical practice: the INSIGHTS-IPF registry. *Eur Respir J* 2015; 46: 186–196.

53. Costabel U, Bendstrup E, Cottin V, *et al.* Pirfenidone in idiopathic pulmonary fibrosis: expert panel discussion on the management of drug-related adverse events. *Adv Ther* 2014; 31: 375–391.

54. Cottin V. Nintedanib: a new treatment for idiopathic pulmonary fibrosis. *Clin Invest* 2015: 1–12.

55. Roth GJ, Binder R, Colbatzky F, *et al.* Nintedanib: from discovery to the clinic. *J Med Chem* 2015; 58: 1053–1063.

56. Wuyts WA, Antoniou KM, Borensztajn K, *et al.* Combination therapy: the future of management for idiopathic pulmonary fibrosis? *Lancet Respir Med* 2014; 2: 933–942.

57. Hilberg F, Roth GJ, Krssak M, *et al.* BIBF 1120: triple angiokinase inhibitor with sustained receptor blockade and good antitumor efficacy. *Cancer Res* 2008; 68: 4774–4782.

58. Grimminger F, Gunther A, Vancheri C. The role of tyrosine kinases in the pathogenesis of idiopathic pulmonary fibrosis. *Eur Respir J* 2015; 45: 1426–1433.

59. Daniels CE, Lasky JA, Limper AH, *et al.* Imatinib treatment for idiopathic pulmonary fibrosis: Randomized placebo-controlled trial results. *Am J Respir Crit Care Med* 2010; 181: 604–610.

60. Wollin L, Wex E, Pautsch A, *et al.* Mode of action of nintedanib in the treatment of idiopathic pulmonary fibrosis. *Eur Respir J* 2015; 45: 1434–1445.

61. Ahluwalia N, Shea BS, Tager AM. New therapeutic targets in idiopathic pulmonary fibrosis. Aiming to rein in runaway wound-healing responses. *Am J Respir Crit Care Med* 2014; 190: 867–878.

62. Wollin L, Maillet I, Quesniaux V, *et al.* Antifibrotic and anti-inflammatory activity of the tyrosine kinase inhibitor nintedanib in experimental models of lung fibrosis. *J Pharmacol Exp Ther* 2014; 349: 209–220.

63. Hostettler KE, Zhong J, Papakonstantinou E, *et al.* Anti-fibrotic effects of nintedanib in lung fibroblasts derived from patients with idiopathic pulmonary fibrosis. *Respir Res* 2014; 15: 157.

64. Rangarajan S, Kurundkar A, Kurundkar D, *et al.* Novel Mechanisms for the Antifibrotic Action of Nintedanib. *Am J Respir Cell Mol Biol* 2016; 54: 51–59.

65. Richeldi L, Costabel U, Selman M, *et al.* Efficacy of a tyrosine kinase inhibitor in idiopathic pulmonary fibrosis. *N Engl J Med* 2011; 365: 1079–1087.

66. Richeldi L, Cottin V, Flaherty KR, *et al.* Design of the INPULSIS trials: two phase 3 trials of nintedanib in patients with idiopathic pulmonary fibrosis. *Respir Med* 2014; 108: 1023–1030.

67. Richeldi L, du Bois RM, Raghu G, *et al.* Efficacy and safety of nintedanib in idiopathic pulmonary fibrosis. *N Engl J Med* 2014; 370: 2071–2082.

68. Cottin V. The impact of emphysema in pulmonary fibrosis. *Eur Respir Rev* 2013; 22: 153–157.

69. Akagi T, Matsumoto T, Harada T, *et al.* Coexistent emphysema delays the decrease of vital capacity in idiopathic pulmonary fibrosis. *Respir Med* 2009; 103: 1209–1215.

70. Richeldi L, Ryerson CJ, Lee JS, *et al.* Relative *versus* absolute change in forced vital capacity in idiopathic pulmonary fibrosis. *Thorax* 2012; 67: 407–411.

71. Zappala CJ, Latsi PI, Nicholson AG, *et al.* Marginal decline in forced vital capacity is associated with a poor outcome in idiopathic pulmonary fibrosis. *Eur Respir J* 2010; 35: 830–836.

72. Suissa S, Ernst P. The INPULSIS enigma: exacerbations in idiopathic pulmonary fibrosis. *Thorax* 2015; 70: 508–510.

73. Costabel U, Inoue Y, Richeldi L, *et al.* Efficacy of nintedanib in idiopathic pulmonary fibrosis across prespecified subgroups in INPULSIS. *Am J Respir Crit Care Med* 2016; 193: 178–185.

74. Raghu G, Rochwerg B, Zhang Y, *et al.* An official ATS/ERS/JRS/ALAT clinical practice guideline: treatment of idiopathic pulmonary fibrosis. an update of the 2011 clinical practice guideline. *Am J Respir Crit Care Med* 2015; 192: e3–19.

75. Noth I, Anstrom KJ, Calvert SB, *et al.* A placebo-controlled randomized trial of warfarin in idiopathic pulmonary fibrosis. *Am J Respir Crit Care Med* 2012; 186: 88–95.

76. Raghu G, Anstrom KJ, King TE Jr, *et al.* Prednisone, azathioprine, and N-acetylcysteine for pulmonary fibrosis. *N Engl J Med* 2012; 366: 1968–1977.

77. Raghu G, Behr J, Brown KK, *et al.* Treatment of idiopathic pulmonary fibrosis with ambrisentan: a parallel, randomized trial. *Ann Intern Med* 2013; 158: 641–649.

78. King TE Jr, Brown KK, Raghu G, *et al.* BUILD-3: a randomized, controlled trial of bosentan in idiopathic pulmonary fibrosis. *Am J Respir Crit Care Med* 2011; 184: 92–99.

79. King TE Jr, Behr J, Brown KK, *et al.* BUILD-1: a randomized placebo-controlled trial of bosentan in idiopathic pulmonary fibrosis. *Am J Respir Crit Care Med* 2008; 177: 75–81.

80. Raghu G, Million-Rousseau R, Morganti A, et al. Macitentan for the treatment of idiopathic pulmonary fibrosis: the randomised controlled MUSIC trial. *Eur Respir J* 2013; 42: 1622–1632.

81. Jackson RM, Glassberg MK, Ramos CF, et al. Sildenafil therapy and exercise tolerance in idiopathic pulmonary fibrosis. *Lung* 2010; 188: 115–123.

82. Zisman DA, Schwarz M, Anstrom KJ, et al. A controlled trial of sildenafil in advanced idiopathic pulmonary fibrosis. *N Engl J Med* 2010; 363: 620–628.

83. Tomioka H, Kuwata Y, Imanaka K, et al. A pilot study of aerosolized N-acetylcysteine for idiopathic pulmonary fibrosis. *Respirology* 2005; 10: 449–455.

84. Homma S, Azuma A, Taniguchi H, et al. Efficacy of inhaled N-acetylcysteine monotherapy in patients with early stage idiopathic pulmonary fibrosis. *Respirology* 2012; 17: 467–477.

85. Martinez FJ, de Andrade JA, Anstrom KJ, et al. Randomized trial of acetylcysteine in idiopathic pulmonary fibrosis. *N Engl J Med* 2014; 370: 2093–2101.

86. Corte TJ, Keir GJ, Dimopoulos K, et al. Bosentan in pulmonary hypertension associated with fibrotic idiopathic interstitial pneumonia. *Am J Respir Crit Care Med* 2014; 190: 208–217.

87. Shulgina L, Cahn AP, Chilvers ER, et al. Treating idiopathic pulmonary fibrosis with the addition of co-trimoxazole: a randomised controlled trial. *Thorax* 2013; 68: 155–162.

88. Raghu G, Martinez FJ, Brown KK, et al. CC-chemokine ligand 2 inhibition in idiopathic pulmonary fibrosis: a phase 2 trial of carlumab. *Eur Respir J* 2015; 46: 1740–1750.

89. Cantin AM, Hubbard RC, Crystal RG. Glutathione deficiency in the epithelial lining fluid of the lower respiratory tract in idiopathic pulmonary fibrosis. *Am Rev Respir Dis* 1989; 139: 370–372.

90. Demedts M, Behr J, Buhl R, et al. IFIGENIA: effects of N-acetylcysteine (NAC) on primary end points VC and DLco. *Eur Respir J* 2004; 24: Suppl. 48, P4078.

91. Oldham JM, Ma SF, Martinez FJ, et al. TOLLIP, MUC5B, and the response to N-acetylcysteine among individuals with idiopathic pulmonary fibrosis. *Am J Respir Crit Care Med* 2015; 192: 1475–1482.

92. Han MK, Bach DS, Hagan PG, et al. Sildenafil preserves exercise capacity in patients with idiopathic pulmonary fibrosis and right-sided ventricular dysfunction. *Chest* 2013; 143: 1699–1708.

93. Lee JS, Collard HR, Anstrom KJ, et al. Anti-acid treatment and disease progression in idiopathic pulmonary fibrosis: an analysis of data from three randomised controlled trials. *Lancet Respir Med* 2013; 1: 369–376.

94. Lee JS, Ryu JH, Elicker BM, et al. Gastroesophageal reflux therapy is associated with longer survival in patients with idiopathic pulmonary fibrosis. *Am J Respir Crit Care Med* 2011; 184: 1390–1394.

95. Wuyts WA, Bonella F, Costabel U, et al. An important step forward, but still a way to go. *Am J Respir Crit Care Med* 2016; 193: 340–341.

96. Wells AU, Kokosi M, Karagiannis K. Treatment strategies for idiopathic interstitial pneumonias. *Curr Opin Pulm Med* 2014; 20: 442–448.

97. Bonella F, Stowasser S, Wollin L. Idiopathic pulmonary fibrosis: current treatment options and critical appraisal of nintedanib. *Drug Des Develop Ther* 2015; 9: 6407–6419.

98. Cordier JF, Cottin V. Neglected evidence in idiopathic pulmonary fibrosis: from history to earlier diagnosis. *Eur Respir J* 2013; 42: 916–923.

99. Schmidt SL, Tayob N, Han MK, et al. Predicting pulmonary fibrosis disease course from past trends in pulmonary function. *Chest* 2014; 145: 579–585.

100. Reichmann WM, Yu YF, Macaulay D, et al. Change in forced vital capacity and associated subsequent outcomes in patients with newly diagnosed idiopathic pulmonary fibrosis. *BMC Pulm Med* 2015; 15: 167.

101. Loveman E, Copley VR, Scott DA, et al. Comparing new treatments for idiopathic pulmonary fibrosis – a network meta-analysis. *BMC Pulm Med* 2015; 15: 37.

102. Ogura T, Taniguchi H, Azuma A, et al. Safety and pharmacokinetics of nintedanib and pirfenidone in idiopathic pulmonary fibrosis. *Eur Respir J* 2015; 45: 1382–1392.

103. Wells A. Combination therapy in idiopathic pulmonary fibrosis: the way ahead will be hard. *Eur Respir J* 2015; 45: 1208–1210.

Disclosures: V. Cottin has received honoraria for participating as an advisory panel member and/or speaker for the following companies: Actelion, Bayer, Biogen Idec, Boehringer Ingelheim, Gilead, GSK, InterMune, Novartis, Pfizer, Roche and Sanofi. He has also received support for attending meetings from GSK. His wife is an employee of Sanofi Pasteur. C. Valenzuela has received honoraria for participating as an advisory panel member and/or speaker for the following companies: Boehringer Ingelheim, Gilead and Roche.

Chapter 17

Symptom management: dyspnoea and cough

Wim A. Wuyts

Emerging information on the pathogenesis of IPF has led to the first specific treatments for this disease. These agents only have an effect on FVC decline, although pirfenidone also has a positive effect on survival. None of these agents seems to significantly alter symptoms that are crucial for patients, such as dyspnoea and cough. Dyspnoea seems to be directly related to disease progression but is also determined by comorbidities such as cardiac disease and PH. Treatment of dyspnoea includes lung transplantation and symptom-based therapies such as supplemental oxygen, pulmonary rehabilitation, the use of opioids and treatment of comorbidities such as PH. Cough is also a cardinal feature of IPF. There are some animal data on the use of pirfenidone, but convincing treatment evidence for both pirfenidone and nintedanib is lacking. Thalidomide and codeine have shown promising effects, but it is obvious that new tools and an innovative trial design will be crucial to detect the activity of new agents on the critical determinants of QoL in patients with IPF.

IPF is a relentless fibrotic disorder characterised by a process of progressive damage to the lung [1]. This leads to the production of pro-fibrotic cytokines, activation of (myo)fibroblasts and the formation of a collagen matrix structure. This gradual formation of scar tissue in the lung leads to architectural distortion and a problematic diffusion of oxygen through the alveoli into the blood vessels. This in turn leads to a progressive dyspnoea, initially only with considerable exertion but later on also occurring at rest. Next to dyspnoea, the disease is characterised by a dry cough, often present before the occurrence of dyspnoea. These symptoms are not specific for IPF but also occur in most of the entities categorised in the group of ILDs [1].

In the last decade, this field has been characterised by a considerable evolution in both diagnosis and treatment [1]. More than 10 years ago, patients were treated with anti-inflammatory agents (high dosage of corticosteroids in combination with azathioprine or other immunosuppressive agents). Recently, it has been shown that the use of high-dose steroids induces increased mortality and an increased number of hospitalisations in comparison with placebo in patients with IPF [2]. As more data have become available on

Unit for Interstitial Lung Diseases, Dept of Pulmonary Medicine, University Hospitals Leuven, Leuven, Belgium.

Correspondence: Wim A. Wuyts, Unit for Interstitial Lung Diseases, Dept of Pulmonary Medicine, University Hospitals Leuven, Herestraat 49, 3000 Leuven, Belgium. E-mail: wim.wuyts@uzleuven.be

Copyright ©ERS 2016. Print ISBN: 978-1-84984-067-5. Online ISBN: 978-1-84984-068-2. Print ISSN: 2312-508X. Online ISSN: 2312-5098.

the key pathogenic processes, it has been recognised that inflammation in IPF seems not to be a key process; rather, a pro-fibrotic environment leads to relentless fibrosis [3]. The emergence of this new pathogenic paradigm has led to the development of new antifibrotic agents. Two of these agents, pirfenidone and nintedanib, are already approved by the US Food and Drug Administration (FDA) and the European Medicines Agency (EMA) for patients with IPF. In clinical trials, both have been shown to slow down the evolution of FVC [4–6], and pirfenidone in particular has been shown to decrease mortality in patients with IPF [6]. Classically, pulmonary function parameters are chosen as end-points of clinical trials, but the parameters used to measure QoL seem not to correlate strictly with PFT outcome parameters.

It is clear that the impact of the disease can be separated into two major components: first, parameters that are correlated with disease progression such as survival and evolution of PFT, and secondly, a set of components that has more to do with QoL, the main representatives of this group being dyspnoea and cough. It is well known that the mean survival in IPF is between 2 and 4 years [1]. However, next to its detrimental effect on survival, IPF is a disease characterised by high morbidity consisting mainly of limited exercise capacity, dyspnoea and cough. In this chapter, we will focus on these problems. Dyspnoea is clearly the major problem that drives patients to look for medical attention [7]; it is regarded as a major determinant of QoL [8] and may even be correlated with death [9].

Another key issue in the daily concerns of patients is cough. Cough is one of the first symptoms in the evolution of IPF. Unfortunately, it is almost never the key to an early diagnosis, although it highly influences QoL. Many patients do not dare to leave home, or go to the theatre for example, with this difficult-to-manage cough [10]. Cough in IPF presents many challenges such as developing tools to determine cough intensity, the relationship with QoL and, last but not least, treatment. It is clear that the management of dyspnoea and cough are among the most important determinants of QoL in IPF and are therefore a key target for treatment.

As already mentioned, one of the major steps forward in the last decade has been the availability of antifibrotic agents, but their effects on QoL in general and dyspnoea in particular have not been clearly determined. The most-used methods to tackle dyspnoea include supplemental oxygen, pulmonary rehabilitation (covered in another chapter of this *Monograph* [11]), medication such as opioids and the treatment of comorbidities. Lung transplantation may be another option for treating dyspnoea (also covered in another chapter of this *Monograph* [11]). For dyspnoea in particular, the current data provide conflicting evidence, and it is relatively difficult for physicians to obtain clear guidance on this important matter. The same is true for cough, where data on the use of specific antifibrotics for treatment are sparse, although opioids can be used to tackle cough.

Thus, it is clear that there is still a major need for further studies that aim to alleviate the crucial QoL determinants for patients with IPF. Until now, most clinical trials have focused on the evolution of PFT and on survival [12], but what really matters for patients is an improvement in their QoL. This can only be done by redesigning future clinical trials in order to change what bothers patients: alleviating dyspnoea and cough. This is not a type of palliative care, which is performed after antifibrotic treatment has failed; rather, it is part of the holistic approach that should be developed in the care of patients with IPF [13].

Dyspnoea

Dyspnoea in IPF

Up to 90% of IPF patients report dyspnoea at the time of diagnosis [7]. Therefore, it is clear that dyspnoea is a major constraint for QoL in IPF patients [8]. In addition, there is a strong correlation between dyspnoea and mortality [9]. Thus, in IPF, dyspnoea is the most common and, for the majority of patients, the most debilitating symptom and the primary driver of QoL impairment [7, 14]. There is therefore an emerging need for symptom-based strategies, next to other goals such as stabilising disease progression (measured using PFTs and mortality).

As dyspnoea in IPF is highly variable and often not always strictly related to the PFTs, some form of standardisation of the measurement of dyspnoea is mandatory. Several methods exist, and we will review some of them. One of the tests often used to quantify dyspnoea is the University of California San Diego (UCSD) Shortness of Breath Questionnaire with a patient-reported outcome; 21 of the 24 items ask respondents to rate the dyspnoea (on a scale of 0–5) they perceived while performing various physical activities during the previous week, together with three ratings on limitations caused by dyspnoea or fear of dyspnoea [15]. The UCSD questionnaire has been validated to determine dyspnoea in IPF patients [16] and has been used as a secondary end-point in most pivotal IPF trials. Another way of determining dyspnoea is the Borg Dyspnoea Index, which measures perceived breathlessness on a scale of 0 (none) to 10 (maximum) [17]. A third method used to quantify limitation in IPF is the Medical Research Council (MRC) dyspnoea scale, which is commonly used to grade the severity of activity limitation caused by dyspnoea in patients with COPD [18, 19]. In IPF, the MRC score has been shown to correlate with PFT, radiographic features, exercise capacity and even prognosis [20–23].

Management of dyspnoea

Several approaches can be taken to treating dyspnoea, such as disease-modifying agents, lung transplantation and finally symptom-based therapy. Below, we will focus on these three topics; other approaches will be discussed in more detail in other chapters of this *Monograph* [11].

Disease-modifying agents

Disease-modifying agents, also called antifibrotic agents, are a relatively new treatment in this field. The two agents that have been approved by the FDA and EMA are pirfenidone and nintedanib. These agents have been shown to alter the decrease in % predicted FVC [4–6], and pirfenidone has also been shown to improve survival [6]. However, it can be argued that the effects of antifibrotic agents on QoL in IPF and on dyspnoea in particular are not clearly proven [24]. There are several possible explanations for the absence of benefit with disease-modifying therapies. First, dyspnoea was not the primary end-point in most of these studies, and most studies were underpowered to evaluate changes in dyspnoea. In addition, most of the dyspnoea metrics used in these studies were developed in non-ILD populations and may not be as accurate or sensitive to change in patients with ILD and IPF in particular [24]. It is clear that in the future there should be a general effort from all stakeholders to develop better tools for measuring dyspnoea and, more importantly, to adapt the design of future clinical trials that might have QoL and dyspnoea in particular as primary end-points.

Lung transplantation

This might be considered as a valuable treatment for dyspnoea. However, lung transplantation implies a high cost and is still hampered by the lack of donor organs and the occurrence of rejection after transplantation. This will be discussed more extensively in a specific chapter of this *Monograph* [11].

Symptom-based therapy

The last possible approach is symptom-based therapy. This comprises several ways to modulate dyspnoea, such as supplemental oxygen, pulmonary rehabilitation, medication and treatment of comorbidities that might influence dyspnoea.

Supplemental oxygen

Oxygen is the most logical solution for treatment of dyspnoea, although many issues are still unclear, specifically in IPF. In the evaluation of the need for oxygen in a patient with IPF, determination of hypoxaemia is crucial. Hypoxaemia is determined as a partial arterial oxygen tension (P_aO_2) of <55 mmHg. In these patients, long-term oxygen therapy (LTOT) is often recommended. This is based on two studies that demonstrated a mortality benefit of LTOT for COPD patients [25, 26]. However, studies on oxygen in IPF patients are sparse, and it is clear that there are no data demonstrating a benefit of supplemental oxygen therapy for all patients with IPF. Those patients who might benefit can be divided into those who benefit from oxygen at rest and those who benefit from oxygen on exertion. The results of these studies are summarised in table 1.

It is likely that IPF patients with resting hypoxaemia will be treated with LTOT, but studies to guide this decision are sparse. One randomised controlled trial reported a favourable effect of oxygen in ILD patients with resting hypoxaemia, but this study was not performed only in patients with IPF (eight IPF, one hypersensitivity pneumonitis and one amiodarone-induced ILD) [27]. These results are encouraging, but so far a mortality benefit has not been proven [28].

The use of oxygen on exertion in IPF is even less clear. By analogy with COPD patients, it seems likely that oxygen might have a beneficial effect on dyspnoea and exercise capacity in patients with IPF. However, straightforward parallels between both diseases can be difficult to make. Two recent studies on ILDs (including IPF) showed inconsistent results. The first study by VISCA et al. [29] suggested that ambulatory oxygen significantly improved 6MWD, oxygen saturation and dyspnoea score in ILD patients, but a slight limitation of this study was that it was not limited to IPF specifically. A second retrospective study was limited to patients with IPF and showed an increase in exercise capacity after the start of ambulatory oxygen [30].

Unfortunately, only one placebo-controlled prospective study has been performed in IPF patients with desaturation on exercise (not at rest) in a crossover design [31]. The authors reported that ambulatory oxygen on exertional dyspnoea in IPF with a flow rate of 4 L·min^{-1} did not improve dyspnoea after a standardised 6MWT. Surprisingly, oxygen did not cause a significant improvement in walk distance, leg fatigue or heart rate. This is in substantial contrast to findings in COPD patients, and adds to the confusion.

Table 1. Studies with oxygen performed in patients with IPF

First author [ref.]	Type of study	Type of hypoxia	Population	Intervention	Tools used	Outcome
SWINBURN [27]	Double blind, randomised	Resting hypoxaemia (hospital inpatients)	Eight IPF, one HP and one amiodarone-induced ILD	4 L O_2 at rest	Sa_{O_2}; VAS dyspnoea score	O_2 saturation increased; dyspnoea score increased; no effect on survival
VISCA [29]	Retrospective	Hypoxia on exertion	52 ILD and 34 IPF, iNSIP patients	O_2 depending on grade of desaturation	Borg dyspnoea score	6MWD increased; Sa_{O_2} increased; dyspnoea score increased
FRANK [30]	Retrospective	Hypoxia on exertion	70 IPF patients only	O_2 uptitration	Sa_{O_2}	6MWD increased; no effect on Borg score
NISHIYAMA [30]	Double blind, placebo controlled, randomised, crossover	Hypoxia on exertion	20 IPF patients	4 $L \cdot min^{-1}$ O_2	Sa_{O_2}; Borg dyspnoea score	Dyspnoea score did not improve; 6MWD did not improve

HP: hypersensitivity pneumonitis; Sa_{O_2}: arterial oxygen saturation; VAS: visual analogue scale; iNSIP: idiopathic NSIP.

Thus, it is clear that the underlying mechanisms for dyspnoea in fibrotic lung diseases are complex. Next to oxygenation, other factors involved might be ventilatory demand, respiratory and peripheral muscle function, and cardiovascular factors [32]. Therefore, results from studies in COPD cannot always be extrapolated to restrictive lung diseases.

These results should also be taken into account when prescribing oxygen for a patient with IPF. It should always be a balance between relief of dyspnoea and the fact that administration of oxygen implies much practical organisation for patients [13], which might lead to less activity and a worsening of health-related QoL for the patient.

Pulmonary rehabilitation

Pulmonary rehabilitation has been studied extensively in COPD, where it has been shown to be an effective treatment, next to pharmacological therapy. In pulmonary fibrosis and especially IPF, data on PH are sparse. A randomised controlled study of 28 subjects found no benefit of pulmonary rehabilitation on dyspnoea [33]. Another study with an uncontrolled study design evaluated dyspnoea in 17 patients after a 12-week home-based pulmonary rehabilitation programme [34]. In the 15 patients who completed the programme, dyspnoea improved, measured as walking distance and QoL. A Cochrane review analysed all available data for pulmonary rehabilitation and IPF [35]. They reported a nonsignificant improvement in dyspnoea in patients with IPF (standardised mean difference 0.56, 95% CI 1.26–0.14).

A recent prospective cohort study investigated 54 patients (22 of whom had IPF) who were included in three pulmonary rehabilitation programmes [36]. Dyspnoea was measured using the UCSD Shortness of Breath Questionnaire. Following rehabilitation, there was a short-term improvement where the majority of patients improved significantly for dyspnoea (65%); however, this was not maintained 6 months after rehabilitation.

Medication

Opioids for dyspnoea. Only two small studies have evaluated the use of opioids for dyspnoea in patients with IPF. The first investigated nebulised morphine in six patients with ILD (three of whom had IPF), but the results showed no significant effect on dyspnoea [37]. The other study, comprising 11 IPF patients, showed a significant decrease in dyspnoea using subcutaneous diamorphine without significant side effects [38]. A useful pragmatic approach has been suggested by the British Thoracic Society (BTS) in their latest guidelines on ILD. They suggest that palliative care services, including opioids for dyspnoea, should be (rather early on) involved, which may lead to a more holistic approach to symptom relief [39].

Colchicine. The effect of colchicine has been assessed in a few studies. A randomised study of 10 patients who were treated with prednisone and colchicine showed a significantly improved dyspnoea score in comparison with those treated with prednisone alone or with a combination of prednisone and cyclophosphamide [40]. However, another open-label study could not find any improvement in 19 subjects treated with prednisone and colchicine [41]. Furthermore, in both studies, no other end-points were improved by this approach, which makes the potential for this treatment rather low. The treatment of IPF with immunosuppressive agents has also been shown to have a deleterious effect on mortality and hospitalisation [2], which makes a combination with steroids very difficult to endorse.

Treatment of comorbidities in IPF

It is clear that the symptoms of IPF are caused by the direct effects of pulmonary fibrosis on the lung architecture. However, it should be emphasised that, as well as these direct effects, comorbidities may also influence symptoms and should be considered for treatment. Possible targets might be concomitant emphysema, as in CPFE, or cardiovascular disease in patients with IPF. The best-studied comorbidity in IPF until now is PH.

PH is an important comorbidity and might be a new target for treatment of pulmonary fibrosis patients. However, a study of the endothelin receptor antagonist bosentan in patients with IPF gave negative results [42].

Another treatment often used in pulmonary arterial hypertension is sildenafil. This has been tested in a few interesting studies in the field of ILD, with dyspnoea as one of the end-points. A randomised controlled trial studying 29 patients with PH, defined as a pulmonary artery systolic pressure of 25–50 mmHg on echocardiography, showed no significant effect of sildenafil on dyspnoea [43]. Another small open-label study (11 patients) with PH detected on right heart catheterisation also showed no effect on dyspnoea, but an improvement in walking distance was found [44]. The largest study, however, was a randomised study in 180 patients with advanced IPF, defined as having a D_{LCO} of <35% pred [45]. Patients were treated for 12 weeks with placebo or sildenafil. Sildenafil improved dyspnoea, some features of QoL, oxygenation and D_{LCO}. A substudy examined 119 of the 180 patients with available echocardiography. In the subgroup of patients with right ventricular dysfunction, sildenafil treatment resulted in better preservation of exercise capacity in comparison with placebo [46].

Because of the lack of proven benefit, sildenafil is not recommended for general use in patients with IPF in the latest American Thoracic Society (ATS)/European Respiratory Society (ERS)/Japanese Respiratory Society (JRS)/Latin American Thoracic Association (ALAT) IPF guidelines [1]. Nevertheless, a recent study at least brings some new hope of altering dyspnoea, even in patients with more advanced disease, as in these patients dyspnoea is the major limitation for QoL [46]. This can only be achieved by performing more studies treating PH in patients with IPF.

Noninvasive ventilatory assistance

One study of 10 patients evaluated noninvasive ventilator assistance during exercise. The authors found an improvement in comparison with no ventilator assistance [47]. Furthermore, exercise tolerance was improved, which might lead to a better QoL. However, this solution is very complex in daily clinical practice, so further research is warranted.

Cough

In a recent survey on palliative care needs for fibrotic ILDs, patients and their caregivers highlighted that cough was a common and highly irritating problem, next to shortness of breath and insomnia. In this study, patients reported that the paroxysms of cough and the considerable effort involved in trying to bring up phlegm were totally exhausting [10]. These major problems often lead to a certain degree of social isolation. In particular, in this study it was shown that healthcare professionals often have a rather limited appreciation of these symptoms.

Cough in IPF

Chronic non-productive cough is a cardinal clinical feature of IPF. Theoretically, cough can also be caused by mechanisms other than IPF such as GERD and airway hyperresponsiveness [48]. In an analysis of 242 IPF patients, it was reported that as many as 84% of patients reported cough, and that this symptom was an independent predictor of disease progression [49]. Moreover, the results showed that cough was increased in subjects with IPF who had lower FVC and DLCO. In this study, there was no correlation of cough with the presence of asthma, COPD, GERD or the use of angiotensin-converting enzyme (ACE) inhibitors. Therefore, the authors speculated that cough in IPF might be produced by either mechanical or chemical stimulation of peripheral cough receptors. Mechanical cough receptors could be stimulated by architectural distortion caused by worsening fibrosis, whereas chemical cough receptors could be stimulated by subclinical inflammation, as shown in several studies [50]. Interestingly, a recent paper found that genetic background can influence cough in patients with IPF, as cough severity was associated with the presence of the minor T allele of the *MUC5B* polymorphism [51]. These findings are highly interesting and may be a possible link between IPF pathogenesis and the occurrence of cough in the majority of IPF patients. There might be several explanations for this interesting observation, such as increased mucus production or mucus clearance. This interesting finding adds to the current knowledge that genetic background may not only predispose for the development of IPF but might also influence disease evolution.

It is crucial to carefully assess other known causes for cough. Common causes of cough could be respiratory or non-respiratory conditions, such as GERD, (viral) infections of the upper respiratory tract, upper airway cough syndrome (also called postnasal drip syndrome), cough-variant asthma, eosinophilic bronchitis, pleural diseases and the use of drugs such as ACE inhibitors [52]. These causes should be meticulously excluded before cough can be attributed to IPF.

The evaluation of cough is crucial in the diagnosis of IPF. One way to evaluate cough in IPF is the Cough Quality of Life Questionnaire, which has been validated for IPF [53], as well as use of a cough visual analogue score.

Management of cough in IPF

As stated before, other causes of cough should be excluded. If there is clear evidence for GERD in an individual patient, this should be treated as suggested in the latest IPF guidelines [1]. However, a benefit of antiacid therapy in IPF has been the subject of substantial discussion [54]. Other treatments that have been suggested are the use of high-dose steroids [55], but there is currently no further evidence to support this practice. When considering this as a possible treatment, one should take into account the fact that high doses of steroids have been shown to increase morbidity and mortality in IPF [2]. There is no evidence to support treatment with bronchodilators or other antiasthma treatment in IPF patients. We will go on to discuss possible suggested treatments for cough in IPF; however, it should be noted that the evidence is very limited.

Disease-modifying agents
Pirfenidone
A study by OKAZAKI *et al.* [56] reported the positive effects of pirfenidone on cough reflex sensitivity in guinea pigs. In a model of aerosolised antigen challenge in sensitised guinea pigs,

pirfenidone was administered intraperitoneally, and 48 h after challenge the number of coughs induced by aerosolised capsaicin was decreased in the treated group in comparison with placebo.

AZUMA et al. [57] performed an exploratory analysis of the Japanese Phase III trial with pirfenidone. In this study, they found significant positive effects on cough in several subpopulations with mild to moderate IPF at week 52.

WIJSENBEEK et al. [58] reported preliminary effects of pirfenidone on cough in a cohort of 19 IPF patients. In 11 of these patients, the clinical cough score decreased after 1 month of pirfenidone treatment (mean reduction −2.2 points) and this remained unchanged in seven patients after 1 year. An observational study of the effect of pirfenidone on cough and QoL in patients with IPF in daily practice is currently ongoing [59]. Furthermore, several real life registries are ongoing, some of which also use scores to monitor cough and the effect of treatment [60].

Thalidomide
One randomised crossover trial investigated the effect of thalidomide on cough in IPF patients [61]. After 12 weeks of thalidomide cough improved significantly.

Thalidomide is, of course, an agent that is known to induce many side effects, such as peripheral neuropathy, venous thromboembolism, skin rash and constipation, but also bowel perforation, which is less common [62].

Currently, this toxicity profile limits use, but it is clear that more studies are necessary to determine the exact balance between potential benefit and side-effects in IPF.

Codeine
Conventional agents such as oral codeine are widely used, especially in the palliative care setting [63], but their effect has never been proven in IPF.

General discussion and conclusion

Both dyspnoea and cough are important symptoms in IPF as they are frequently reported and interfere dramatically with QoL. It is clear that major progress is being made in the treatment of IPF and of dyspnoea in particular. Several aspects of dyspnoea can be treated by disease-modifying agents, lung transplantation and symptom-based therapy. To date, disease-modifying agents have shown a limited direct impact on dyspnoea, and lung transplantation is not always an option; therefore, symptom-based therapy is becoming an important alternative. There are limited studies on the use of supplemental oxygen specifically in the IPF population [26–32]. However, taking into account these few studies, together with the large amount of evidence in other fields such as COPD, the available data suggest that supplemental oxygen might be useful in IPF. For patients with persistent resting hypoxaemia (P_{aO_2} <55 mmHg or <60 mmHg with PH) and who are breathless, continuous oxygen should be provided. If the patient is still active and regularly leaves home, ambulatory oxygen might also be beneficial. For patients who are breathless on exertion and have a desaturation on exertion (<90%), ambulatory oxygen should be considered if this leads to improved exercise capacity or reduced breathlessness [39]. It is clear that there is still a high need for new trials in this specific subpopulation. Opioids seem to be widely used, but the evidence for their effectiveness is limited. Another solution tested is assisted ventilation on exertion [48]; however, this is rather impractical, even more than the use of oxygen on exercise. Another area that should be emphasised is the presence of comorbidities that might influence symptoms and should be considered for treatment. The best-studied comorbidity in IPF is PH, and there are some encouraging findings with sildenafil that warrant further investigation with PH treatment in these patients [43–47]. PH is an important cofactor of pulmonary fibrosis; however, it is not clear whether it is a driver or a result of the fibrotic process. What is clear is that treatment of comorbidities is an interesting target for new treatments of pulmonary fibrosis, so more studies should be performed, such as in IPF patients with concomitant emphysema and cardiovascular disease.

On closer analysis, several aspects of dyspnoea are still unclear, so it seems likely that the pathogenesis consists of a complex interplay between pulmonary, cardiac, neurological and psychological factors. A reason to support this is the encouraging effect of pulmonary rehabilitation, which seems to have a positive effect on dyspnoea, although without any real proof of a positive effect on pulmonary function; however, pulmonary rehabilitation seems to have more of an effect on cardiovascular function and muscle function.

Concerning cough, it is clear that the way studies with antifibrotic agents have been designed means that they cannot be used to detect whether these agents are active in supressing cough in IPF, although several pre-clinical and small studies suggest that there might be an effect [4–6]. Currently, opioids are used to treat cough, but the evidence, specifically in IPF, is sparse. A small trial suggested some effect of thalidomide in treating cough in IPF [62]. Codeine is widely used, but specific studies are lacking.

In conclusion, it is clear that for patients with IPF, dyspnoea and cough are the core components of the impact of the disease. However, we have no specific tools to adequately treat these symptoms. It is clear that there is an urgent need for specific studies in this field, and dyspnoea and cough are important targets for future treatment.

References

1. Raghu G, Rochwerg B, Zhang Y, *et al.* An Official ATS/ERS/JRS/ALAT Clinical Practice Guideline: Treatment of Idiopathic Pulmonary Fibrosis. An Update of the 2011 Clinical Practice Guideline. *Am J Respir Crit Care Med* 2015; 192: e3–e19.
2. The Idiopathic Pulmonary Fibrosis Clinical Research Network. Prednisone, azathioprine, and N-acetylcysteine for pulmonary fibrosis. *N Engl J Med* 2012; 366: 1968–1977.
3. Wuyts WA, Agostini C, Antoniou KM, *et al.* The pathogenesis of pulmonary fibrosis: a moving target. *Eur Respir J* 2013; 41: 1207–1218.
4. Noble PW, Albera C, Bradford WZ, *et al.* Pirfenidone in patients with idiopathic pulmonary fibrosis (CAPACITY): two randomised trials. *Lancet* 2011; 377: 1760–1769.
5. Richeldi L, du Bois RM, Raghu G, *et al.* Efficacy and safety of nintedanib in idiopathic pulmonary fibrosis. *N Engl J Med* 2014; 370: 2071–2082.
6. King TE Jr, Bradford WZ, Castro-Bernardini S, *et al.* A phase 3 trial of pirfenidone in patients with idiopathic pulmonary fibrosis. *N Engl J Med* 2014; 370: 2083–2092.
7. Bjoraker JA, Ryu JH, Edwin MK, *et al.* Prognostic significance of histopathologic subsets in idiopathic pulmonary fibrosis. *Am J Respir Crit Care Med* 1998; 157: 199–203.
8. Swigris JJ, Kuschner WG, Jacobs SS, *et al.* Health-related quality of life in patients with idiopathic pulmonary fibrosis: a systematic review. *Thorax* 2005; 60: 588–594.
9. King TE Jr, Schwarz MI, Brown K, *et al.* Idiopathic pulmonary fibrosis: relationship between histopathologic features and mortality. *Am J Respir Crit Care Med* 2001; 164: 1025–1032.
10. Bajwah S, Higginson IJ, Ross JR, *et al.* The palliative care needs for fibrotic interstitial lung disease: a qualitative study of patients, informal caregivers and health professionals. *Palliat Med* 2013; 27: 869–876.

11. Kenn K, Gloeckl R, Heinzelmann I, *et al.* Nonpharmacological interventions: rehabilitation, palliative care and transplantation. *In*: Costabel U, Crestani B, Wells AU, eds. Idiopathic Pulmonary Fibrosis (ERS Monograph). Sheffield, European Respiratory Society, 2016; pp. 230–242.

12. Raghu G, Collard HR, Anstrom KJ, *et al.* Idiopathic pulmonary fibrosis: clinically meaningful primary end-points in phase 3 clinical trials. *Am J Respir Crit Care Med* 2012; 185: 1044–1048.

13. Wuyts WA, Peccatori FA, Russell AM. Patient-centred management in idiopathic pulmonary fibrosis: similar themes in three communication models. *Eur Respir Rev* 2014; 23: 231–238.

14. Swigris JJ, Gould MK, Wilson SR. Health-related quality of life among patients with idiopathic pulmonary fibrosis. *Chest* 2005; 127: 284–294.

15. Eakin EG, Resnikoff PM, Prewitt LM, *et al.* Validation of a new dyspnea measure: the UCSD Shortness of Breath Questionnaire. University of California, San Diego. *Chest* 1998; 113: 619–624.

16. Swigris JJ, Han M, Vij R, *et al.* The UCSD shortness of breath questionnaire has longitudinal construct validity in idiopathic pulmonary fibrosis. *Respir Med* 2012; 106: 1447–1455.

17. Ries AL. Minimally clinically important difference for the UCSD Shortness of Breath Questionnaire, Borg Scale, and Visual Analog Scale. *COPD* 2005; 2: 105–110.

18. Fletcher CM, Elmes PC, Fairbairn AS, *et al.* The significance of respiratory symptoms and the diagnosis of chronic bronchitis in a working population. *Br Med J* 1959; 2: 257–266.

19. Bestall JC, Paul EA, Garrod R, *et al.* Usefulness of the Medical Research Council (MRC) dyspnoea scale as a measure of disability in patients with chronic obstructive pulmonary disease. *Thorax* 1999; 54: 581–586.

20. Kozu R, Jenkins S, Senjyu H. Evaluation of activity limitation in patients with idiopathic pulmonary fibrosis grouped according to Medical Research Council dyspnea grade. *Arch Phys Med Rehabil* 2014; 95: 950.

21. Papiris SA, Daniil ZD, Malagari K, *et al.* The Medical Research Council dyspnea scale in the estimation of disease severity in idiopathic pulmonary fibrosis. *Respir Med* 2005; 99: 755–761.

22. Mura M, Ferretti A, Ferro O, *et al.* Functional predictors of exertional dyspnea, 6-min walking distance and HRCT fibrosis score in idiopathic pulmonary fibrosis. *Respiration* 2006; 73: 495–502.

23. Nishiyama O, Taniguchi H, Kondoh Y, *et al.* A simple assessment of dyspnoea as a prognostic indicator in idiopathic pulmonary fibrosis. *Eur Respir J* 2010; 36: 1067–1072.

24. Ryerson CJ, Donesky D, Pantilat SZ, *et al.* Dyspnea in idiopathic pulmonary fibrosis: a systematic review. *J Pain Symptom Manage* 2012; 43: 771–782.

25. Nocturnal Oxygen Therapy Trial Group. Continuous or nocturnal oxygen therapy in hypoxemic chronic obstructive lung disease: a clinical trial. *Ann Intern Med* 1980; 93: 391–398.

26. Medical Research Working Council. Long term domiciliary oxygen therapy in chronic hypoxic cor pulmonale complicating chronic bronchitis and emphysema. Report of the Medical Research Council Working Party. *Lancet* 1981; 317: 681–686.

27. Swinburn CR, Mould H, Stone TN, *et al.* Symptomatic benefit of supplemental oxygen in hypoxemic patients with chronic lung disease. *Am Rev Respir Dis* 1991; 143: 913–915.

28. Crockett AJ, Cranston JM, Antic N. Domiciliary oxygen for interstitial lung disease. *Cochrane Database Syst Rev* 2001; 3: CD002883.

29. Visca D, Montgomery A, de Lauretis A, *et al.* Ambulatory oxygen in interstitial lung disease. *Eur Respir J* 2011; 38: 987–990.

30. Frank RC, Hicks S, Duck AM, *et al.* Ambulatory oxygen in idiopathic pulmonary fibrosis: of what benefit? *Eur Respir J* 2012; 40: 269–270.

31. Nishiyama O, Miyajima H, Fukai Y, *et al.* Effect of ambulatory oxygen on exertional dyspnea in IPF patients without resting hypoxemia. *Respir Med* 2013; 107: 1241–1246.

32. Parshall MB, Schwartzstein RM, Adams L, *et al.* An official American Thoracic Society statement: update on the mechanisms, assessment, and management of dyspnea. *Am J Respir Crit Care Med* 2012; 185: 435–452.

33. Nishiyama O, Kondoh Y, Kimura T, *et al.* Effects of pulmonary rehabilitation in patients with idiopathic pulmonary fibrosis. *Respirology* 2008; 13: 394–399.

34. Ozalevli S, Karaali H, Ilgin D, *et al.* Effect of home-based pulmonary rehabilitation in patients with idiopathic pulmonary fibrosis. *Multidiscip Respir Med* 2010; 5: 31–37.

35. Holland A, Hill C. Physical training for interstitial lung disease. *Cochrane Database Syst Rev* 2008; 4: CD006322.

36. Ryerson CJ, Cayou C, Topp F, *et al.* Pulmonary rehabilitation improves long-term outcomes in interstitial lung disease: a prospective cohort study. *Respir Med* 2014; 108: 203–210.

37. Harris-Eze AO, Sridhar G, Clemens RE, *et al.* Low-dose nebulized morphine does not improve exercise in interstitial lung disease. *Am J Respir Crit Care Med* 1995; 152: 1940–1945.

38. Allen S, Raut S, Woollard J, *et al.* Low dose diamorphine reduces breathlessness without causing a fall in oxygen saturation in elderly patients with end-stage idiopathic pulmonary fibrosis. *Palliat Med* 2005; 19: 128–130.

39. Bradley B, Branley HM, Egan JJ, *et al.* Interstitial lung disease guideline: the British Thoracic Society in collaboration with the Thoracic Society of Australia and New Zealand and the Irish Thoracic Society. *Thorax* 2008; 63: Suppl. 5, v1–v58.

40. Fiorucci E, Lucantoni G, Paone G, *et al.* Colchicine, cyclophosphamide and prednisone in the treatment of mild-moderate idiopathic pulmonary fibrosis: comparison of three currently available therapeutic regimens. *Eur Rev Med Pharmacol Sci* 2008; 12: 105–111.

41. Selman M, Carrillo G, Salas J, *et al.* Colchicine, D-penicillamine, and prednisone in the treatment of idiopathic pulmonary fibrosis: a controlled clinical trial. *Chest* 1998; 114: 507–512.

42. King TE Jr, Brown KK, Raghu G, *et al.* BUILD-3: a randomized, controlled trial of bosentan in idiopathic pulmonary fibrosis. *Am J Respir Crit Care Med* 2011; 184: 92–99.

43. Jackson RM, Glassberg MK, Ramos CF, *et al.* Sildenafil therapy and exercise tolerance in idiopathic pulmonary fibrosis. *Lung* 2010; 188: 115–123.

44. Collard HR, Anstrom KJ, Schwarz MI, *et al.* Sildenafil improves walk distance in idiopathic pulmonary fibrosis. *Chest* 2007; 131: 897–899.

45. Idiopathic Pulmonary Fibrosis Clinical Research Network, Zisman DA, Schwarz M, *et al.* A controlled trial of sildenafil in advanced idiopathic pulmonary fibrosis. *N Engl J Med* 2010; 363: 620–628.

46. Han MK, Bach DS, Hagan PG, *et al.* Sildenafil preserves exercise capacity in patients with idiopathic pulmonary fibrosis and right-sided ventricular dysfunction. *Chest* 2013; 143: 1699–1708.

47. Moderno EV, Yamaguti WP, Schettino GP, *et al.* Effects of proportional assisted ventilation on exercise performance in idiopathic pulmonary fibrosis patients. *Respir Med* 2010; 104: 134–141.

48. Brown KK. Chronic cough due to chronic interstitial pulmonary diseases: ACCP evidence-based clinical practice guidelines. *Chest* 2006; 129: 180S–185S.

49. Ryerson CJ, Abbritti M, Ley B, *et al.* Cough predicts prognosis in idiopathic pulmonary fibrosis. *Respirology* 2011; 16: 969–975.

50. Veeraraghavan S, Latsi PI, Wells AU, *et al.* BAL findings in idiopathic nonspecific interstitial pneumonia and usual interstitial pneumonia. *Eur Respir J* 2003; 22: 239–244.

51. Scholand MB, Wolff R, Crossno PF, *et al.* Severity of cough in idiopathic pulmonary fibrosis is associated with MUC5 B genotype. *Cough* 2014; 10: 3.

52. Chung KF. Approach to chronic cough: the neuropathic basis for cough hypersensitivity syndrome. *J Thorac Dis* 2014; Suppl. 7, S699–S707.

53. Lechtzin N, Hilliard ME, Horton MR. Validation of the Cough Quality-of-Life Questionnaire in patients with idiopathic pulmonary fibrosis. *Chest* 2013; 143: 1745–1749.

54. Kilduff CE, Counter MJ, Thomas GA, *et al.* Effect of acid suppression therapy on gastroesophageal reflux and cough in idiopathic pulmonary fibrosis: an intervention study. *Cough* 2014; 10: 4.

55. Hope-Gill BD, Hilldrup S, Davies C, *et al.* A study of the cough reflex in idiopathic pulmonary fibrosis. *Am J Respir Crit Care Med* 2003; 168: 995–1002.

56. Okazaki A, Ohkura N, Fujimura M, *et al.* Effects of pirfenidone on increased cough reflex sensitivity in guinea pigs. *Pulm Pharmacol Ther* 2013; 26: 603–608.

57. Azuma A, Taguchi Y, Ogura T, *et al.* Exploratory analysis of a phase III trial of pirfenidone identifies a subpopulation of patients with idiopathic pulmonary fibrosis as benefiting from treatment. *Respir Res* 2011; 12: 143.

58. Wijsenbeek MS, Van Beek FT, Geel AL. Pirfenidone in daily clinical use in patients with idiopathic pulmonary fibrosis in the Netherlands. *Am J Respir Crit Care Med* 2013; 187: A4340.

59. Erasmus Medical Center. The effect of pirfenidone on cough in patients with idiopathic pulmonary fibrosis (Cough-IPF). NCT02009293. http://clinicaltrials.gov/ct2/show/NCT02009293. Date last updated: December 8, 2013. Date last accessed: December 8, 2013.

60. Wuyts W, Bondue B, Slabbynck H, *et al.* PROOF-registry: a prospective observational registry to describe the disease course and outcomes of idiopathic pulmonary fibrosis patients in a real-world clinical setting. *Am J Respir Crit Care Med* 2015; 191: A2506.

61. Horton MR, Santopietro V, Matthew L, *et al.* Thalidomide for the treatment of cough in idiopathic pulmonary fibrosis. *Ann Intern Med* 2012; 157: 398–406.

62. Ghobrial IM, Rajkumar SV. Management of thalidomide toxicity. *J Support Oncol* 2003; 1: 194–205.

63. Hansen-Flaschen J. Advanced lung disease. Palliation and terminal care. *Clin Chest Med* 1997; 18: 645–655.

Disclosures: W.A. Wuyts reports receiving a grant from Intermune and travel grants from Boehringer Ingelheim and Bayer AG, outside the submitted work.

Chapter 18

Nonpharmacological interventions: rehabilitation, palliative care and transplantation

Klaus Kenn[1,2], Rainer Gloeckl[1,3], Inga Heinzelmann[1] and Nikolaus Kneidinger[4]

Only a limited number of pharmacological treatments are available for IPF patients. However, a variety of nonpharmacological options are beneficial in such patients. Pulmonary rehabilitation is one of the most effective nonpharmacological interventions used to increase exercise capacity, reduce dyspnoea, and improve QoL. Furthermore, long-term oxygen therapy and, in some patients, even nocturnal noninvasive ventilation may be supportive in reducing the burden of disease. Lung transplantation (LTx) can be the most effective treatment in highly selected patients with IPF. However, early consideration for LTx and close monitoring of disease progression are mandatory because of the highly variable nature of the disease.

Although IPF patients report symptoms of psychosocial stress, including anxiety and depression, palliative care is delayed or even neglected because of various reasons, such as discomfort with discussing end of life fears.

Thus, all nonpharmacological options should be implemented as early as possible when treating IPF patients.

Beside symptoms of severe dyspnoea, patients with chronic lung diseases suffer from reduced exercise capacity and QoL, and increased risk of mortality. Consequences of chronic lung disease, as described by the WHO in the International Classification of Functioning, Disability and Health (ICF), include a reduction of participation in physical activities and social events. The ICF provides the basis for pulmonary rehabilitation programmes that have been shown to be highly effective in patients with COPD, improving patients' psychological and physical condition. In COPD, the therapeutic effectiveness of pulmonary rehabilitation is reflected in the highest level of evidence, *i.e.* grade A [1]. There is growing evidence that pulmonary rehabilitation is also beneficial in patients with IPF, which has led to its recommendation in the current ATS/ERS statement on pulmonary rehabilitation [2].

[1]Dept of Respiratory Medicine and Pulmonary Rehabilitation, Schoen Klinik Berchtesgadener Land, Schoenau am Koenigssee, Germany. [2]Dept of Pulmonary Rehabilitation, University of Marburg, Marburg, Germany. [3]Dept for Prevention, Rehabilitation and Sports Medicine, Klinikum Rechts der Isar, Technische Universität München (TUM), Munich, Germany. [4]Dept of Internal Medicine V, Comprehensive Pneumology Center (CPC-M), University of Munich, Member of the German Center for Lung Research (DZL), Munich, Germany.

Correspondence: Klaus Kenn, Dept of Respiratory Medicine and Pulmonary Rehabilitation, Schoen Klinik Berchtesgadener Land, Malterhoeh 1, 83471 Schoenau am Koenigssee, Germany. E-mail: kkenn@schoen-kliniken.de

Pulmonary rehabilitation comprises a comprehensive, multimodal intervention; this includes patient-tailored therapies that promote long-term adherence to health-enhancing behaviours, including a physically active lifestyle. The main components of pulmonary rehabilitation programmes are exercise training, pharmaceutical treatment, education and motivation, breathing therapy, smoking cessation, and psychosocial support. These therapeutic components differ individually and are dependent on the patient's specific health status and personal goals.

Physical exercise training

Patients with chronic respiratory diseases often suffer from muscle dysfunction related to skeletal muscle fibre shift from oxidative (type I) to glycolytic (type II) fibres, reduced capillarisation, and impaired oxidative energy metabolism. Therefore, physical exercise, which has shown to reverse some of this dysfunction, is one of the major components of pulmonary rehabilitation. In particular, muscle wasting can be reduced with both endurance and resistance exercise. The conventional training modality for endurance training in patients with respiratory diseases is at least 20 min of continuous exercise at 60–70% of the individual's peak work rate, determined by maximal incremental exercise testing, 3–5 times per week. An alternative and well-established modality in severe COPD is high-intensity interval training. This is characterised by alternating 30 s of exercise at 100% of the individual's peak work rate with 30 s of rest for a period of at least 12 min. Intervals can be adapted to ratios such as 40:20 s or 20:40 s to make exercise more or less intense. In patients with severe dyspnoea and low exercise capacity who are not able to cycle continuously for at least 10 min, interval training has been shown to be more feasible than continuous training [3]. Both modalities seem to be equally effective in improving exercise performance [4].

In addition, long-term oxygen therapy (LTOT) is important to ensure safe training conditions in patients with chronic respiratory failure.

Education

To optimise adherence, education is necessary to increase patients' knowledge about self- and exacerbation management, smoking cessation, and especially a physically active lifestyle. Behavioural change programmes are in most cases mandatory to improve compliance with home-based physical activity and/or exercise training programmes. Therefore, it is essential to arrange an individually targeted programme for patients to ease the transition from supervised pulmonary rehabilitation to their home environment.

Psychosocial support

Anxiety, depression, and panic disorders are common in patients with chronic respiratory diseases. Patients with advanced lung diseases often also suffer from "end of life fears". Pulmonary rehabilitation is effective in reducing these and other psychological disorders and therefore significantly increases health-related QoL.

Pulmonary rehabilitation in IPF patients

Physical deconditioning likely plays a similar role in IPF as it does in other chronic respiratory diseases, such as COPD [5–7]. Avoidance of physical activities that provoke dyspnoea and fatigue [8] may be an important key factor of physical deconditioning and exercise intolerance. Even if IPF and COPD are entities with very different pathophysiological mechanisms in many respects, they lead to similar limitations for patients' everyday life. Mounting evidence has suggested that pulmonary rehabilitation may result in meaningful benefits in exercise capacity and QoL in patients with IPF [2]. Since patients with IPF show limited response to conventional pharmacological treatment [9], pulmonary rehabilitation as a nonpharmacological approach may be an effective alternative and supplemental therapy. Because exercise capacity has been recognised as a crucially important prognostic factor in IPF and is positively related to ease of performing activities of daily living [10, 11], pulmonary rehabilitation should mainly focus on increasing physical performance in these patients.

Benefits

Three small randomised controlled trials have shown improvements in functional exercise tolerance, dyspnoea, and QoL after 8–12 weeks of pulmonary rehabilitation in patients with IPF [12–14]. However, the magnitude of these improvements was smaller than that generally seen in patients with COPD [1]. Disease severity of IPF may also play an important role in improving exercise capacity after pulmonary rehabilitation, although findings are inconsistent. Kozu et al. [15] enrolled 65 IPF patients (mean FVC: 65% predicted) in an 8-week pulmonary rehabilitation programme. Individuals with mild-to-moderate IPF underwent a supervised outpatient programme, whereas individuals with severe IPF participated in an unsupervised, home-based programme that included a visit from a home care provider every 2 weeks. In this study, only patients with mild IPF improved their 6MWD significantly, whereas patients with severe IPF showed almost no improvement. Huppmann et al. [16] investigated a specialised and comprehensive 4-week inpatient pulmonary rehabilitation programme in a subgroup of 202 patients with IPF (mean FVC: 53% predicted). The improvement in 6MWD after pulmonary rehabilitation was 45 m (range: 130–236 m), approximately 15% of the baseline value (p<0.001). Of all the variables tested (age, sex, BMI, smoking history, use of LTOT, baseline FVC, baseline 6MWD, and baseline dyspnoea), only baseline 6MWD was a significant predictor of change in 6MWD. Mean improvement in 6MWD was higher in patients with low baseline 6MWD. Therefore, in patients with advanced IPF, providing pulmonary rehabilitation in a multimodal and specialised centre under close supervision seems a more effective strategy.

In a randomised controlled trial carried out by Jackson et al. [17], IPF patients could maintain improvements in exercise capacity 3 months after pulmonary rehabilitation. Holland et al. [13] investigated the long-term effects of pulmonary rehabilitation in 34 IPF patients. Six months after the conclusion of pulmonary rehabilitation, there were no differences between the pulmonary rehabilitation and control groups for any of the outcome variables. This may reflect the challenges involved in providing pulmonary rehabilitation for rapidly progressive diseases such as IPF. A major aim of pulmonary rehabilitation in IPF patients must be to instruct and motivate patients to maintain home-based follow-up training modalities to retain the benefits of pulmonary rehabilitation [18].

Exercise training regimes

Most exercise protocols for IPF patients use a combination of endurance and resistance training modalities similar to those recommended for patients with COPD [3]. Endurance training is usually performed on a stationary cycle ergometer or as a walking programme at an intensity of 50–80% of maximal exercise capacity for 10–30 min per session [12, 15, 19, 20]. Strength training should focus on major muscle groups with three sets of 8–12 repetitions at the highest tolerated load [2]. Other complementary training modalities, such as interval endurance training [4], neuromuscular electrical muscle stimulation [21], inspiratory muscle training [22], t'ai chi [23], or whole body vibration training [24], could also be useful in IPF.

To the authors' knowledge, exercise-related adverse events in IPF patients have not been reported [25].

Supplemental oxygen

IPF-specific guidelines include a strong recommendation for the use of LTOT in patients with clinically significant resting hypoxaemia [26]. It is still unknown if LTOT in patients who are only hypoxaemic during exertion improves survival [26]. Furthermore, whether the effect of LTOT is on exercise capacity or exertional dyspnoea in these patients remains controversial [27, 28].

Noninvasive ventilation

The use of nocturnal noninvasive inspiratory positive pressure ventilation (NIPPV) is uncommon in patients with ILD. DREHER et al. [29] investigated the effects of NIPPV in ILD patients with hypercapnia during inpatient pulmonary rehabilitation. Twenty-nine hypercapnic patients were included in the intervention group receiving NIPPV, with eight patients listed for lung transplantation; 319 patients without hypercapnia served as a comparison group. NIPPV was initiated in the first days of pulmonary rehabilitation and was performed at night for 7.2 h, with a mean inspiratory and expiratory pressure of 23.8 mbar and 5.3 mbar, respectively. After 25 days, both patient groups significantly improved exercise capacity and QoL (mental score of the SF-36). However, the increase in 6MWD was significantly more pronounced in the intervention group receiving nocturnal NIPPV (+64 m versus +43 m). Only the intervention group showed a relevant reduction of dyspnoea after pulmonary rehabilitation. Therefore, NIPPV initiated during an inpatient, supervised pulmonary rehabilitation setting seems to be feasible, safe, and beneficial even in hypercapnic ILD patients.

Benefits of pulmonary rehabilitation before and after lung transplantation

Three studies investigated the effect of pulmonary rehabilitation before lung transplantation and included IPF patients among others. An average improvement in 6MWD of 46 m to 72 m was significant despite differences in research settings [16, 30, 31]. Additionally, QoL, measured with the SF-36 questionnaire, was shown to significantly increase after pulmonary rehabilitation in these studies. All trials clearly demonstrated the efficacy of pulmonary rehabilitation even in patients with end-stage ILDs.

To the authors' knowledge, until now, no literature investigating the effects of pulmonary rehabilitation in ILD patients following lung transplantation has been published.

Summary

Pulmonary rehabilitation can be an effective intervention in patients with IPF to improve exercise tolerance, QoL, and exertional dyspnoea. Exercise training is the most important component of pulmonary rehabilitation in IPF. Since IPF is known as a heterogeneous disorder in terms of disease progression, response to therapy, and prognosis [26], the optimal timing of pulmonary rehabilitation in the disease trajectory is still unknown and requires further elaboration [32].

Palliative care

Definition

According to the WHO, palliative care is "an approach that improves the QoL of patients and their families facing the problems associated with life-threatening illness, through the prevention and relief of suffering by means of early identification and impeccable assessment and treatment of pain and other problems, physical, psycho-social and spiritual" [33].

Palliative care is only mentioned briefly in the current IPF guidelines and its potential role in the treatment of IPF patients is not well described. The recently published update of the guidelines by RAGHU et al. [34] also does not add any further information.

Lack of evidence and clinical perspective

Although palliative care is well established in cancer patients, it has not been integrated in the standard therapy for patients with chronic lung diseases, such as IPF. This is surprising considering the poor prognosis of IPF patients; their median survival of between 3 and 5 years from the time of diagnosis is worse than several malignant diseases.

Currently, literature regarding palliative care of patients with IPF is almost completely lacking. Thus, it is not possible to present a comprehensive overview of the evidence. An ATS clinical policy statement [26] suggested initiating palliative care as soon as patients with respiratory diseases become symptomatic. Clinical practice may differ between countries depending on cultural influences and different national healthcare systems.

IPF patients, including those with advanced disease, are reluctant to initiate discussions with healthcare professionals with regard to fears about death and dying [35]. A recent retrospective analysis by LINDELL et al. [36] showed that out of 404 patients who died from IPF between 2000 and 2012, only 14% had a formal palliative care referral. Of these, 71% were referred within 1 month, 18% within 6 months, and 11% within 12 months before death occurred. This referral pattern agrees with observations in metastatic lung cancer patients; the introduction of palliative care within 12 weeks after diagnosis leads to improvement in QoL and mood compared to patients receiving standard care [37].

There are several reasons for the delay or neglect in starting palliative care, including the discomfort of physicians, caregivers, and family members in discussing end of life fears and the belief that discussing these subjects may diminish hope of recovery. However, along with dyspnoea, cough, and fatigue, IPF patients typically report symptoms of psychosocial stress, including anxiety and depression [36]. AKHTAR *et al.* [38] observed that 49% of 118 IPF patients were suffering from depression. Surprisingly, only nine were identified as having psychological symptoms and were administered antidepressant therapy. In another study involving 34 ILD patients, DE VRIES *et al.* [39] observed that 24% patients suffered from depression.

In a small study conducted by HOLLAND *et al.* [40], 18 ILD patients (nine with IPF) participated in in-depth interviews about living with ILD. The majority of the nine patients with IPF expected their condition to be progressive and eventually fatal. Almost all had looked up information on the Internet and most of the participants were interested in receiving information on planning for end of life. No relationship with the stage of the disease was observed. The researchers concluded that pulmonary rehabilitation is an ideal opportunity to inform patients and discuss prognosis and end of life scenarios. We have observed remarkable reductions in anxiety and depression after comprehensive pulmonary rehabilitation, even without participation in a specific psychotherapeutic intervention (unpublished data).

Future perspectives

There are very few data on palliative care in IPF patients, reflecting a general tentativeness in considering palliative care routinely in daily practice. Despite clear recommendations, physicians and patients seem to avoid discussing topics that may make them feel uncomfortable during their communications. However, data show that patients search for support independently (*e.g.* on the Internet) and specifically search for information about disease progression and death. This is comparable with experiences when treating COPD patients. It is imperative that practitioners learn to address these topics as soon as the IPF diagnosis is made.

Perhaps, the alternative term "supportive care", with its more positive connotation, should be adopted. Within supportive care, patients need to know early on that practitioners are equally interested in discussing and resolving their symptoms (*i.e.* dyspnoea, fatigue, and cough) and psychological condition as they are discussing lung function parameters. This may include discussing the use of prescription medications (*e.g.* low-dose morphine) in cases of increasing and/or intolerable dyspnoea. The regular practice of supportive care in IPF may help prevent patients from developing negative thoughts, especially imagining unrealistic and highly frightful end of life scenarios. However, in selected patients, lung transplantation may be the last resort.

Transplantation

Despite current advances in pharmacological treatments, lung transplantation remains the ultimate treatment option for selected patients with IPF. Recently, the dismal prognosis and progressive nature of IPF have been taken into account in most transplant allocation systems, thus significantly reducing waiting list mortality. Whereas the survival benefit of lung transplantation has clearly been demonstrated in patients with IPF, their outcome after lung transplantation tends to be worse than in patients with other end-stage lung diseases. Both single (SLTx) and bilateral (BLTx) lung transplantation have been successfully performed. While recent data favour BLTx for improved long-term survival, multiple factors have to be considered when selecting the procedure of choice. Furthermore, shortage of donor lungs is a universal problem that has to be taken into account.

Candidate identification

Even though the natural history of the disease is highly variable, patients with histological or radiographic evidence of UIP should be considered for lung transplantation irrespective of vital capacity [41]. Early identification of potential lung transplant candidates might be of benefit, especially in patients with rapidly progressive disease, since at the time of diagnosis the course of the disease is hard to predict. However, despite the strong recommendation to provide lung transplantation for appropriate patients with IPF [26], there are still potential lung transplant candidates who are not considered for transplantation [42]. Although not all patients would be eligible for or willing to undergo transplantation, detailed information should be provided to every potential lung transplant candidate.

On initial consideration, patients must undergo a number of medical tests as part of the pre-transplant evaluation to rule out any contraindications and identify problems that may have an impact on the postoperative course. The International Society for Heart & Lung Transplantation (ISHLT) has defined absolute and relative contraindications; these are discussed in the most recent guidelines for the selection of lung transplant candidates and are generally applicable in end-stage lung disease [41]. Pre-transplant evaluation is recommended for clinically stable patients, but not as a rescue strategy for critically ill patients.

IPF is associated with a number of comorbidities, which are discussed in a separate chapter of this *Monograph* [43]. These comorbidities might have a significant impact on the course of the disease and/or the postoperative outcome and should be specifically assessed in the context of transplant evaluation.

Patients with IPF are more susceptible to coronary artery disease (CAD) than patients with other end-stage lung diseases [44]. CAD has a substantial impact on postoperative outcome in patients with IPF [45] and therefore must be investigated as part of the transplant evaluation. According to the ISHLT guidelines, CAD not amenable to percutaneous coronary intervention or bypass grafting, or associated with significant impairment of left ventricular function, is regarded as an absolute contraindication to lung transplantation [41].

Whereas PH is associated with increased mortality in patients with IPF [46], the effect of PH on survival after lung transplantation seems to be largely nonsignificant [47, 48]. However, in the presence of PH most transplant centres now favour BLTx over SLTx to avoid perfusion asymmetry leading to haemodynamic instability and primary graft dysfunction. Thus, early graft-related mortality should be reduced in patients with IPF and concomitant PH.

Patients with IPF also tend to be overweight. An extremely high or low BMI is also an independent risk factor for mortality after lung transplantation [49]. Obese patients with IPF have a higher 90-day mortality risk [50]. Overweight patients tend to have low functional capacity; reducing body weight and/or improving functional capacity tend to lead to better outcomes. Therefore, early dietary advice and referral to pulmonary rehabilitation, which target healthy weight loss and improve functional capacity, should be included in the pre-transplant evaluation [30].

After exclusion of any potential contraindications and detailed explanation of obligations and responsibilities, an optimal time point for listing must be established. It is important to consider that the duration between listing to transplantation can differ significantly from patient to patient due to a number of factors, including the variable nature of the disease.

Furthermore, a limited window of opportunity exists to refer IPF patients for lung transplantation and patients with IPF have the highest waiting list mortality rates among all lung transplant candidates [51, 52].

Because baseline measures are often of limited usefulness, continuous disease monitoring is mandatory to identify disease progress and patients at risk for a worse outcome. This is discussed in a separate chapter of the *Monograph* [53].

Various prognostic factors have been reported that identify patients with poor survival. Based on these features, the ISHLT recommends the guidelines for transplantation shown in table 1.

Further features associated with increased mortality in IPF that should be taken into account are baseline dyspnoea [54, 55] and changes of dyspnoea over time [56], cough [57], the presence of PH [46, 58], a change in D_{LCO} [26], exacerbations [59], and increased levels of partial pressure of carbon dioxide [5]. Furthermore, on approval of two new drugs (pirfenidone and nintedanib) for the treatment of IPF, treatment failure might become another indication for early placement on the waiting list. However, the timing of listing also depends on the individual patient and the referring physician's estimation of survival prospects.

Allocation

Allocation systems vary around the world and depend on geographical conditions, accumulated waiting time, or urgency criteria. Individually or in combination, they are used to guide allocation. Centre-based regional distribution is common in some European countries while others place emphasis on waiting period, urgency, or prospective transplant benefit [60].

In 2005, the United Network for Organ Sharing (UNOS) implemented the lung allocation score (LAS) in the United States. In 2011, the Eurotransplant foundation adopted LAS for the allocation of donor lungs in some European countries.

LAS is used to prioritise waiting list candidates based on a combination of waiting list urgency and estimated post-transplant survival to assess the prospective survival benefit [45]. Consequently, a drop in waiting list mortality in general [60] and especially for patients with IPF has been reported [61]. Implementation of LAS has resulted in an increased number of IPF patients receiving a lung transplant and IPF has become the most common indication for lung transplantation [60, 62, 63].

Table 1. International Society for Heart and Lung Transplantation recommendations for lung transplantation in IPF patients

Timing for referral
  Histological or radiographic evidence of UIP regardless of lung function
Timing for listing
  Decline in D_{LCO} of <39% predicted
  Decline in FVC ≥10% during 6 months of follow-up
  A decrease in pulse oximetry below 88% during a 6MWT
  Honeycombing on HRCT (fibrosis score of >2)

Data from [78].

Type of procedure

Both SLTx and BLTx are successfully performed in patients with IPF. While historically SLTx has been the procedure of choice, recently worldwide more than half of lung transplant candidates with IPF receive a BLTx [63]. Some centres provide SLTx for older patients or patients with comorbidities to reduce the risk of short-term mortality. Younger patients, however, might profit from larger lung volumes and should not be affected by problems arising from the remaining native lung. Hence, it is not clear whether SLTx or BLTx provide the best outcome.

Retrospective studies investigating transplantation outcome are often limited by a selection bias and randomised trials are not available. Therefore, in the current updated ATS/ERS/ JRS/ALAT clinical practice guidelines on the treatment of IPF, no recommendations exist with regard to the procedure of choice in lung transplant recipients with IPF [34].

Existing cohort studies have reported conflicting observations [48, 64–67]. Two analyses of data from the UNOS registry failed to show any survival advantage for BLTx over SLTx after adjusting for baseline characteristics [66, 67]. The second analysis, however, provided evidence that SLTx confers short-term survival benefit but results in more long-term complications, whereas BLTx confers complications over the short-term but long-term survival benefit [67].

Recently, SCHAFFER et al. [48] conducted a large exploratory analysis of the UNOS registry data, which incorporated the implementation of LAS. BLTx was associated with better graft survival than SLTx in patients with IPF after using propensity score analysis to control for potential confounding factors.

In conclusion, a decision on the type of procedure must be made individually, on a case-by-case basis, using an exhaustive and multidisciplinary approach. Disease severity, recipient age, existing comorbidities, nutritional and functional status, PH, and centre experience must all be taken into account. Moreover, severe cough and sputum production, which are difficult to quantify, sometimes warrant consideration of BLTx. Finally, waiting list time is generally longer for BLTx recipients and this should be considered in the case of rapid progressive disease. Patients listed for a BLTx only are generally at greater risk of dying while on the transplant list, and are less likely to receive a lung transplant than patients listed for SLTx or both [61].

Shortage of donor organs is a worldwide problem. Accordingly, the decision to give a BLTx to a single patient rather than to give SLTx to two patients must be considered carefully. It is critical to understand in which IPF patients a BLTx is necessary and in which IPF patients SLTx may be preferable [68].

Outcome and surveillance

Several studies have shown that lung transplantation confers survival benefit for patients with IPF [52, 69–71]. However, patients with IPF have the lowest survival of all lung transplant recipients [72]. Patients with IPF tend to have more infectious complications compared to patients with other end-stage lung diseases [73, 74]. Additionally, they are more susceptible to pulmonary embolism [75], which at least partially explains the observed survival differences.

In patients with IPF who undergo SLTx, progression of fibrosis in the native lung might continue after transplantation. The native lung is not protected from further deterioration, despite aggressive immunomodulatory treatment after transplantation [76, 77]. A further decrease of lung volumes can occur and may be misinterpreted as chronic allograft dysfunction. Moreover, after SLTx a debilitating cough might limit QoL and thus must be addressed when present. Finally, shrinkage of the native lung might lead to an increase of the relative size of the allograft with potential elongation of the main bronchus, which in turn can contribute to large airway disease.

Summary

Lung transplantation provides an effective treatment option in highly selected patients with IPF. However, early consideration and referral and close monitoring of disease progression are mandatory due to the highly variable nature of the disease. At the time of first objective progression or when poor prognosis is present, active placement on the waiting list should be performed. The window for active listing and transplantation to provide maximal transplant benefit is limited and requires optimal preparation. The procedure of choice has to be established in a multidisciplinary approach taking various variables into account. Close post-transplant monitoring is mandatory to achieve maximum benefits for long-term survival and provide QoL for the patient.

Conclusion

In patients with IPF, only a limited number of pharmacological treatments are available. However, some nonpharmacological options are beneficial to IPF patients. Pulmonary rehabilitation is certainly one of the most effective nonpharmacological interventions used to increase exercise capacity, reduce dyspnoea, and improve QoL in IPF patients. Furthermore, LTOT and in some patients even NIPPV may be supportive in reducing disease burden. Patients with very advanced disease should not be the only ones to be referred to palliative care programmes to reduce anxieties and end of life fears.

LTx provides an effective treatment option in highly selected patients with IPF. However, early consideration for LTx and close monitoring of disease progression are mandatory due to the highly variable nature of the disease. Taking this into account, there is still an unmet need to further prove the efficacy of pulmonary rehabilitation prior to LTx to establish this as a mandatory intervention for LTx candidates, as it is already the case in several healthcare systems.

References

1. McCarthy B, Casey D, Devane D, *et al.* Pulmonary rehabilitation for chronic obstructive pulmonary disease. *Cochrane Database Syst Rev* 2015; 2: CD003793.
2. Spruit MA, Singh SJ, Garvey C, *et al.* An official American Thoracic Society/European Respiratory Society statement: key concepts and advances in pulmonary rehabilitation. *Am J Respir Crit Care Med* 2013; 188: e13–e64.
3. Gloeckl R, Marinov B, Pitta F. Practical recommendations for exercise training in patients with COPD. *Eur Respir Rev* 2013; 22: 178–186.
4. Gloeckl R, Halle M, Kenn K. Interval *versus* continuous training in lung transplant candidates: a randomized trial. *J Heart Lung Transplant* 2012; 31: 934–941.
5. Holland AE. Exercise limitation in interstitial lung disease – mechanisms, significance and therapeutic options. *Chron Respir Dis* 2010; 7: 101–111.

6. Swigris JJ, Kuschner WG, Jacobs SS, *et al.* Health-related quality of life in patients with idiopathic pulmonary fibrosis: a systematic review. *Thorax* 2005; 60: 588–594.

7. Caminati A, Bianchi A, Cassandro R, *et al.* Walking distance on 6-MWT is a prognostic factor in idiopathic pulmonary fibrosis. *Respir Med* 2009; 103: 117–123.

8. Nakayama M, Bando M, Araki K, *et al.* Physical activity in patients with idiopathic pulmonary fibrosis. *Respirology* 2015; 20: 640–646.

9. Rafii R, Juarez MM, Albertson TE, *et al.* A review of current and novel therapies for idiopathic pulmonary fibrosis. *J Thorac Dis* 2013; 5: 48–73.

10. Lederer DJ, Arcasoy SM, Wilt JS, *et al.* Six-minute-walk distance predicts waiting list survival in idiopathic pulmonary fibrosis. *Am J Respir Crit Care Med* 2006; 174: 659–664.

11. Swigris JJ, Swick J, Wamboldt FS, *et al.* Heart rate recovery after 6-min walk test predicts survival in patients with idiopathic pulmonary fibrosis. *Chest* 2009; 136: 841–848.

12. Nishiyama O, Kondoh Y, Kimura T, *et al.* Effects of pulmonary rehabilitation in patients with idiopathic pulmonary fibrosis. *Respirology* 2008; 13: 394–399.

13. Holland AE, Hill CJ, Conron M, *et al.* Short term improvement in exercise capacity and symptoms following exercise training in interstitial lung disease. *Thorax* 2008; 63: 549–554.

14. Vainshelboim B, Oliveira J, Yehoshua L, *et al.* Exercise training-based pulmonary rehabilitation program is clinically beneficial for idiopathic pulmonary fibrosis. *Respiration* 2014; 88: 378–388.

15. Kozu R, Jenkins S, Senjyu H. Effect of disability level on response to pulmonary rehabilitation in patients with idiopathic pulmonary fibrosis. *Respirology* 2011; 16: 1196–1202.

16. Huppmann P, Sczepanski B, Boensch M, *et al.* Effects of inpatient pulmonary rehabilitation in patients with interstitial lung disease. *Eur Respir J* 2013; 42: 444–453.

17. Jackson RM, Gómez-Marín OW, Ramos CF, *et al.* Exercise limitation in IPF patients: a randomized trial of pulmonary rehabilitation. *Lung* 2014; 192: 367–376.

18. Rammaert B, Leroy S, Cavestri B, *et al.* Home-based pulmonary rehabilitation in idiopathic pulmonary fibrosis. *Rev Mal Respir* 2011; 28: e52–e57.

19. Holland AE, Hill CJ, Glaspole I, *et al.* Predictors of benefit following pulmonary rehabilitation for interstitial lung disease. *Respir Med* 2012; 106: 429–435.

20. Kozu R, Senjyu H, Jenkins SC, *et al.* Differences in response to pulmonary rehabilitation in idiopathic pulmonary fibrosis and chronic obstructive pulmonary disease. *Respiration* 2011; 81: 196–205.

21. Sillen MJ, Speksnijder CM, Eterman RM, *et al.* Effects of neuromuscular electrical stimulation of muscles of ambulation in patients with chronic heart failure or COPD: a systematic review of the English-language literature. *Chest* 2009; 136: 44–61.

22. Gosselink R, De Vos J, van den Heuvel SP, *et al.* Impact of inspiratory muscle training in patients with COPD: what is the evidence? *Eur Respir J* 2011; 37: 416–425.

23. Wu W, Liu X, Wang L, *et al.* Effects of Tai Chi on exercise capacity and health-related quality of life in patients with chronic obstructive pulmonary disease: a systematic review and meta-analysis. *Int J Chron Obstruct Pulmon Dis* 2014; 9: 1253–1263.

24. Gloeckl R, Heinzelmann I, Kenn K. Whole body vibration training in patients with COPD: a systematic review. *Chron Respir Dis* 2015; 12: 212–221.

25. Holland A, Hill C. Physical training for interstitial lung disease. *Cochrane Database Syst Rev* 2008; 4: CD006322.

26. Raghu G, Collard HR, Egan JJ, *et al.* An official ATS/ERS/JRS/ALAT statement: idiopathic pulmonary fibrosis: evidence-based guidelines for diagnosis and management. *Am J Respir Crit Care Med* 2011; 183: 788–824.

27. Hallstrand TS, Boitano LJ, Johnson WC, *et al.* The timed walk test as a measure of severity and survival in idiopathic pulmonary fibrosis. *Eur Respir J* 2005; 25: 96–103.

28. Nishiyama O, Miyajima H, Fukai Y, *et al.* Effect of ambulatory oxygen on exertional dyspnea in IPF patients without resting hypoxemia. *Respir Med* 2013; 107: 1241–1246.

29. Dreher M, Ekkernkamp E, Schmoor C, *et al.* Pulmonary rehabilitation and noninvasive ventilation in patients with hypercapnic interstitial lung disease. *Respiration* 2015; 89: 208–213.

30. Florian J, Rubin A, Mattiello R, *et al.* Impact of pulmonary rehabilitation on quality of life and functional capacity in patients on waiting lists for lung transplantation. *J Bras Pneumol* 2013; 39: 349–356.

31. Kenn K, Gloeckl R, Soennichsen A, *et al.* Predictors of success for pulmonary rehabilitation in patients awaiting lung transplantation. *Transplantation* 2015; 99: 1072–1077.

32. Dowman L, McDonald CF, Hill C, *et al.* The benefits of exercise training in interstitial lung disease: protocol for a multicentre randomised controlled trial. *BMC Pulm Med* 2013; 13: 8.

33. WHO Definition of Palliative Care. www.who.int/cancer/palliative/definition/en/. Date last accessed: January 20, 2016.

34. Raghu G, Rochwerg B, Zhang Y, *et al.* An official ATS/ERS/JRS/ALAT clinical practice guideline: treatment of idiopathic pulmonary fibrosis. An update of the 2011 clinical practice guideline. *Am J Respir Crit Care Med* 2015; 192: e3–e19.

35. Gardiner C, Gott M, Small N, *et al.* Living with advanced chronic obstructive pulmonary disease: patients concerns regarding death and dying. *Palliat Med* 2009; 23: 691–697.

36. Lindell KO, Liang Z, Hoffman LA, *et al.* Palliative care and location of death in decedents with idiopathic pulmonary fibrosis. *Chest* 2015; 147: 423–429.

37. Temel JS, Greer JA, Muzikansky A, *et al.* Early palliative care for patients with metastatic non-small-cell lung cancer. *N Engl J Med* 2010; 363: 733–742.

38. Akhtar AA, Ali MA, Smith RP. Depression in patients with idiopathic pulmonary fibrosis. *Chron Respir Dis* 2013; 10: 127–133.

39. De Vries J, Kessels BL, Drent M. Quality of life of idiopathic pulmonary fibrosis patients. *Eur Respir J* 2001; 17: 954–961.

40. Holland AE, Fiore JF Jr, Goh N, *et al.* Be honest and help me prepare for the future: what people with interstitial lung disease want from education in pulmonary rehabilitation. *Chron Respir Dis* 2015; 12: 93–101.

41. Orens JB, Estenne M, Arcasoy S, *et al.* International guidelines for the selection of lung transplant candidates: 2006 update – a consensus report from the Pulmonary Scientific Council of the International Society for Heart and Lung Transplantation. *J Heart Lung Transplant* 2006; 25: 745–755.

42. Behr J, Kreuter M, Hoeper MM, *et al.* Management of patients with idiopathic pulmonary fibrosis in clinical practice: the INSIGHTS-IPF registry. *Eur Respir J* 2015; 46: 186–196.

43. Kreuter M, Brunnemer E, Ehlers-Tenenbaum S, *et al.* Other comorbidities. *In*: Costabel U, Crestani B, Wells AU, eds. Idiopathic Pulmonary Fibrosis (ERS Monograph). Sheffield, European Respiratory Society, 2016; pp. 186–195.

44. Hubbard RB, Smith C, Le Jeune I, *et al.* The association between idiopathic pulmonary fibrosis and vascular disease: a population-based study. *Am J Respir Crit Care Med* 2008; 178: 1257–1261.

45. Egan TM, Murray S, Bustami RT, *et al.* Development of the new lung allocation system in the United States. *Am J Transplant* 2006; 6: 1212–1227.

46. Lettieri CJ, Nathan SD, Barnett SD, *et al.* Prevalence and outcomes of pulmonary arterial hypertension in advanced idiopathic pulmonary fibrosis. *Chest* 2006; 129: 746–752.

47. Hayes D Jr, Higgins RS, Black SM, *et al.* Effect of pulmonary hypertension on survival in patients with idiopathic pulmonary fibrosis after lung transplantation: an analysis of the United Network of Organ Sharing registry. *J Heart Lung Transplant* 2015; 34: 430–437.

48. Schaffer JM, Singh SK, Reitz BA, *et al.* Single- *vs* double-lung transplantation in patients with chronic obstructive pulmonary disease and idiopathic pulmonary fibrosis since the implementation of lung allocation based on medical need. *JAMA* 2015; 313: 936–948.

49. Lederer DJ, Wilt JS, D'Ovidio F, *et al.* Obesity and underweight are associated with an increased risk of death after lung transplantation. *Am J Respir Crit Care Med* 2009; 180: 887–895.

50. Gries CJ, Bhadriraju S, Edelman JD, *et al.* Obese patients with idiopathic pulmonary fibrosis have a higher 90-day mortality risk with bilateral lung transplantation. *J Heart Lung Transplant* 2015; 34: 241–246.

51. Hosenpud JD, Bennett LE, Keck BM, *et al.* Effect of diagnosis on survival benefit of lung transplantation for end-stage lung disease. *Lancet* 1998; 351: 24–27.

52. De Meester J, Smits JM, Persijn GG, *et al.* Listing for lung transplantation: life expectancy and transplant effect, stratified by type of end-stage lung disease, the Eurotransplant experience. *J Heart Lung Transplant* 2001; 20: 518–524.

53. Milger K, Behr J. Monitoring. *In*: Costabel U, Crestani B, Wells AU, eds. Idiopathic Pulmonary Fibrosis (ERS Monograph). Sheffield, European Respiratory Society, 2016; pp. 106–121.

54. Manali ED, Stathopoulos GT, Kollintza A, *et al.* The Medical Research Council chronic dyspnea score predicts the survival of patients with idiopathic pulmonary fibrosis. *Respir Med* 2008; 102: 586–592.

55. Nishiyama O, Taniguchi H, Kondoh Y, *et al.* A simple assessment of dyspnoea as a prognostic indicator in idiopathic pulmonary fibrosis. *Eur Respir J* 2010; 36: 1067–1072.

56. Collard HR, King TE Jr, Bartelson BB, *et al.* Changes in clinical and physiologic variables predict survival in idiopathic pulmonary fibrosis. *Am J Respir Crit Care Med* 2003; 168: 538–542.

57. Ryerson CJ, Abbritti M, Ley B, *et al.* Cough predicts prognosis in idiopathic pulmonary fibrosis. *Respirology* 2011; 16: 969–975.

58. Nadrous HF, Pellikka PA, Krowka MJ, *et al.* Pulmonary hypertension in patients with idiopathic pulmonary fibrosis. *Chest* 2005; 128: 2393–2399.

59. Collard HR, Moore BB, Flaherty KR, *et al.* Acute exacerbations of idiopathic pulmonary fibrosis. *Am J Respir Crit Care Med* 2007; 176: 636–643.

60. Gottlieb J, Greer M, Sommerwerck U, *et al.* Introduction of the lung allocation score in Germany. *Am J Transplant* 2014; 14: 1318–1327.

61. Nathan SD, Shlobin OA, Ahmad S, *et al.* Comparison of wait times and mortality for idiopathic pulmonary fibrosis patients listed for single or bilateral lung transplantation. *J Heart Lung Transplant* 2010; 29: 1165–1171.

62. Yusen RD, Shearon TH, Qian Y, *et al.* Lung transplantation in the United States, 1999–2008. *Am J Transplant* 2010; 10: 1047–1068.

63. Yusen RD, Christie JD, Edwards LB, *et al.* The registry of the International Society for Heart and Lung Transplantation: thirtieth adult lung and heart-lung transplant report–2013; focus theme: age. *J Heart Lung Transplant* 2013; 32: 965–978.

64. Meyer DM, Edwards LB, Torres F, et al. Impact of recipient age and procedure type on survival after lung transplantation for pulmonary fibrosis. *Ann Thorac Surg* 2005; 79: 950–957.

65. De Oliveira NC, Osaki S, Maloney J, et al. Lung transplant for interstitial lung disease: outcomes for single *versus* bilateral lung transplantation. *Interact Cardiovasc Thorac Surg* 2012; 14: 263–267.

66. Force SD, Kilgo P, Neujahr DC, et al. Bilateral lung transplantation offers better long-term survival, compared with single-lung transplantation, for younger patients with idiopathic pulmonary fibrosis. *Ann Thorac Surg* 2011; 91: 244–249.

67. Thabut G, Christie JD, Ravaud P, et al. Survival after bilateral versus single-lung transplantation for idiopathic pulmonary fibrosis. *Ann Intern Med* 2009; 151: 767–774.

68. Kistler KD, Nalysnyk L, Rotella P, et al. Lung transplantation in idiopathic pulmonary fibrosis: a systematic review of the literature. *BMC Pulm Med* 2014; 14: 139.

69. Geertsma A, Ten Vergert EM, Bonsel GJ, et al. Does lung transplantation prolong life? A comparison of survival with and without transplantation. *J Heart Lung Transplant* 1998; 17: 511–516.

70. Charman SC, Sharples LD, McNeil KD, et al. Assessment of survival benefit after lung transplantation by patient diagnosis. *J Heart Lung Transplant* 2002; 21: 226–232.

71. Thabut G, Mal H, Castier Y, et al. Survival benefit of lung transplantation for patients with idiopathic pulmonary fibrosis. *J Thorac Cardiovasc Surg* 2003; 126: 469–475.

72. Christie JD, Edwards LB, Kucheryavaya AY, et al. The registry of the International Society for Heart and Lung Transplantation: 29th adult lung and heart-lung transplant report – 2012. *J Heart Lung Transplant* 2012; 31: 1073–1086.

73. de Perrot M, Chaparro C, McRae K, et al. Twenty-year experience of lung transplantation at a single center: influence of recipient diagnosis on long-term survival. *J Thorac Cardiovasc Surg* 2004; 127: 1493–1501.

74. Vicente R, Morales P, Ramos F, et al. Perioperative complications of lung transplantation in patients with emphysema and fibrosis: experience from 1992–2002. *Transplant Proc* 2006; 38: 2560–2562.

75. Nathan SD, Barnett SD, Urban BA, et al. Pulmonary embolism in idiopathic pulmonary fibrosis transplant recipients. *Chest* 2003; 123: 1758–1763.

76. Wahidi MM, Ravenel J, Palmer SM, et al. Progression of idiopathic pulmonary fibrosis in native lungs after single lung transplantation. *Chest* 2002; 121: 2072–2076.

77. Grgic A, Lausberg H, Heinrich M, et al. Progression of fibrosis in usual interstitial pneumonia: serial evaluation of the native lung after single lung transplantation. *Respiration* 2008; 76: 139–145.

78. Weill D, Benden C, Corris PA, et al. A consensus document for the selection of lung transplant candidates: 2014 – an update from the Pulmonary Transplantation Council of the International Society for Heart and Lung Transplantation. *J Heart Lung Transplant* 2015; 34: 1–15.

Disclosures: None declared.

Chapter 19

Key patients' needs: a patient's perspective

Derek Ross

Although the needs of IPF patients vary, some are cited frequently. Needs are being met differently in various centres but satisfaction, unsurprisingly, is highest at the specialist centres. Communication and information is an overarching theme. This ensures that informed decisions are made interactively, such that the patient feels they have participated fully.

The important specific needs include the following. 1) Reducing under, or inconclusive, diagnosis, and speeding up the diagnostic process. 2) Better prognostic information. 3) Clearer articulation of the severity of the patient's IPF and its interaction with various aspects of their QoL. 4) Integrated care, ideally with one, easily accessible, point of contact, managing all aspects of the patient journey. 5) Quick approval of effective new drugs. 6) The opportunity to participate in clinical trials. 7) Understanding the criteria for lung transplantation, their personal chances of receiving a transplant, and confidence that access is determined fairly.

The inclusion of a patient contribution in a professional medical publication reflects the contemporary trend towards greater patient focus. It is hoped that this material might offer an alternative insight into the disease and help clinicians ensure that they fully incorporate patient needs into their everyday practice.

This perspective is based only on my personal experience and that of other patients, as expressed in those support and focus groups with which I have been involved at the Royal Brompton Hospital (RBH) in London. Patients will have different individual needs and patient views as to how needs are met will be different in other centres.

Patients generally appreciate that their needs, both real and perceived, must be set in the context that both skills and resources vary by country and medical institution. Needs will require prioritisation; it follows that some may go unmet or be partially met. Furthermore, not all needs should be met by doctors; some are appropriately met by other medical professionals, nonmedical specialists, charities and support groups.

First contact

Starting at the beginning, I was diagnosed in 2010, aged 60, with mild IPF. I was fortunate because this was by chance. A scan taken for an unrelated reason indicated the lung

Correspondence: derek_a_ross@msn.com

problem. I was able to access a specialist centre (RBH) and within a few months I had a video-assisted thoracic surgical (VATS) biopsy. Following interpretation of the biopsy, my specialist (Professor Wells) explained that the multidisciplinary team had reached the conclusion of IPF.

This is probably the first unmet need for many prospective patients; one that they will not be aware of and arguably the most serious, under-diagnosis. It seems that many patients will not be aware that they have IPF. In my case, if I had not had a scan for a quite different purpose, I would not have recognised the change in lung function for maybe 2–3 years, and even then might not refer to a doctor, believing that the loss of function was age related. Even a general health check might not have revealed the condition because, at the time, my doctors could not hear any velcro crackles and my FVC was not significantly below normal. It was the RBH specialist lung function laboratory that identified an abnormally low transfer capacity (DLCO). Some mechanism for picking up the signs of possible IPF would meet this need, but the cost-effectiveness of such mechanisms is something that experts would need to assess.

Although this was not my experience, it is likely that some patients will not receive a conclusive diagnosis. I have sometimes seen a description of the multidisciplinary team approach, drawing on the CT scan, the VATS biopsy and the other indications, as the "gold standard". My specialist has, however, cautioned that, in his view, there is no gold standard. Accordingly, it would appear to follow that inconclusive diagnosis, as well as misdiagnosis, are high risks. Patients receiving inconclusive information are obviously left in an unsatisfactory and potentially stressful predicament, but presumably this will be unavoidable until science finds a more definitive process. I understand that revised diagnostic criteria have been published and a layman would assume that this is a valuable advance, but I am also aware that it has important limitations that should be addressed [1].

A second unmet need relates to the speed to reach diagnosis. I was privileged to get accurate information to identify the appropriate centre and consultant, and was able to access their services quickly, resulting in a rapid diagnosis. However, many patients report that, having gone to their doctor with symptoms, reaching the diagnosis can be protracted. It seems likely that this process might even miss some IPF patients. There is thus an unmet need in these circumstances, particularly for early referral to a specialist centre. Those patients who have not had such access, unsurprisingly, seem to be generally less satisfied with their care [2].

Issues to consider therefore include: 1) training of general practitioners in identifying possible IPF, and 2) timely access to specialist centres and multidisciplinary teams.

Diagnosis: delivery and consequences

The next step chronologically was receiving the diagnosis. My diagnosis was delivered by a consultant who had done this many times before, and was able to tailor the words and tone to his assessment of me as an individual. Some patients have mentioned that their diagnosis was delivered in, at best, an unprepared and, at worst, an unsympathetic manner. Obviously this discussion, a routine one for the consultant, is life-changing for the patient, so it must be prepared and be given adequate time. The shock will inevitably mean that the patient will forget many questions that he or she needs to ask. Accordingly, the patient should be given the opportunity for a follow-up consultation shortly thereafter, when the information has sunk in, to discuss the implications, preferably with the same consultant.

At my consultation the pros and cons of the various drug combinations were clearly explained. At the time, pirfenidone was not generally available in the UK and the consensus was the old "triple therapy". I was grateful that my consultant did not just give me a prescription and expect me to accept that this was unquestioningly the right approach. He was candid about the unproven merits of the various treatments and combinations. So when, for example, I felt uncomfortable about the immunosuppressant, we reached an agreement that we would start with just low-dose steroids and NAC. With the benefit of hindsight and the results of subsequent studies, this may well have been the wisest choice.

When it became available, we later discussed the merits of pirfenidone, and I am now taking this also. Other patients have mentioned that their treatment was given to them without going through such a collaborative process. For medical conditions where the treatment is clearly defined then it is understandable that doctors will see little utility in having a long discussion about their treatment recommendation. However, for IPF, where so little is understood, it is important to be participative, setting out the merits, disadvantages, side-effects, uncertainties, *etc.*, and guiding the patient towards a regime which is medically appropriate but which also makes sense intuitively to a lay person.

In this regard, I understand that there are now two drugs proven to slow IPF progression but which work on different pathways, *i.e.* pirfenidone and nintedanib. Patients naturally want to know which is best for them. Again I understand that the science about which pathways are relevant for a particular patient, and therefore which drug to use, or indeed whether both should be combined, is a question as yet unanswered. Patients are therefore left in a position of wondering whether the alternative drug might be more effective or if the combination would be better still. This uncertainty could arguably be regarded as an unmet need.

Looking back to my diagnostic consultation, I believe I would have benefitted from being given some written material about IPF, what I could expect, frequently asked questions, *etc.* I am not aware that any such document currently exists in the UK. This is rather surprising. The patient will also be aware of the time pressures on senior medical professionals and may be reluctant to want to take up their time with questions that are important to the patient but which may be regarded as routine. Accordingly, access to further information should be explained. This should include the contact details for a named staff member, such as a specialist IPF nurse, who can answer the most common questions. Other ideas in this regard are mentioned below.

Management process

After diagnosis the patient will come to terms with the condition and react individually. Naturally there will be an initial emotional response which may require support. The emotion will also change over time and hence so will the appropriate support [3].

After diagnosis patients will then also interact with the system at regular intervals for monitoring the progression. At the RBH this was typically every 6 months, although in the last couple of years it has moved out to around 9 months. Patients report that in some countries the follow-ups are more frequent and one assumes there will be instances where the period may be longer.

Some patients report that they feel their care would be better if they had continuity of care, where possible seeing the same consultant at each visit. There is some merit in this desire. Patients will often feel more comfortable by establishing a personal rapport and be reassured that the consultant is familiar with their condition. In my case, I usually see a different doctor at each visit but do not feel this to be a serious problem. This is because, providing the notes are adequate, there is also merit in seeing different doctors; they will often give a slightly different perspective. In coming to terms with a disease of such uncertainty, getting as many varied perspectives as possible is, in my judgement, helpful, but some patients will not share this view. Needless to say when different doctors see patients, they should have enough time to read the notes thoroughly. This has not been an issue at RBH, but some patients elsewhere have reported that they have been exasperated when needing to repeat to different doctors the same information each time they visit, when of course it is, or should be, in the notes.

At the RBH, the clinic is busy and the doctors need to get through their list efficiently. Nonetheless I have never felt unreasonably rushed. This does not appear to be the position universally across all centres; some patients reporting hurried consultations. Patients obviously appreciate the economic trade-offs, but it is of course one of many examples where demand for resource is almost limitless. In an environment where professional resource must be deployed efficiently, patients also have a responsibility to prepare for the consultation, knowing in advance their objectives for the meeting and marshalling their questions logically such that they can exploit limited time effectively. Maybe there is a need for some information for patients on how to get the most from the time with the consultant?

Although my experience has been of good quality care, there are aspects of the system within which the professionals work that are of concern, and which have been reported by others. It is of vital importance for patients that the system for approving new medications is efficient and fast; however, the current approach is anything but. All sorts of reasons are doubtless advanced for the delays but the bottom line is that, when facing possibly a short survival period, many patients cannot afford to wait.

There is also the issue of access to the existing therapies. In the UK, for example, the system for assessing eligibility is based on a detailed and rigorous cost–benefit analysis. This is probably appropriate from a public interest and finance standpoint. Whilst rational in theory, the outcome is that the criteria for whether a particular patient receives the drug may not be sensible. For example, one drug has a criteria for a range of FVCs, but D_{LCO} is not included, and I understand there are other inconsistencies. Clinicians tell me that there are patients they are sure would benefit from certain drugs, but they are excluded because of the application of inflexible rules.

Another aspect of treatment that needs examination is the approach to transplantation. Again, this is not relevant to me as I know I am too old to be considered. I am aware, however, that many IPF patients are unclear about transplantation and therefore whether this might be a possibility for them. I have also been told that access, in the UK, to transplantation for IPF patients is less favourable than for other lung conditions. I do not know what the position is in other countries. Patients need to feel that they are being treated fairly in terms of transplant eligibility and access.

Management responsibilities

During the progression of my IPF I needed personally to manage the various services and specialisms, such as reflux and microaspiration experts, pH technicians, hernia surgeons, osteopenia experts (regarding long-term steroid and antireflux therapies), pulmonary rehabilitation, physiotherapists, *etc*. Not all patients will have the information or the confidence to take ownership of the management process.

For example, knowing that my consultant held a longstanding view of the role of reflux, I arranged to see a pH and manometry specialist, then a gastroenterologist and then a gastric surgeon to do a fundoplication, and again back to recheck pH and manometry. I have no idea whether reflux was contributing to my disease, because the procedure was quite recent, but it seemed sensible to eliminate one possible factor, particularly as the surgery was straightforward. Similarly, because of the long-term use of prednisolone and pantoprazole, I needed to organise a bone density scan which indeed identified an issue that required appropriate treatment. I also arranged a course of pulmonary rehabilitation (see below) which I found helpful.

Other patients might need a more integrated approach to include matters, such as psychological support or oxygen services.

It would be helpful if there could be one point of contact responsible for integrating the medical services because the specialists do not always liaise well with each other, particularly if they work at different institutions. The default position is that the patient must take the initiative and will probably need personally to manage the integration.

In the UK, the professional best placed to undertake this sort of project management role is the patient's general practitioner (GP). However, the GP service is under considerable strain, and most GPs do not have the time to keep all of their patients under close and continuous review. Possibly the IPF specialist nurse might be able to take on this job, but equally they will often have a large number of patients to cover, and this sort of liaison and management is time-consuming. I suspect that the need for a single point of contact for patient management is a need that will continue unmet, at least in the UK, without some additional resource and possibly organisational redesign. Again, I am not able to comment on the situation in other countries.

Regarding communication, patients nowadays have an expectation that they will be able to use the communication medium of their choice to interface with the appropriate professionals. The question arises as to which contact details should be given, such as E-mail, direct dial or even mobile telephone numbers, *etc*. Some of these channels may not always be practical, or indeed acceptable, to the medical professionals. There therefore needs to be an open and frank discussion between patients and professionals about what is appropriate, such that patient expectations can be set at a realistic level.

Severity and prognosis

Patients do not have any generally agreed benchmark with which to measure the severity of their condition. Of course they have their own experience and qualitative assessment of their QoL (see below). I am aware of attempts to develop a scale of severity, some metrics combining various lung function statistics (*e.g.* the composite physical index) and some quantitative QoL measures. The QoL methodologies are, for obvious reasons, generally based on questionnaires, so the output is highly subjective. Turning these qualitative results into quantitative measures that can be integrated with the clinical metrics seems like a difficult exercise.

The most important question for the patient is "how long have I got?" Patients generally appreciate that there is no confident answer possible. It ought, however, to be possible to offer some prognosis probabilities. Doubtless expert readers will have scientifically robust views on how this objective could be achieved, but without wishing to prejudge the methodology, the conversation might be along the lines of: 1) "On a scale of, say, 1 to 5, with each point objectively defined by various specific measures, what is the severity of my IPF?", 2) "Over the next, say, 5 years what is the yearly probability of dying for a patient currently at this point on the scale?" and 3) "How do these probabilities change with therapies such as pirfenidone or nintedanib?".

Patients appreciate that there may be difficulties in collecting, validating and analysing sufficient data to use such a methodology confidently. Nonetheless there is much publicity about "big data" and its potentially transformative role. Accordingly, there are contemporary expectations that it should be possible to share sufficient data internationally and meet the need of patients for better guidance on the state of their disease and its possible progression. There are many lifestyle and financial decisions that patients need to make that would be greatly facilitated if more confidence could be introduced into the prognosis. Patients would generally understand the necessary caveats.

Pulmonary rehabilitation

Throughout my life I have tried to maintain a reasonable level of fitness and understand that it is important to maintain this even as my lung function deteriorates [4]. It can be difficult for patients to understand that exercise, which obviously cannot change their lung fibrosis, is nonetheless beneficial in other ways, so this effect needs to be carefully explained [5, 6].

I certainly benefitted from some guidance specifically tailored to my condition by arranging a course of pulmonary rehabilitation. The challenge, however, is to maintain the exercise regime. Some patients have experienced patchy availability of these services however.

Living with IPF

Relevant advice and information at the right stage on how to live with IPF is important. I have been able to find adequate information on self-management of breathlessness, cough, fatigue, worry, *etc.*, but it has been a piecemeal process. I note that this subject has been of increasing focus, so doubtless more insights into QoL issues will emerge [7–10].

Patient interactions with clinicians at their regular reviews are, quite appropriately, focussed on the medical issues such as disease progression; however, helping patients understand, possibly even anticipate, the key challenges of living with the disease should be integrated as far as is practical [11].

Palliative and end-of-life care

I have little experience of this matter other than in relation to management of cough where I have been able to obtain effective advice from the RBH. Other patients report varied information and access to controlling IPF symptoms, such as sleep quality [12].

End-of-life care is something that patients generally fear, so such referrals must be communicated with care. There is a serious risk that the patient will interpret the message, no matter how well intentioned, as code that their doctor can do no more and will now be abandoning them to their inevitable death.

Communication and information

An overarching issue at each stage of the patient's journey concerns communication and information [13]. In addition to the initial information needed at the point of diagnosis, referred to above, there is a need for information at the appropriate time in respect of many other matters. These include the answers to worrying end-of-life questions such as "How will I die?", "Will it be painful or distressing?", "What is the role of palliative care?", *etc.*

Additionally, there will be some basic questions of concern. These include questions about the chances and criteria for lung transplantation, how to control cough, how to avoid infections, how to recognise and what to do about acute exacerbations, how to avoid stress, and how and when to take medications, particularly if the patient has other conditions being medicated concurrently. There seems to be an unmet need in most of these areas.

With regard to the last point above, patients report that doctors and pharmacists sometimes give inconsistent information about how and when to take drugs. This is tied up with a general concern, or even fear, about adverse interactions, when patients are taking many different drugs for IPF and other conditions. There is sometimes a lack of information about side-effects and how to manage them. An easy way of meeting this need is for patients to be given a schedule consolidating all the drugs they take. This should be annotated with all the important information needed, including how and when to take them, possible interactions, and side-effects. Naturally, the schedule should be agreed by the doctor and the pharmacist.

Mentioned above is the potentially greater use of technology. It is likely that many patient needs can cost-effectively be met, at least in part, by greater use of appropriate technology. For example, using web-based video consulting, more communication by E-mail and more dissemination of information to patients by, say, webinars. Many patients would value such facilities.

The unmet need for better information might also be addressed by setting up a virtual library. Patients could then simply access the self-help resources as and when required. This would be an appropriate project for one of the IPF or general lung condition charities, but might be most cost-effective if undertaken globally at one central hub.

The most comprehensive source of information that I have found is the US charity, the Pulmonary Fibrosis Foundation (www.pulmonaryfibrosis.org). I have often used their material, particularly the educational resources, such as the webinars. They also have a helpline (PFF

Patient Communication Center) available by E-mail and telephone. The scale of the help and information available in the USA is unsurprising given the size and homogeneity of the region. The obvious route for other countries would appear to be to leverage these existing resources.

Role of patient support groups and charities

In addition to individual self-help, support groups can also play a role, reinforcing the message that the patient is not alone and giving an opportunity for discussion of mutually interesting subjects. As with all such support groups, their success, or otherwise, reflects the input of the membership. Patients report that their satisfaction with support groups is therefore patchy. A support group will not succeed without the energy and commitment of its members; it may require only one enthusiast to achieve success. Nonetheless, some initial set-up assistance, again possibly from the hospital or the relevant charities, might be the catalyst needed. If an IPF patient support group proves itself, then it would be appropriate for the related institution also to contribute. This could be, for example, by providing a venue plus medical and other speakers on subjects, such as latest research results, drug trial information, exercise, use of oxygen, insurance and travel arrangements, *etc.*

There is sometimes an unmet need concerning information and support for living with severe IPF. Patients will vary in how positive they feel about living life to the fullest possible. These are not primarily medical issues but, more often, practical ones, such as those mentioned above, where support groups and charities would be well positioned to help.

In addition to patient support, the charities also have an important role in raising awareness of IPF, lobbying policy and decision makers, particularly budget holders, encouraging and potentially supporting research.

Research

Patients will from time to time be asked to participate in research and individuals must make their own decisions [14]. Researchers need to sign up patients and therefore patients generally report that the process works well, with good quality communication and explanations about the project, including the nature of the patient's involvement. What does not always work so well is the communication after the project. Patients would not sign up unless they were interested in the utility of the research, but sometimes they do not get feedback on the results. This need can be met quite simply. For example, at the RBH the research team produces a regular newsletter on their projects and results. This team also organises a seminar from time to time, at which research participants and other interested parties can hear direct from the researchers and the medical professionals about the results and implications of their work. The most senior consultants in the ILD department give presentations; it is apparent that patients appreciate that these professionals are prepared to invest valuable time communicating this feedback.

Carers

Throughout the process, some patients will also have carers or loved ones participating. Their needs, whilst not directly the responsibility of the medical professionals, ought reasonably to be considered, although this is not the subject matter of this chapter.

Table 1. Summary of patient needs and related issues

The diagnosis process, under- and inconclusive diagnosis, and speed
Access to specialist centres and multidisciplinary teams
Training in the delivery of the diagnosis of a terminal condition with uncertain timescales,
  including understanding the effect of the message on the psychology of the patient
Training in how to reach agreement with the patient, if appropriate, on the best treatment regime
Access to a follow-up consultation, preferably with the same consultant, to ask further questions
Ensuring adequate time for the consultation
If seeing the patient for the first time, devoting sufficient time to read the notes
Better guidance on prognosis
Access to a nurse specialist to provide ongoing information, support and referral as necessary to
  other specialists, such as pulmonary rehabilitation, pharmacists, psychologists, counsellors,
  palliative care, charities and support groups
Integrated management, ideally with one point of contact
Efficient and convenient communication channels, including the appropriate use of technology
Faster, more efficient, approval of new drugs
Easy and consistent access to pulmonary rehabilitation
Equitable approach to eligibility for transplantation

Conclusion

It is hoped that the above inventory of personal experiences is a helpful reminder of the matters which are important to patients. Patients will have expectations as well as needs, some reasonable, others less so, and therefore compromises are inevitable. Clearly many patients' needs can only be met with advances in medical science and some will be constrained by budgetary considerations. Others, however, can be achieved more readily. An overarching theme is the need for the right information to be communicated at the right time and in an appropriate format.

Table 1 provides a summary of patient needs and related issues, and table 2 provides examples of information needs. The European IPF Patient Organisations have published a useful document which summarises many of the issues dealt with in this chapter [15].

Table 2. Examples of information needs

Leaflets and answers to frequently asked questions when the diagnosis is delivered
Information on which of the two current drugs in use, or a combination, would have the greatest
  effect in slowing progression
Drug interactions, how and when to take the various drugs
Symptom control, including cough, fatigue and sleep problems
Managing the medical system, including how to get the best out of a consultation
Dealing with stress
Identifying infections, when to use antibiotics
Recognising and knowing what to do about acute exacerbations
Support groups
Nonmedical information, such as travel, insurance and financial matters
Lung transplantation
Use of oxygen
Palliative and end-of-life care

References

1. Wells AU. The revised ATS/ERS/JRS/ALAT diagnostic criteria for IPF – practical implications. *Respir Res* 2013; 14: Suppl. 1, S2.
2. Schoenheit G, Becattelli I, Cohen AH. Living with idiopathic pulmonary fibrosis: an in-depth qualitative survey of European patients. *Chron Respir Dis* 2011; 183: 788–824.
3. Giot C, Maronati M, Becattelli I, *et al*. Idiopathic pulmonary fibrosis: an EU patient perspective survey. *Curr Respir Med Rev* 2013; 9: 112–119.
4. Spruit MA, Singh SJ, Garvey C, *et al*. An official American Thoracic Society/European Respiratory Society statement: key concepts and advances in pulmonary rehabilitation. *Am J Respir Crit Care Med* 2013; 188: e13–e64.
5. Nici L, ZuWallack R, Wouters E, *et al*. On pulmonary rehabilitation and the flight of the bumblebee. *Eur Respir J* 2006; 28: 461–462.
6. Troosters T, Spruit MA, Franssen FME. ERS Vision 'Take the Active Option'. http://www.ersvision.org/videos/ take-the-active-option Date last accessed: January 29, 2016.
7. De Vries J, Kessels BL, Drent M. Quality of life in idiopathic pulmonary fibrosis patients. *Eur Respir J* 2001; 17: 954–961.
8. Swigris JJ, Kuschner WG, Jacobs SS, *et al*. Health-related quality of life in patients with idiopathic pulmonary fibrosis: a systematic review. *Thorax* 2005; 60: 588–594.
9. Martinez TY, Pereira CA, dos Santos ML, *et al*. Evaluation of the short-form 36-item questionnaire to measure health-related quality of life in patients with idiopathic pulmonary fibrosis. *Chest* 2000; 117: 1627–1632.
10. Swigris JJ, Stewart AL, Gould MK, *et al*. Patients' perspectives on how idiopathic pulmonary fibrosis affects the quality of their lives. *Health Qual Life Outcomes* 2005; 3: 61.
11. Duck A, Spencer LG, Bailey S, *et al*. Perceptions, experiences and needs of patients with idiopathic pulmonary fibrosis. *J Adv Nurs* 2015; 71: 1055–1065.
12. Krishnan V, McCormack MC, Mathai SC, *et al*. Sleep quality and health-related quality of life in idiopathic pulmonary fibrosis. *Chest* 2008; 134: 693–698.
13. Collard H, Tino G, Noble PW, *et al*. Patient experiences with pulmonary fibrosis. *Respir Med* 2007; 101: 1350–1354.
14. Russell A-M, Sprangers MA, Wibberley S, *et al*. The need for patient-centred clinical research in idiopathic pulmonary fibrosis. *BMC Med* 2015; 13: 240.
15. European IPF Patient Organisations. European Idiopathic Pulmonary Fibrosis (IPF) Patient Charter. http://www. ipfcharter.org/wp-content/uploads/2014/08/European-IPF-Patient-Charter_English_Final_12.05.2014_English_ clean.pdf.

Disclosures: None declared.

Chapter 20

Key ongoing issues in trial design

Mark G. Jones and Luca Richeldi

Recently significant progress has been made in the therapeutic targeting of IPF. This has culminated in the worldwide approval of the first antifibrotic therapies, nintedanib and pirfenidone. Whilst an important first step, patients continue to progress and better therapies are urgently required. However, there is an increasing number of potential obstacles in the design of new trials; at the same time, new potential opportunities are emerging from the advancement of our scientific knowledge. The recent advances in our understanding of genetics, biomarkers and study design are particularly relevant. In this chapter, we discuss future priorities if we are to continue to increase the length and QoL of patients with IPF, and describe some possible approaches to increase the efficiency of future trials.

Despite (or maybe partly because of) the recent approval of two antifibrotic therapies for the treatment of IPF, nintedanib and pirfenidone, intense clinical research activity is ongoing worldwide [1]. In particular, a number of early-phase trials are currently enrolling patients (figure 1), although some of them were designed before approval of current antifibrotic drugs and, therefore, have been almost invariably modified in order to allow background therapies and make recruitment feasible. However, a key question remains unanswered: which trial design will best enable future putative antifibrotic therapies to demonstrate efficacy in an era of approved therapies? The aim of this chapter is to illustrate and discuss some of the most significant factors that will need to be considered in the design of ongoing and future IPF clinical trials.

Genetics

Pulmonary fibrosis has probably been one of the areas of respiratory medicine with the most impressive recent advances in understanding how genetic background might impact on not just an individual's risk of developing IPF but also their prognosis and potentially even their response to pharmacological therapy. Genome-wide association studies have now identified more than a dozen common genetic variants associated with IPF risk [2, 3]. In particular, a common single-nucleotide polymorphism (SNP) (rs35705950) in the promoter region of the gene encoding mucin 5B (*MUC5B*) has been significantly associated in multiple independent studies as the risk variant with the largest genetic effect on the development of both familial and sporadic forms of IPF (OR 4–8 per allele) [2–8]. *MUC5B* encodes a mucin 5B precursor

National Institute for Health Research Southampton Respiratory Biomedical Research Unit and Clinical and Experimental Sciences, University of Southampton, Southampton, UK.

Correspondence: Luca Richeldi, National Institute for Health Research Southampton Respiratory Biomedical Research Unit, Mailpoint 813, E Level, South Academic Block, University Hospital Southampton NHS Foundation Trust, Tremona Road, Southampton SO16 6YD, UK. E-mail: L.Richeldi@soton.ac.uk

Copyright ©ERS 2016. Print ISBN: 978-1-84984-067-5. Online ISBN: 978-1-84984-068-2. Print ISSN: 2312-508X. Online ISSN: 2312-5098.

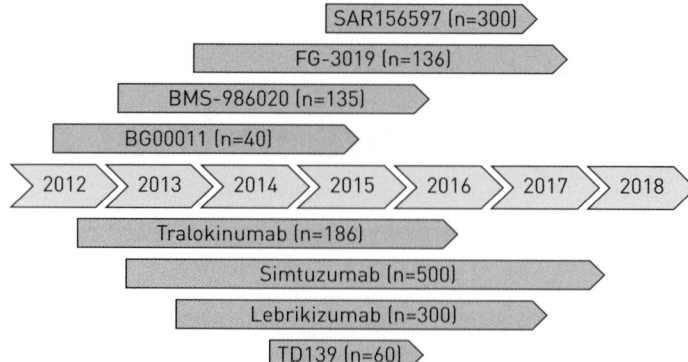

Figure 1. Ongoing phase II randomised clinical trials in IPF, with estimated numbers of patients enrolled and timeframes (from clinicaltrials.gov).

protein that contributes to airway mucus production and may have an important role in lung host defense [9, 10]. Additional work identified that the *MUC5B* polymorphism, in addition to being a risk factor for development of IPF, might have prognostic implications, as those with the common T allele have a higher rate of survival, with the 7% of patients with the TT genotype having a very low risk of death and the 28–34% of patients with the GG genotype having the highest risk of death [11]. This finding requires prospective validation, although in keeping with the proposed prognostic correlation was the identification in UK patients with IPF that the minor T allele was associated with less rapidly progressive decline in lung function [7]. These recent findings might be crucially relevant for the design of future IPF clinical trials and, to date, no trial has addressed the potential impact of genetic factors on efficacy results with particular consideration of survival rates.

Whilst *MUC5B* has been most studied, a number of other common polymorphisms have been identified as potential prognostic polymorphisms. A novel variant of Toll-interacting protein (TOLLIP), an important regulator of innate immune responses acting downstream from the Toll-like receptors, has been found to be associated with IPF susceptibility and progression. IPF patients that carry the minor alleles of associated *TOLLIP* SNPs have decreased TOLLIP expression in lung tissue. Individuals who develop IPF despite having the protective *TOLLIP* minor allele of rs5743890 were found to have an increased mortality risk (hazard ratio (HR) 1.72, 95% CI 1.24–2.38; p=0.0012) [3].

PANTHER-IPF (Prednisone, Azathioprine, and *N*-Acetylcysteine: a Study that Evaluates Response in Idiopathic Pulmonary Fibrosis) was a three-arm study, sponsored by the IPFnet in the USA, which compared the efficacy of so-called triple therapy (prednisolone, azathioprine and NAC) with NAC alone and with placebo. Following a planned efficacy and safety interim analysis, the triple-therapy arm was halted. Although the absolute numbers of events were relatively small compared with the placebo arm (n=78), statistically significant increased risks of death (11% *versus* 1%), all-cause hospitalisation (29% *versus* 8%) and treatment-related serious adverse events (31% *versus* 9%) were seen. The placebo and NAC monotherapy arms continued as a two-arm study, and identified no difference with respect to preservation of FVC in patients with IPF [12]. These trials informed the recent American Thoracic Society (ATS)/European Respiratory Society (ERS)/Japanese Respiratory Society/ Latin American Thoracic Society guidelines on the treatment of IPF, where a strong recommendation against the use of triple therapy and a conditional recommendation against the use NAC monotherapy were made [13].

Interestingly, in a recent *post hoc* analysis of patients participating in the PANTHER-IPF clinical trial, the response of individuals to NAC was correlated with their genetic variants within *TOLLIP* and *MUC5B* [14]. This identified a significant interaction between NAC therapy and polymorphisms within the *TOLLIP* SNP rs3750920. In patients with a TT genotype, NAC therapy was associated with a significant reduction in composite end-point risk (HR 0.14, 95% CI 0.02–0.83; p=0.03). However, in patients with a CC genotype, a nonsignificant increase in composite end-point risk (HR 3.23, 95% CI 0.79–13.16; p=0.10) was identified. Interpretation of this putative association must recognise that the study was exploratory and had multiple limitations: it was a *post hoc* analysis of a negative clinical trial, less than half of study participants consented to genetic analysis, the number of patients within each analysis subgroup was small and multiple analyses were undertaken. However, it was the first study to suggest that the genetic background of a patient might have a meaningful impact on potential benefit or potential harm of any putative antifibrotic therapy, and provides a clear rationale for a prospective genotype-stratified clinical trial of NAC to confirm this finding. In any case, future trials will need to consider the role of genetic factors both in disease progression (*i.e.* the impact on study end-points) and differential response to investigational drug (both in terms of efficacy and safety). It is therefore clear that all future clinical trials must control, and perhaps even consider stratifying, for the presence of prognosis-modifying genetic variants. However, whether these findings will ultimately translate to clinical practice is yet to be determined, and robust prospective studies are required to better understand whether genetic factors may influence the diagnosis and treatment of IPF.

Biomarkers

A number of recent papers have discussed that biomarkers have the potential to significantly facilitate multiple steps in drug development in IPF [15–17]. However, although numerous potential biomarkers have been studied so far, as yet, none has been prospectively validated, and so there are significant hurdles to overcome. A particular focus of recent studies has been to identify molecular biomarkers to stratify patients with IPF prognostically. This might have a potential impact on the design of future IPF trials. In particular, the approach of using drug-related biomarkers to enrich trials for "responders" is attractive.

A recent example of this strategy has been published by SAINI *et al.* [18], who quantified the $\alpha_V\beta_6$-integrin, an epithelium-restricted molecule implicated in multiple models of lung fibrosis. Histological analyses of $\alpha_V\beta_6$-integrin expression of 43 lung tissue sections of patients with pulmonary fibrosis identified that the 33% of patients classified as having the highest $\alpha_V\beta_6$-integrin expression were at increased risk of death and the 7% with very low expression the lowest risk of death, leading to the hypothesis that these represent distinct endotypes of disease [18]. A phase II trial of STX-100 (Biogen Idec, Cambridge, MA, USA), a humanised monoclonal antibody against the $\alpha_V\beta_6$-integrin, is in progress (NCT01371305, clinicaltrials.gov). A further example is represented by the study in which CHIEN *et al.* [19] measured lysyl oxidase-like 2 (LOXL2), which has been proposed to promote collagen cross-linking in fibrosis, in serum from two small, independent cohorts of patients with IPF. They identified a consistent association of higher LOXL2 levels correlating with disease progression. A large phase IIb trial of simtuzumab (Gilead Sciences, Foster City, CA, USA), a humanised monoclonal antibody against LOXL2, is in progress (NCT01362231), which will inform our understanding of these findings.

These novel findings are all supportive of the concept of molecular biomarkers of IPF, although whether they ultimately have utility, diagnostically, prognostically or theragnostically, requires prospective longitudinal studies. The PROFILE (Prospective Observation of Fibrosis in the Lung Clinical Endpoints) study, the largest prospective, multicentre, observational cohort study of patients with IPF to date, identified that several matrix metalloproteinase-degraded protein fragments (neoepitopes) are increased in the serum of patients with IPF compared to age-matched healthy controls, and that a change in neoepitope concentration over only 3 months may be predictive of subsequent outcome [20]. Whilst requiring external validation, the identification of neoepitopes potentially predicting outcome could have utility to shorten early phase clinical trials. However, validation of this finding, or of any putative biomarker, must occur in a new IPF landscape where a patient would be anticipated to commence an antifibrotic therapy at time of diagnosis. Prospective observational longitudinal studies of patients receiving antifibrotic therapy are therefore essential to identify and understand the role of biomarkers in facilitating ongoing progress in drug development.

Patient selection

The use of the terms possible, probable and definite IPF within current international consensus guidelines for IPF demonstrates the challenge that persists in the diagnosis of IPF and, hence, patient selection for clinical trials [21]. The recent phase III trials of nintedanib and pirfenidone aimed to enrol homogeneous populations of patients, although radiological diagnostic entry criteria differed. In the ASCEND (Assessment of Pirfenidone to Confirm Efficacy and Safety in Idiopathic Pulmonary Fibrosis) trials of pirfenidone, a radiological diagnosis of IPF was made according to current ATS/ERS consensus guidelines, and required the presence of honeycomb lung destruction on HRCT [22]. In the INPULSIS trials of nintedanib, a radiological diagnosis of IPF was made on HRCT if, in the absence of atypical features, there was either honeycomb lung destruction or traction bronchiectasis, and a reticular abnormality consistent with fibrosis was present with a basal and peripheral predominance [23]. According to the current consensus guidelines, in patients within the INPULSIS trials without honeycomb lung destruction (*i.e.* without radiologically definite IPF), a diagnostic lung biopsy should be required to inform the diagnosis of IPF. Both radiological criteria identified patients where antifibrotic therapy was efficacious, thus advancing our understanding of the disease behaviour of these radiological patterns of disease and providing valuable data for future patient selection criteria.

Patients with an FVC <50% predicted, considered to have more "severe" disease, were not included within these trials. Both nintedanib and pirfenidone received regulatory approval in the USA without any FVC threshold [1]. It is therefore anticipated that "real world" observational data may soon increase our understanding of disease behaviour and tolerability of antifibrotic therapy within this patient cohort, thus informing future trial designs for this group of patients who have clear unmet medical needs.

Study design

The worldwide approval of two novel antifibrotic therapies for the treatment of IPF was a landmark moment; however, at least two significant questions remain unanswered. First, although it has been speculated that efficacy for both compounds is a result of pleiotropic mechanisms of actions, this is uncertain, and a better understanding of why these treatments have proven efficacious is required. Secondly, it is unknown whether treatment response is homogenous or whether specific individuals differ in response, for example, as a consequence of identified common IPF genetic polymorphisms, as yet unrecognised pharmacogenetic factors or divergent mechanistic pathways of fibrosis. To address such questions, which have the potential to inform our knowledge of future study design, collaborative, multicentre, prospective cohorts with longitudinal clinical data collection and systematic biobanking will be extremely useful. In this context, it is very promising that initial attempts are ongoing to amalgamate and coordinate national IPF trials.

There are now multiple putative candidate antifibrotic therapies. One particular challenge to their development is that the relevance of pre-clinical models of IPF to patients remains uncertain. No animal model has similarities to the histopathological features or progressive nature of IPF, so screening of potential compounds is challenging [24]. Although pre-clinical models of both nintedanib and pirfenidone demonstrated efficacy, many therapeutic candidates with similar pre-clinical data in animal models have not translated (or even potentially caused harm) to patients with IPF [25]. A clear priority is therefore the development of better pre-clinical models of IPF; whilst potentially advancing our understanding of mechanisms of disease, this may also facilitate the study of novel therapeutics in isolation but also, as future trials may be additive to current antifibrotic therapies, provide insight into a putative antifibrotics' actions in the presence of pirfenidone or nintedanib. The development of better animal models may facilitate this, such as humanised models of lung fibrosis, or the use of more advanced cell culture systems using disease relevant tissue or cells. One possible approach was demonstrated by BOOTH et al. [26], who developed a methodology to prepare acellular lung matrices using human lung tissue, providing a more physiological environment for cell culture in vitro.

Recent reviews have identified the progress that has been made in clinical trial design in IPF, culminating in robust, large-scale phase III clinical trials demonstrating therapeutic efficacy [25, 27, 28]. COLLARD et al. [29] highlighted key considerations for future clinical trials in IPF, emphasising the importance of input from all relevant stakeholders in clinical trial design. As long-term, placebo-controlled trials will no longer be ethical, the challenge is how to conduct feasible, safe clinical trials with the optimum chance of demonstrating efficacy.

Following a period of debate, FVC was accepted as a clinically relevant primary efficacy measure in IPF, and in placebo-controlled trials, this enabled demonstration of efficacy of both pirfenidone and nintedanib for regulatory approval [1]. As a new era of clinical trials commences, a particular challenge will be the selection of a new primary end-point with sufficient power to enable a feasible study size for late-phase clinical trials, which are anticipated to be either in combination with the standard of care (pirfenidone or nintedanib) or head-to-head. Recruitment of patients to combination therapy studies with the aim of demonstrating an additive or synergistic therapeutic benefit is likely to be most feasible; however, identifying superiority using a primary end-point of FVC alone within such trials may not be possible. Furthermore, issues of tolerability of combination therapy and the management of standard-of-care therapy (for example, changes in therapy from pirfenidone to nintedanib or vice versa) during a clinical trial will require careful trial design and robust data handling methodologies. As both nintedanib and pirfenidone roughly halve the rate of decline in lung function compared to placebo, demonstrating efficacy above this standard of care might require unrealistic patient numbers or study durations, given the proportionally reduced changes in the rate of FVC decline now possible [22, 23]. One approach to facilitating such trials is the use of composite end-points. Recently, DURHEIM et al. [30] identified that the combination of hospital admission and categorical changes in FVC might be a clinically relevant composite end-point. This highlights that ongoing *post hoc* analyses from previous clinical trials will be invaluable in designing future clinical trials. Whilst such composite end-points may be an essential tool to enable the design of studies with realistic patient recruitment and duration, how such end-points would correlate with long-term clinical outcome is currently uncertain.

Although nintedanib and pirfenidone demonstrated a reduction in the rate of lung function decline, neither has clear evidence of a symptomatic benefit for patients. As discussed by RUSSELL *et al.* [31], a priority must be the development of a pulmonary fibrosis-specific patient-reported outcome tool. Validation of a disease-specific questionnaire would provide an important option for future clinical trials to understand better the effect of a therapeutic agent on symptomatology.

Conclusion

The clinical trial landscape of putative IPF therapies has been transformed by the worldwide approval of the first antifibrotic therapies, nintedanib and pirfenidone. At the same time, our knowledge of genetics, biomarkers and clinical trial design has advanced significantly. If we are to continue to increase the length and quality of life of patients with IPF, we must embrace this new era with innovative trial design integrating ongoing scientific advances.

References

1. Karimi-Shah BA, Chowdhury BA. Forced vital capacity in idiopathic pulmonary fibrosis – FDA review of pirfenidone and nintedanib. *N Engl J Med* 2015; 372: 1189–1191.
2. Fingerlin TE, Murphy E, Zhang W, *et al.* Genome-wide association study identifies multiple susceptibility loci for pulmonary fibrosis. *Nature Genet* 2013; 45: 613–620.
3. Noth I, Zhang Y, Ma S-F, *et al.* Genetic variants associated with idiopathic pulmonary fibrosis susceptibility and mortality: a genome-wide association study. *Lancet Respir Med* 2013; 1: 309–317.
4. Seibold MA, Wise AL, Speer MC, *et al.* A common *MUC5B* promoter polymorphism and pulmonary fibrosis. *N Engl J Med* 2011; 364: 1503–1512.
5. Hunninghake GM, Hatabu H, Okajima Y, *et al.* *MUC5B* promoter polymorphism and interstitial lung abnormalities. *N Engl J Med* 2013; 368: 2192–2200.
6. Peljto AL, Selman M, Kim DS, *et al.* The *MUC5B* promoter polymorphism is associated with IPF in a Mexican cohort but is rare among Asian ancestries. *Chest* 2015; 147: 460–464.
7. Stock CJ, Sato H, Fonseca C, *et al.* Mucin 5B promoter polymorphism is associated with idiopathic pulmonary fibrosis but not with development of lung fibrosis in systemic sclerosis or sarcoidosis. *Thorax* 2013; 68: 436–441.
8. Zhang Y, Noth I, Garcia JGN, *et al.* A variant in the promoter of *MUC5B* and idiopathic pulmonary fibrosis. *N Engl J Med* 2011; 364: 1576–1577.
9. Roy MG, Livraghi-Butrico A, Fletcher AA, *et al.* *Muc5b* is required for airway defence. *Nature* 2015; 505: 412–416.
10. Molyneaux PL, Cox MJ, Willis-Owen SAG, *et al.* The role of bacteria in the pathogenesis and progression of idiopathic pulmonary fibrosis. *Am J Respir Crit Care Med* 2014; 190: 906–913.
11. Peljto AL, Zhang Y, Fingerlin TE, *et al.* Association between the *MUC5B* promoter polymorphism and survival in patients with idiopathic pulmonary fibrosis. *JAMA* 2013; 309: 2232–2239.
12. The Idiopathic Pulmonary Fibrosis Clinical Research Network. Randomized trial of acetylcysteine in idiopathic pulmonary fibrosis. *N Engl J Med* 2014; 370: 2093–2101.
13. Raghu G, Rochwerg B, Zhang Y, *et al.* An official ATS/ERS/JRS/ALAT clinical practice guideline: treatment of idiopathic pulmonary fibrosis. An update of the 2011 clinical practice guideline. *Am J Respir Crit Care Med* 2015; 192: e3–e19.
14. Oldham JM, Ma S-F, Martinez FJ, *et al.* TOLLIP, MUC5B and the response to *N*-acetylcysteine among individuals with idiopathic pulmonary fibrosis. *Am J Respir Crit Care Med* 2015; 192: 1475–1482.

15. Ley B, Brown KK, Collard HR. Molecular biomarkers in idiopathic pulmonary fibrosis. *Am J Physiol Lung Cell Mol Physiol* 2014; 307: L681–L691.
16. van den Blink B, Wijsenbeek MS, Hoogsteden HC. Serum biomarkers in idiopathic pulmonary fibrosis. *Pulm Pharmacol Ther* 2010; 23: 515–520.
17. Kass DJ, Flynn M, Baker E. Idiopathic pulmonary fibrosis biomarkers: clinical utility and a way of understanding disease pathogenesis. *Current Biomark Find* 2015; 5: 21–33.
18. Saini G, Weinreb PH, Violette SM, *et al.* $\alpha_V\beta_6$ integrin may be a potential prognostic biomarker in interstitial lung disease. *Eur Respir J* 2015; 46: 486–494.
19. Chien JW, Richards TJ, Gibson KF, *et al.* Serum lysyl oxidase-like 2 levels and idiopathic pulmonary fibrosis disease progression. *Eur Respir J* 2014; 43: 1430–1438.
20. Jenkins RG, Simpson JK, Saini G, *et al.* Longitudinal change in collagen degradation biomarkers in idiopathic pulmonary fibrosis: an analysis from the prospective, multicentre PROFILE study. *Lancet Respir Med* 2015; 3: 462–472.
21. Raghu G, Collard HR, Egan JJ, *et al.* An official ATS/ERS/JRS/ALAT statement: idiopathic pulmonary fibrosis: evidence-based guidelines for diagnosis and management. *Am J Respir Crit Care Med* 2011; 183: 788–824.
22. King TE Jr, Bradford WZ, Castro-Bernardini S, *et al.* A phase 3 trial of pirfenidone in patients with idiopathic pulmonary fibrosis. *N Engl J Med* 2014; 370: 2083–2092.
23. Richeldi L, Bois du RM, Raghu G, *et al.* Efficacy and safety of nintedanib in idiopathic pulmonary fibrosis. *N Engl J Med* 370: 2071–2082.
24. Moore BB, Hogaboam CM. Murine models of pulmonary fibrosis. *Am J Physiol Lung Cell Mol Physiol* 2007; 294: L152–L160.
25. Jones MG, Fletcher S, Richeldi L. Idiopathic pulmonary fibrosis: recent trials and current drug therapy. *Respiration* 2013; 86: 353–363.
26. Booth AJ, Hadley R, Cornett AM, *et al.* Acellular normal and fibrotic human lung matrices as a culture system for *in vitro* investigation. *Am J Respir Crit Care Med* 2012; 186: 866–876.
27. Collard HR. Where do we go from here? Clinical drug development in idiopathic pulmonary fibrosis. 2015; 45: 1218–1220.
28. O'Riordan T, Smith V, Raghu G. Development of novel agents for idiopathic pulmonary fibrosis: progress in target selection and clinical trial design. *Chest* 2015; 148: 1083–1092.
29. Collard HR, Bradford WZ, Cottin V, *et al.* A new era in idiopathic pulmonary fibrosis: considerations for future clinical trials. *Eur Respir J* 2015; 46: 243–249.
30. Durheim MT, Collard HR, Roberts RS, *et al.* Association of hospital admission and forced vital capacity endpoints with survival in patients with idiopathic pulmonary fibrosis: analysis of a pooled cohort from three clinical trials. *Lancet Respir Med* 2015; 3: 388–396.
31. Russell A-M, Sprangers MA, Wibberley S, *et al.* The need for patient-centred clinical research in idiopathic pulmonary fibrosis. *BMC Med* 2015; 13: 240.

Disclosures: L. Richeldi is a member of the advisory boards of InterMune, Medimmune, Roche and Takeda; has acted as a consultant to Biogen Idec, Sanofi-Aventis and ImmuneWorks; has received a speaker's fee from Shionogi; and is a member of the steering committee of Boehringer Ingelheim.

Chapter 21

Perspectives for the future

Toby M. Maher[1,2] and Paolo Spagnolo[3]

The recent establishment of two effective therapies for IPF is a remarkable achievement for patients and clinicians alike. However, the unmet medical need for patients with IPF remains substantial, and a number of issues need to be urgently addressed if we are to move IPF research forward. One such priority is the establishment of well-characterised cohorts of patients with standardised, comprehensive and longitudinally collected clinical and biological data. Equally important are the establishment of centralised open-access biorepositories of samples from patients (and appropriate controls), the validation of an IPF-specific patient-reported outcome tool, and the development and validation of biomarkers to facilitate the design and efficiency of future therapeutic trials. Several pharmacological agents with high potential are currently being tested in trials and many more are ready to be evaluated in the near future. However, only through a continued, concerted partnership between all stakeholders will the ultimate goal of curing patients with this terrible disease be achieved.

O ver the past decade, important new insights into the pathobiology of IPF, coupled with improved disease definition and standardised diagnostic criteria, have allowed a number of high-quality, large, global, randomised controlled clinical trials of pharmacological interventions to be undertaken and successfully completed in IPF. This massive effort on the part of patients, the IPF medical community and the pharmaceutical industry has led to the approval of two effective anti-fibrotic therapies; pirfenidone and nintedanib. However, there remain several areas of urgent unmet need for those with IPF, as well as further opportunities to advance the field to improve delivery of care to this patient group. In this chapter, we discuss what we see as the major priority areas and directions for future clinical research in IPF over the coming 5 to 10 years.

Establishing national/international cohorts of phenotypically and geographically well-defined patients with IPF

As a rare and orphan disease, IPF is difficult to study even within referral centres and regional collaborative networks [1]. Several prospective IPF registries exist, but they often

[1]National Institute for Health Research Biomedical Research Unit, Royal Brompton Hospital, London, UK. [2]National Heart and Lung Institute, Imperial College, London, UK. [3]Medical University Clinic, Canton Hospital Baselland and University of Basel, Liestal, Switzerland.

Correspondence: Toby M. Maher, National Heart and Lung Institute, Imperial College, Sir Alexander Fleming Building, Exhibition Road, London, SW7 2AZ, UK. E-mail: t.maher@imperial.ac.uk use different methodologies, which makes it difficult for them to be combined. A global IPF registry, however, would improve our understanding of disease behaviour, inform on clinical impact and cost-effectiveness of specific therapeutic approaches (particularly with regard to patient adherence, resource utilisation and safety) and help establish and implement best practices [2]. In addition, a global IPF registry would create a stable and strong foundation for more efficient and affordable clinical trials, facilitate the collection of biological samples for testing and validation of biomarkers, and provide a platform for collaboration among stakeholders (patients, clinicians, professional respiratory societies, industry, governments and advocacy groups). The clinical trial network model has been successful in other rare diseases (*e.g.* cystic fibrosis) and has recently been endorsed by the US National Cancer Institute through the development of an institute-wide clinical research network. RYERSON *et al.* [3] recently proposed a 5-year plan to create a global registry of patients with IPF. They identified five major steps for the development of such a registry: 1) create a network of highly motivated IPF centres at an international level; 2) secure funding; 3) define clear objectives and establish priorities; 4) determine core data elements based on registry objectives; and 5) identify problems and verify test procedures before expanding the registry to additional sites.

Developing centralised open-access biorepositories of tissue from patients with IPF and appropriate controls

The direct study of patient data and tissues is central to accelerating progress in understanding the pathobiology of human disease. Historically, a number of obstacles have hampered the set-up and implementation of biorepositories, including; heterogeneity in acquisition and storage of biologic specimens; difficulties in securing specific informed consent; privacy, confidentiality and data protection; controlling data access; guaranteed accessibility to biospecimens for outside research groups; benefit sharing; commercialisation; intellectual property rights; and genetic discrimination [4]. Moreover, in the case of a complex and heterogeneous condition such as IPF, research utilising patient data and tissue samples is often hindered by the lack of well-phenotyped and clinically annotated samples [5]. The most efficient and effective way to overcome these limitations is to prospectively collect biological samples, along with linked longitudinal clinical data, from carefully characterised patients using universally applied standardised operating procedures for sample collection, processing and storage. While such an effort will clearly require substantial investment in terms of financial resources, infrastructure and personnel, a biorepository is critical for addressing gaps in our understanding of the disease [6, 7]. In this regard, recent evidence suggesting that the genetic make-up of patients with IPF may determine their response to therapy [8] underscores the importance of pharmacogenetics in IPF and supports systematic biological sample collection so that genetic subgroups predisposed to treatment-related benefit or harm can be identified. Ideally, any biorepository should also include control subjects selected from the same source population as the case subjects [9]. While enrolling the correct control group will require considerable planning and investment, enrolling either the wrong control group or no control group could jeopardise the success of biomarker discovery programmes [10]. More discussion between all stakeholders needs to occur regarding standardisation of sample collection and agreement to make biorepositories open access, which in turn needs to be balanced against the differing regulatory frameworks between territories. However, we believe that the transformational potential of such a biorepository warrants the effort required to deliver such a project.

Use of bioinformatics and systems biology to better understand disease pathogenesis and improve diagnosis

Despite the existence of clear guidelines, the diagnosis of IPF (and other ILDs) is frequently challenging. The currently accepted gold standard for diagnosis is multidisciplinary team assessment of clinical, radiological and, where necessary, histopathological data. It is well recognised, however, that many facets of current ILD diagnosis have major flaws. Each aspect of the diagnostic process is plagued by problems of inter- and intra-observer variability in the reporting of specific findings. In addition to this, surgical lung biopsy is an invasive procedure that carries an appreciable risk of causing significant morbidity and even mortality. In this regard, recent data support the role of bronchoscopic lung cryobiopsy in the evaluation of patients with suspected IPF [11]. Indeed, TOMASSETTI et al. [11] showed that the integrated and dynamic addition of bronchoscopic lung cryobiopsy data to clinical and HRCT data increased the diagnostic confidence level in a large proportion of such cases. Most notably, bronchoscopic lung cryobiopsy was safe and well tolerated compared to surgical lung biopsy. However, the diagnostic accuracy of bronchoscopic lung cryobiopsy compared to surgical lung biopsy, which would require an intra-patient comparison of the two procedures, has not been formally assessed. Finally, it is recognised that in a significant minority of patients the final diagnosis only becomes clear over time. This most frequently occurs when ILD predates the development of an overt connective tissue disease [12, 13]. These inherent challenges in diagnosis often delay treatment, create uncertainty about optimal therapy in individual cases and frequently result in exclusion from clinical trials.

Current disease phenotyping relies on a small number of clinical features. What remains unknown is the relative weight, or prior probability, that should be assigned to any individual clinical feature when diagnosing IPF or other fibrotic ILDs and, importantly, how much emphasis should be applied to any given factor when determining prognosis or choice of therapy. The application of "big data" statistical approaches to large data sets is revolutionising disease understanding [14]. The use of clinical bioinformatics techniques has brought about novel disease insights in a range of cancers (as exemplified by the Cancer Genome Atlas) and psychiatric disorders [15–17]. Small scale studies suggest there are measurable differences in whole lung transcriptome profile [18–20], frequency of specific genetic polymorphisms [21] and blood cytokine levels [22] between individuals with fibrotic ILD of differing aetiologies. There has, however, been no attempt to rigorously apply a systems biology approach to better understand disease behaviour in fibrotic ILD [23]. Development of disease registries and biorepositories, coupled with the application of both omics-based technology and emerging big data bioinformatics and systems biology tools, promises to transform diagnosis, classification and disease understanding in IPF. The potential for this emerging field to influence future therapeutic developments in IPF should provide added impetus to the drive to develop open-access registries and biorepositories.

Developing a new paradigm for acute exacerbation of IPF

Approximately 10% of IPF patients experience idiopathic episodes of acute respiratory worsening termed acute exacerbation of IPF that result in substantial morbidity and mortality [24, 25]. The diagnostic criteria for acute exacerbation of IPF proposed by the IPF Clinical Research Network (i.e. worsening of dyspnoea within the previous 30 days, new bilateral opacities on HRCT of the chest, no evidence of infection by endotracheal or

BAL analysis and exclusion of other alternative causes) have considerably improved our understanding of a previously under-recognised and under-appreciated aspect of the natural history of IPF [26]. However, aetiology, pathogenesis, management and prognosis of these life-threatening events remain poorly defined. Notably, emerging data show that many acute exacerbations of IPF are in fact not idiopathic (*i.e.* they appear to have identifiable triggers including infection and micro-aspiration); yet, acute exacerbation of IPF and acute respiratory worsening of known causes share similar clinical characteristics and outcome [27, 28], suggesting that acute exacerbation of IPF, as currently defined, may be an artificial construct [29]. Management is largely supportive, and most patients receive high-dose corticosteroids and empiric antibiotics, although there is no robust data to support their use [30]. Future research is desperately needed to further advance our knowledge of acute exacerbation of IPF.

The future of IPF treatment

The development pathway for novel treatments for IPF has been complex and difficult for several reasons, including: incomplete understanding of disease pathogenesis; unpredictable clinical course; lack of validated biomarkers; low clinical predictive value of animal models of pulmonary fibrosis; and the need to perform large clinical trials of long duration to obtain evidence of efficacy [31]. Nonetheless, recent advances in translational medicine combined with the information on end-point and patient selection, generated by clinical trials completed over the preceding decade, have led to an unprecedented increase in the number of drug development programmes specifically targeting IPF [32]. Despite the recent approval of two novel anti-fibrotic agents, both of which slow functional decline and disease progression in patients with IPF (*e.g.* pirfenidone and nintedanib) [33, 34], additional therapies capable of modifying the natural history and dismal prognosis of IPF are urgently needed. A selection of the compounds in most advanced development for IPF are listed below and summarised in table 1.

PRM-151

PRM-151 (Promedior, Inc., Lexington, MA, USA) is a recombinant form of human pentraxin-2, a protein that is specifically active at sites of tissue injury. PRM-151 binds to Fc-γ receptors on monocytes and induces their differentiation into regulatory macrophages, thus promoting epithelial healing and resolution of scarring. In a multiple ascending dose, phase 1 study in patients with IPF, PRM-151 was safe and well tolerated, and demonstrated a trend towards improvement in pulmonary function and circulating levels of surfactant protein D and VEGF at 8 weeks [35]. PRM-151 is currently being tested in IPF in a phase 2 randomised, placebo-controlled trial (NCT02550873, clinicaltrials.gov).

IW001

Ongoing adaptive immune response against autoantigens is thought to play an important role in disease progression in some patients with IPF [36]. Type V collagen is a minor collagen normally confined within the lung interstitium and, therefore, hidden from the immune system. Lung injury may lead to Type V collagen exposure, making it available for activation of an autoimmune response [37], which may result in abnormal lung remodelling and fibrotic changes [38, 39]. In a phase 1 study (NCT01199887, clinicaltrials.gov), IW001 (ImmuneWorks, Inc., Indianapolis, IN, USA), an orally available compound that induces

Table 1. Therapeutic compounds currently in development for IPF

Target	Putative role in IPF	Mechanism of action	Developmental phase and status	Clinical trial identifier	Drug code
Galectin-3	Mediator of TGF-β-induced lung fibrosis	Galectin-3 inhibitor	Phase I/II; recruiting	NCT02257177	TD139
Type V collagen	Autoimmune response to collagen V leading to fibrosis	Inductor of immune tolerance to collagen V	Phase I; completed	NCT01199887	IW001
Pentraxin-2	Antifibrotic and anti-inflammatory	Recombinant human pentraxin-2	Phase Ib; completed	NCT02550873	PRM151
LPA receptor	Epithelial cell apoptosis, endothelial cell leak and fibroblast accumulation	LPA receptor inhibitor	Phase II; recruiting	NCT01766817	BMS-986020
Integrin $\alpha_v\beta_6$	TGF-β activation	$\alpha_v\beta_6$ inhibitor	Phase II; recruiting	NCT01371305	STX-100
CTGF	Major profibrotic cytokine	CTGF inhibitor	Phase II; recruiting	NCT01890265	FG-3019
IL-13	Myofibroblast differentiation and collagen deposition	IL-13 inhibitor	Phase II; recruiting	NCT01872689	Lebrikizumab
IL-4 and IL-13	Myofibroblast differentiation and collagen deposition	IL-4 and IL-13 inhibitor	Phase II; completed	NCT02345070	SAR156597
LOXL2	Cross-linking of type-1 collagen molecules	LOXL2 inhibitor	Phase II; recruiting	NCT01769196	Simtuzumab
IL-13	Myofibroblast differentiation and collagen deposition	IL-13 inhibitor	Phase II; recruiting	NCT01629667 and NCT02036580	Tralokinumab

LPA: lysophosphatidic acid; CTGF: connective tissue growth factor; IL: interleukin; LOXL2: lysyl oxidase-like 2.

immune tolerance to Type V collagen, was safe and well tolerated, and showed a trend towards stabilisation of FVC and metalloproteinase-7 levels in anti-Type V collagen antibody-positive patients with IPF [40].

TD139

Galectin-3, a galactoside binding lectin, has been shown to play a central role in fibrosis development and progression through the activation of macrophages and recruitment and activation of myofibroblasts [41]. TD139 (Galecto Biotech AB, Copenhagen, Denmark) is a specific inhibitor of the galactoside binding pocket of galectin-3 formulated for inhalation. Safety and tolerability of TD139 in patients with IPF are currently being evaluated in a phase 1b/2a trial (NCT02257177, clinicaltrials.gov).

BMS-986020

Lysophosphatidic acid (LPA) is a proinflammatory and profibrotic mediator released by platelets following epithelial damage [42], and LPA receptor 1 (LPA1) contributes to the development of IPF by inducing epithelial cell apoptosis, fibroblast recruitment and vascular leak [43, 44]. The safety and efficacy of BMS-986020 (Bristol-Myers Squibb, New York, NY, USA), a selective antagonist of LPA1, is currently being assessed in patients with IPF in a phase 2 trial (NCT01766817, clinicaltrials.gov).

FG-3019

It is a monoclonal antibody directed against connective tissue growth factor, a key mediator of tissue fibrosis. Safety and tolerability of FG-3019 (FibroGen, Inc., San Francisco, CA, USA) in patients with IPF have been evaluated in a phase 2 dose escalation, open-label study. Data from the first dose cohort (15 mg·kg^{-1} *i.v.* every 3 weeks) have been published in the form of an abstract [45]. 53 subjects were enrolled and treated. Overall, FG-3019 was safe and well tolerated. The majority of patients (27 (71%) out of the 38 who had acceptable data at week 48) experienced improvement or a <5% decline in FVC % predicted at week 48. In addition, improved or stable lung fibrosis as measured by quantitative HRCT was observed in more than half of subjects. On average, patients with improved or stable fibrosis also had improved pulmonary function. A randomised, placebo-controlled phase 2 trial in patients with IPF is currently enrolling participants (NCT01890265, clinicaltrials.gov).

Lebrikizumab

Lebrikizumab (Hoffmann-La Roche, Basel, Switzerland) is a humanised monoclonal antibody against IL-13. Lebrikizumab inhibits IL-13 signalling through the type 2 IL-4 receptor (IL-4R), which is composed of IL-13 receptor (IL-13R)α1 and IL-4Rα. IL-13 shares functional redundancy with IL-4 because of shared receptor use at the type 2 IL-4R. *In vitro*, IL-13 stimulates fibroblast proliferation and induces CCL6/C10, a chemotactic factor for mononuclear phagocytes, which in turn are an important source of mediators of extracellular matrix synthesis [46]. *In vivo*, IL-13 overexpression results in increased fibrosis in mice in response to bleomycin. In addition, elevated blood levels of T-helper cell-2 inflammation, including IL-13, are associated with accelerated functional decline and mortality in patients with IPF [22, 47]. Lebrikizumab (as both monotherapy and combination therapy with pirfenidone background therapy) is currently being tested in patients with IPF in a phase 2b study (NCT01872689, clinicaltrials.gov).

Tralokinumab

Tralokinumab (MedImmune LLC, Gaithersburg, MD, USA) is a human IL-13-neutralising antibody. Tralokinumab prevents IL-13 interaction at both IL-13Rα1 and IL-13Rα2, but is unable to block IL-4 signalling. The role of IL-13Rα2 remains unclear, but it might act as a decoy to regulate IL-13 activity. The IL-13 pathway is significantly enhanced in biopsy samples from IPF patients who exhibit a rapidly progressive disease course compared with patients with a slower rate of lung function decline [48]. Inhibition of human IL-13 by tralokinumab has been shown to attenuate established lung fibrosis and promote alveolar epithelial repair in a humanised severe combined immunodeficiency mouse model of IPF [48]. Safety, tolerability and effectiveness of multiple doses of tralokinumab are being evaluated in phase 2 studies (NCT01629667 and NCT02036580, clinicaltrials.gov, the latter only in Japanese patients), which are ongoing but currently not recruiting patients.

SAR156597

IL-4, a cytokine structurally related to IL-13, has been implicated in the abnormal fibroblast proliferation in IPF [49], and targeting of IL-13 and IL-4 receptors modulates the proliferative properties of human lung fibroblasts [50]. SAR156597 (Sanofi S.A., Paris, France) is a humanised bispecific antibody that neutralises circulating IL-4 and IL-13. In a phase 1 study in patients with IPF, SAR156597 has been shown to be generally safe and well tolerated [51]. The safety and efficacy of two dose levels of SAR156597 administered subcutaneously for 52 weeks in patients with IPF are currently being tested in a randomised, double-blind, placebo-controlled phase 2 study (NCT02345070, clinicaltrials.gov).

Simtuzumab

The secretory activity and differentiation of fibroblasts are influenced by the matrix on which they reside. Indeed, a fibrotic matrix has been suggested to represent a self-perpetuating stimulus to collagen production and progression of fibrosis [52]. Simtuzumab (Gilead Sciences, Foster city, CA, USA) is a humanised monoclonal antibody that allosterically inhibits lysyl oxidase-like 2 (LOXL2), a matrix-associated enzyme that crosslinks collagen. LOXL2 protein expression is observed in the fibroblastic foci and collagenous regions of diseased IPF lung tissue [53] and serum LOXL2 levels are associated with increased risk for IPF disease progression [54]. Moreover, in the bleomycin-induced mouse model of pulmonary fibrosis, inhibition of LOXL2 resulted in markedly decreased TGF-β pathway signalling, probably by decreasing matrix tension, a stimulus for TGF-β activation [53]. The safety and efficacy of simtuzumab in patients with IPF are being evaluated in a phase 2 study (NCT01769196, clinicaltrials.gov), which is ongoing but currently not recruiting patients.

STX-100

STX-100 (Biogen Idec, Weston, MA, USA) is a monoclonal antibody against the integrin $\alpha_v\beta_6$, which plays an important role in promoting and maintaining fibrogenesis and epithelial injury by mediating TGF-β activation [55]. In murine bleomycin-induced pulmonary fibrosis, partial inhibition of $\alpha_v\beta_6$ effectively inhibits TGF-β activation, epithelial injury and tissue fibrosis [56], whereas complete inhibition of TGF-β through gene deletion causes excessive inflammation in many organs, including the lungs [57]. The safety and tolerability of subcutaneously administered multiple escalating doses of STX-100 in patients with IPF are being evaluated in a phase 2 study, which is currently recruiting participants.

Mesenchymal stem cells

Mesenchymal stem cells (MSCs) are multipotent stromal cells capable of transdifferentiation, clonality and self-renewal. MSC properties also include immunomodulation, epithelial repair and secretion of growth factors [58]. MSCs have been shown to ameliorate inflammation and mitigate parenchymal remodelling in bleomycin-induced pulmonary fibrosis [59], but the bleomycin model only partially recapitulates the complex pathobiology of IPF [60]. Therefore, the application of MSCs in patients with IPF is controversial and under studied [61]. In a small cohort of patients with IPF (n=14), Tzouvelekis et al. [62] have shown that endobronchial infusion of autologous adipose derived stem cells is not associated with serious adverse events. However, despite their acceptable safety profile, there is only limited, weak preclinical data to support the use of MSCs in IPF. In addition, because of their mesenchymal origin, MSCs may potentially differentiate into a fibroblast phenotype, thus promoting fibrosis [63]. Other unanswered questions include the timing (early or advanced disease) and optimal route of administration (intravenous or endobronchial), source of MSCs (e.g. adipose tissue, bone marrow or umbilical cord), frequency of infusions and appropriate primary end-points to show benefit. As of November 2015, there are three ongoing clinical trials evaluating the safety of either autologous (NCT01919827 and NCT02135380, clinicaltrials.gov) or allogenic (NCT02013700, clinicaltrials.gov) MSCs in patients with IPF.

The future of clinical trials in IPF: biomarker and cohort enrichment strategies

In IPF drug development there is an unmet need for clinical trial design to establish robust proof of efficacy for novel agents in small phase 2 studies of brief duration [31]. Indeed, the TOMORROW (To Improve Pulmonary Fibrosis with BIBF-1120) trial, which can be viewed as a benchmark phase 2 study in IPF, enrolled >400 patients who were treated with one of four escalating doses of nintedanib (50 mg once a day and 50 mg, 100 mg or 150 mg all twice a day) or placebo for 52 weeks [64]. The most realistic approach for reducing the size of phase 2 studies would be the development of biomarkers, which can be proteins found in blood, body fluid or tissue, physiological measures such as FVC, or imaging measures (e.g. quantitative radiology) [23, 65]. Biomarkers have the potential to improve the efficiency of clinical trials in IPF because they may: 1) identify patients at higher risk of disease progression, thereby increasing the chance of recording any positive drug effects with smaller sample size (cohort enrichment approach); 2) act as substitutes for an accepted clinical end-point (e.g. surrogates); or 3) identify subsets of patients more likely to respond to a specific therapy while sparing others significant side-effects and adverse events [66]. In this regard, it has been shown that ~25% of patients with IPF (those carrying the TOLLIP rs3750920 TT genotype), may benefit from NAC therapy, whereas those with the rs3750920 CC genotype may be more susceptible to treatment-related harm [8]. Such "predictive" cohort enrichment is particularly suitable for conditions like IPF that may encompass multiple distinct pathobiological subgroups [14, 67]. Indeed, a recent study by

WILKES *et al.* [40] suggests that therapy directed at modulating the immune response to collagen V might preferentially benefit a subgroup of IPF patients with elevated autoantibody levels to collagen V [40]. Cohort enrichment has been used successfully in a number of diseases including cancer (where it has been incorporated into the concept of precision medicine), and is strongly encouraged in clinical trials of IPF [68].

The availability of two effective drugs will have substantial implications for future research on the natural history of IPF, at least in patients with mild-to-moderate functional impairment. Indeed, conducting placebo-controlled studies in this patient population will prove impractical and/or unethical; however, those patients who may choose not to take, may not have access to or may stop taking nintedanib or pirfenidone due to intolerance or disease progression, may be challenging to identify and unrepresentative of the general IPF population [2]. Therefore, natural history studies might be limited to patients with severe physiological impairment who are at increased risk for acute exacerbation, hospitalisation and mortality [69].

Although the regulatory approval of pirfenidone and nintedanib is for use in all IPF patients regardless of functional impairment, clinical trials in IPF have mainly enrolled highly selected patients with relatively preserved lung function and a lack of significant comorbidities. Many patients are also excluded due to their age or prominent emphysema, whereas rapid progressors often fail inclusion criteria by the time of gaining access to trials. Instead, recruitment of patients with severe physiological impairment (*i.e.* FVC <50% and/or baseline DLCO <35%) may provide an opportunity for prognostic cohort enrichment in a trial powered for hospitalisation and mortality, as this sub-group has been shown to experience these outcomes at an increased rate [69, 70].

Development and selection of more robust and clinically meaningful end-points for clinical trials

The recent approval of pirfenidone and nintedanib for the treatment of IPF has substantial implications for the design and conduct of future late phase clinical trials. It is now ethically unacceptable to conduct longer term (*i.e.* >3 or 6 months) trials in which treatment-naïve patients in one limb receive only placebo and are thus denied effective anti-fibrotic therapy. Instead, trialists will have to perform either active comparator studies (*e.g.* the compound under study is compared head-to-head against an approved agent) or, alternatively, the new agent (or matching placebo) can be added to standard-of-care (which in the majority of cases will comprise anti-fibrotic therapy). However, using current end-points, such studies are likely to require large sample sizes and/or long duration in order to maintain adequate statistical power and to compensate for the probable reduction in disease progression and thus magnitude of treatment effect seen when compared to historical true placebo-controlled trials [31].

The ideal primary end-point in any clinical trials should be reliable, reproducible, clinically meaningful, predictive of outcome, responsive to treatment effect, equally applicable to all patients and easy to measure; yet, none of the outcomes utilised in clinical trials of IPF meets all these criteria. Pirfenidone and nintedanib have both been approved based on their favourable effect on change in FVC, but controversy remains on how best to handle missing data, especially in patients who die [71]. Possible approaches include: 1) calculating the slope of decline in lung function over the study period using statistical modelling;

2) performing categorical analyses of FVC decline (usually using a 10% threshold as this magnitude of decline in FVC is considered a clinically significant event) [72]; or 3) using a composite progression-free survival end-point. Proposed components of such a composite include: a pre-specified categorical change in FVC (usually a 10% decline), death, hospitalisation and categorical change in 6MWD. Ideal components of such an end-point should be clinically relevant and should ideally capture distinct pathophysiological domains of disease progression. The major downside of such time-to-event end-points is that the frequency with which end-point events are captured is determined by the frequency with which the component (*e.g.* FVC) is measured [73–75]. Although composite end-points have several advantages (*e.g.* reduction of the required sample size and study duration through increase in the overall event rate), results based on such end-points may be misleading when "driven" by the most frequent, but perhaps least important, of its constituents [76, 77]. Furthermore, there is no consensus on what constitutes a clinically significant prolongation of time to disease progression [78]. Survival is probably the only indisputable end-point in a deadly disease like IPF, but a properly powered mortality study in patients with mild-to-moderate functional impairment is impracticable due to the number of patients and length of trial needed [79]. Mortality studies might be best suited for patients with more severe physiological impairment as this would reduce the sample size requirements while offering the advantage of higher event rates, larger treatment response and shorter trial duration [69, 79]. However, the disease is not well characterised in this patient population and there are insufficient reliable data to estimate the appropriate sample size and study duration [79]. A fourth approach to IPF clinical trial end-points is to develop biomarkers that act as surrogate measures of therapeutic response. Ideally, any such biomarker should provide an earlier and more sensitive read out than existing clinical measures. The recent observation that neo-epitopes reflective of collagen degradation map with disease progression in IPF gives hope that these markers may have value as measures of treatment response [65]. However, this remains to be tested in prospective intervention studies. IPF is a biologically heterogeneous disease that involves multiple complex and interactive mechanisms, the relative importance of which may vary among individual patients. Therefore, a panel of biomarkers (rather than a single one) reflecting activity across a range of biologically distinct pathways may be more likely to be informative in guiding treatment decisions and advancing patient care.

Developing an IPF-specific patient-reported outcome tool

A patient-centred approach requires strategies that place the patient at the heart of research (*i.e.* giving regard to the individual before the condition) to ensure that research questions address what is important to patients, whilst respecting each individual's health beliefs, values and judgments [80]. This can be achieved through patient involvement at all levels from research design and study conduct to data dissemination. The Patient-Centred Outcomes Research Institute (Washington, DC, USA) strives to generate reliable data that patients, caregivers and practitioners can use to make informed decisions and to assess the value of healthcare options [81]. Notably, studies funded by the Patient-Centred Outcomes Research Institute are evaluated according to three components such as financial accountability, level of adherence to the principles of patient-centeredness (defined as relevant, pragmatic, feasible and participatory), and whether they make a difference to healthcare quality outcomes. In this new era of IPF research a more patient-centred approach is urgently needed.

A patient-reported outcome is defined as any report of the status of a patient's health condition that comes directly from the patient, without interpretation of the patient's response by a clinician or anyone else. In clinical trials of IPF, self-reported measures of how patients feel and function in their daily lives have been included, at best as lower-tier end-points mainly due to the lack of IPF-specific tools, scarcity of longitudinal data to support validity, and uncertainty regarding the significance of score values or minimally important differences [82]. However, it is only through self-reporting that aspects most meaningful to patients, such as symptom frequency and severity, physical functional status, level of independence, social functioning and psychological state can be reliably captured.

Currently, there is only one IPF-specific patient-reported outcome (ATAQ-I (A Tool to Assess QoL in IPF)) [83], which still needs to be validated prospectively. The St George's Respiratory Questionnaire (SGRQ) and, in particular an IPF-specific modified version (SGRQ-IPF), is an acceptable patient-reported outcome for health-related QoL [84]. However, the SGRQ was originally developed for use in patients with COPD and asthma, and studies assessing this tool in IPF are limited. The change in the SGRQ total score from baseline over the 52-week treatment period was one of the key secondary end-points in the INPULSIS-1 and INPULSIS-2 trials [34]. In INPULSIS-2, nintedanib treatment was associated with a significantly smaller increase in the SGRQ total score (consistent with less deterioration in health-related QoL) compared with placebo (2.80 points in the nintedanib group *versus* 5.48 points in the placebo group; p=0.02), whereas in INPULSIS-1 there was no significant between-group difference in terms of health-related QoL (4.34 points in the nintedanib group *versus* 4.39 points in the placebo group; p=0.97).

The University of California San Diego Shortness of Breath Questionnaire (UCSD SOBQ) [85] was used as a secondary outcome measure in the CAPACITY-1, CAPACITY-2 and ASCEND trials. Originally developed for chronic lung disease [85], the UCSD SOBQ needs to be prospectively validated in IPF [86]. No significant treatment group differences in dyspnoea were noted in either of the CAPACITY studies [87]. Similarly, analysis of UCSD SOBQ scores showed no significant between-group difference in dyspnoea at week 52 in the ASCEND trial. Indeed, the end-point of an increase of $\geqslant 20$ points (indicating worsening) on the dyspnoea score or death occurred in 81 (29.1%) patients in the pirfenidone group and in 100 (36.1%) patients in the placebo group (relative reduction 19.3%; p=0.16) [33].

The prognostic value of the Medical Research Council dyspnoea scale (a five-item questionnaire) as an outcome measure in IPF is supported by several studies [88–90]. In addition, the Medical Research Council score is an independent predictor of anxiety and depression in patients with ILD [91], but has not been validated prospectively in patients with IPF.

Conclusion

IPF is no longer an untreatable disease but, despite the advent of effective anti-fibrotic treatments, there remains an urgent need for novel therapeutics with greater efficacy and better tolerability. Without these, individuals with IPF will continue to progress towards respiratory failure and death, albeit at a slower rate than in the past. Progress in our understanding of disease pathobiology coupled with the experience gained from clinical trials performed in the past decade will probably facilitate more rational selection of therapeutic targets and more efficient trial design. Novel biomarkers will hopefully facilitate clinical decision making and will provide a measurement of treatment response for the individual patient whilst also enabling a personalised approach to therapy in this multipathway disease. We believe that continued concerted effort by patients, clinicians, academics, professional respiratory societies, industry, governments and advocacy groups is the way forward in IPF research.

References

1. Spagnolo P, du Bois RM, Cottin V. Rare lung disease and orphan drug development. *Lancet Respir Med* 2013; 1: 479–487.
2. Collard HR, Bradford WZ, Cottin V, *et al*. A new era in idiopathic pulmonary fibrosis: considerations for future clinical trials. *Eur Respir J* 2015; 46: 243–249.
3. Ryerson CJ, Corte TJ, Collard HR, *et al*. A global registry for idiopathic pulmonary fibrosis: the time is now. *Eur Respir J* 2014; 44: 273–276.
4. McGuire AL, Caulfield T, Cho MK. Research ethics and the challenge of whole-genome sequencing. *Nat Rev Genet* 2008; 9: 152–156.
5. White ES, Brown KK, Collard HR, *et al*. Open-access biorepository for idiopathic pulmonary fibrosis. The way forward. *Ann Am Thorac Soc* 2014; 11: 1171–1175.
6. Jenkins G, Blanchard A, Borok Z, *et al*. In search of the fibrotic epithelial cell: opportunities for a collaborative network. *Thorax* 2012; 67: 179–182.
7. Blackwell TS, Tager AM, Borok Z, *et al*. Future directions in idiopathic pulmonary fibrosis research. An NHLBI workshop report. *Am J Respir Crit Care Med* 2014; 189: 214–222.
8. Oldham JM, Ma SF, Martinez FJ, *et al*. TOLLIP, MUC5B and the response to N-acetylcysteine among individuals with idiopathic pulmonary fibrosis. *Am J Respir Crit Care Med* 2015; 192: 1475–1482.
9. Wacholder S, McLaughlin JK, Silverman DT, *et al*. Selection of controls in case-control studies. I. Principles. *Am J Epidemiol* 1992; 135: 1019–1028.
10. Lederer DJ. Embracing complex diseases. The case for an idiopathic pulmonary fibrosis biorepository. *Ann Am Thorac Soc* 2014; 11: 1248–1249.
11. Tomassetti S, Wells AU, Costabel U, *et al*. Bronchoscopic lung cryobiopsy increases diagnostic confidence in the multidisciplinary diagnosis of idiopathic pulmonary fibrosis. *Am J Respir Crit Care Med* 2015; [In press; DOI: 10.1164/rccm.201504-0711OC].
12. Strange C, Highland KB. Interstitial lung disease in the patient who has connective tissue disease. *Clin Chest Med* 2004; 25: 549–559.
13. Mittoo S, Gelber AC, Christopher-Stine L, *et al*. Ascertainment of collagen vascular disease in patients presenting with interstitial lung disease. *Respir Med* 2009; 103: 1152–1158.
14. Maher TM. Beyond the diagnosis of idiopathic pulmonary fibrosis: the growing role of systems biology and stratified medicine. *Curr Opin Pulm Med* 2013; 19: 460–465.
15. Schwarz E, Leweke FM, Bahn S, *et al*. Clinical bioinformatics for complex disorders: a schizophrenia case study. *BMC Bioinformatics* 2009; 10: Suppl 12, S6.
16. Sedgewick AJ, Benz SC, Rabizadeh S, *et al*. Learning subgroup-specific regulatory interactions and regulator independence with PARADIGM. *Bioinformatics* 2013; 29: i62–i70.
17. Cancer Genome Atlas Research Network. Comprehensive molecular characterization of clear cell renal cell carcinoma. *Nature* 2013; 499: 43–49.
18. Selman M, Pardo A, Barrera L, *et al*. Gene expression profiles distinguish idiopathic pulmonary fibrosis from hypersensitivity pneumonitis. *Am J Respir Crit Care Med* 2006; 173: 188–198.
19. Selman M, Carrillo G, Estrada A, *et al*. Accelerated variant of idiopathic pulmonary fibrosis: clinical behavior and gene expression pattern. *PLoS One* 2007; 2: e482.
20. Kim SY, Diggans J, Pankratz D, *et al*. Classification of usual interstitial pneumonia in patients with interstitial lung disease: assessment of a machine learning approach using high-dimensional transcriptional data. *Lancet Respir Med* 2015; 3: 473–482.
21. Fingerlin TE, Murphy E, Zhang W, *et al*. Genome-wide association study identifies multiple susceptibility loci for pulmonary fibrosis. *Nat Genet* 2013; 45: 613–620.
22. Herazo JD, Gibson KF, Juan-Guardela B, *et al*. Peripheral blood monuclear cells gene expression patterns predict mortality in patients with idiopathic pulmonary fibrosis. *Am J Respir Crit Care Med* 2011; 183: A5306.
23. Maher TM. PROFILEing idiopathic pulmonary fibrosis: rethinking biomarker discovery. *Eur Respir Rev* 2013; 22: 148–152.

24. Agarwal R, Jindal SK. Acute exacerbation of idiopathic pulmonary fibrosis: a systematic review. *Eur J Intern Med* 2008; 19: 227–235.

25. Maher TM, Whyte MK, Hoyles RK, *et al.* Development of a consensus statement for the definition, diagnosis, and treatment of acute exacerbations of idiopathic pulmonary fibrosis using the Delphi Technique. *Adv Ther* 2015; [In press; DOI: 10.1007/s12325-015-0249-6].

26. Collard HR, Moore BB, Flaherty KR, *et al.* Acute exacerbations of idiopathic pulmonary fibrosis. *Am J Respir Crit Care Med* 2007; 176: 636–643.

27. Song JW, Hong SB, Lim CM, *et al.* Acute exacerbation of idiopathic pulmonary fibrosis: incidence, risk factors and outcome. *Eur Respir J* 2011; 37: 356–363.

28. Collard HR, Yow E, Richeldi L, *et al.* Suspected acute exacerbation of idiopathic pulmonary fibrosis as an outcome measure in clinical trials. *Respir Res* 2013; 14: 73.

29. Ryerson CJ, Cottin V, Brown KK, *et al.* Acute exacerbation of idiopathic pulmonary fibrosis: shifting the paradigm. *Eur Respir J* 2015; 46: 512–520.

30. Raghu G, Rochwerg B, Zhang Y, *et al.* An Official ATS/ERS/JRS/ALAT Clinical Practice Guideline: Treatment of Idiopathic Pulmonary Fibrosis. An Update of the 2011 Clinical Practice Guideline. *Am J Respir Crit Care Med* 2015; 192: e3–19.

31. O'Riordan TG, Smith V, Raghu G. Development of novel agents for idiopathic pulmonary fibrosis: progress in target selection and clinical trial design. *Chest* 2015; 148: 1083–1092.

32. Spagnolo P, Maher TM, Richeldi L. Idiopathic pulmonary fibrosis: recent advances on pharmacological therapy. *Pharmacol Ther* 2015; 152: 18–27.

33. King TE Jr, Bradford WZ, Castro-Bernardini S, *et al.* A phase 3 trial of pirfenidone in patients with idiopathic pulmonary fibrosis. *N Engl J Med* 2014; 370: 2083–2092.

34. Richeldi L, du Bois RM, Raghu G, *et al.* Efficacy and safety of nintedanib in idiopathic pulmonary fibrosis. *N Engl J Med* 2014; 370: 2071–2082.

35. Van Den Blink B, Burggraaf J, Morrison LD, *et al.* A phase I study of PRM-151 in patients with idiopathic pulmonary fibrosis. *Am J Respir Crit Care Med* 2013; 187: A5707.

36. Kahloon RA, Xue J, Bhargava A, *et al.* Patients with idiopathic pulmonary fibrosis with antibodies to heat shock protein 70 have poor prognoses. *Am J Respir Crit Care Med* 2013; 187: 768–775.

37. Sumpter TL, Wilkes DS. Role of autoimmunity in organ allograft rejection: a focus on immunity to type V collagen in the pathogenesis of lung transplant rejection. *Am J Physioly Lung Cell Mol Physiol* 2004; 286: L1129–L1139.

38. Vittal R, Mickler EA, Fisher AJ, *et al.* Type V collagen induced tolerance suppresses collagen deposition, TGF-beta and associated transcripts in pulmonary fibrosis. *PloS One* 2013; 8: e76451.

39. Parra ER, Teodoro WR, Velosa AP, *et al.* Interstitial and vascular type V collagen morphologic disorganization in usual interstitial pneumonia. *J Histochem Cytochem* 2006; 54: 1315–1325.

40. Wilkes DS, Chew T, Flaherty KR, *et al.* Oral immunotherapy with type V collagen in idiopathic pulmonary fibrosis. *Eur Respir J* 2015; 45: 1393–1402.

41. Nishi Y, Sano H, Kawashima T, *et al.* Role of galectin-3 in human pulmonary fibrosis. *Allergol Int* 2007; 56: 57–65.

42. Watterson KR, Lanning DA, Diegelmann RF, *et al.* Regulation of fibroblast functions by lysophospholipid mediators: potential roles in wound healing. *Wound Repair Regen* 2007; 15: 607–616.

43. Tager AM, LaCamera P, Shea BS, *et al.* The lysophosphatidic acid receptor LPA1 links pulmonary fibrosis to lung injury by mediating fibroblast recruitment and vascular leak. *Nat Med* 2008; 14: 45–54.

44. Xu MY, Porte J, Knox AJ, *et al.* Lysophosphatidic acid induces αvβ6 integrin-mediated TGF-β activation *via* the LPA2 receptor and the small G protein G α_q. *Am J Pathol* 2009; 174: 1264–1279.

45. Raghu G, Scholand MB, De Andrade J, *et al.* Safety and efficacy of anti-CTGF monoclonal antibody FG-3019 for treatment of idiopathic pulmonary fibrosis (IPF): results of Phase 2 clinical trial two years after initiation. *Am J Respir Crit Care Med* 2014; 189: A1429.

46. Belperio JA, Dy M, Burdick MD, *et al.* Interaction of IL-13 and C10 in the pathogenesis of bleomycin-induced pulmonary fibrosis. *Am J Respir Cell Mol Biol* 2002; 27: 419–427.

47. Herazo-Maya JD, Noth I, Duncan SR, *et al.* Peripheral blood mononuclear cell gene expression profiles predict poor outcome in idiopathic pulmonary fibrosis. *Sci Transl Med* 2013; 5: 205ra136.

48. Murray LA, Zhang H, Oak SR, *et al.* Targeting interleukin-13 with tralokinumab attenuates lung fibrosis and epithelial damage in a humanized SCID idiopathic pulmonary fibrosis model. *Am J Respir Cell Mol Biol* 2014; 50: 985–994.

49. Jakubzick C, Choi ES, Joshi BH, *et al.* Therapeutic attenuation of pulmonary fibrosis *via* targeting of IL-4- and IL-13-responsive cells. *J Immunol* 2003; 171: 2684–2693.

50. Jakubzick C, Choi ES, Carpenter KJ, *et al.* Human pulmonary fibroblasts exhibit altered interleukin-4 and interleukin-13 receptor subunit expression in idiopathic interstitial pneumonia. *Am J Pathol* 2004; 164: 1989–2001.

51. Kingwell K. InterMune and Boehringer blaze trails for idiopathic pulmonary fibrosis drugs. *Nat Rev Drug Discov* 2014; 13: 483–484.

52. Klingberg F, Chow ML, Koehler A, *et al.* Prestress in the extracellular matrix sensitizes latent TGF-β1 for activation. *J Cell Biol* 2014; 207: 283–297.

53. Barry-Hamilton V, Spangler R, Marshall D, *et al.* Allosteric inhibition of lysyl oxidase-like-2 impedes the development of a pathologic microenvironment. *Nat Med* 2010; 16: 1009–1017.

54. Chien JW, Richards TJ, Gibson KF, *et al.* Serum lysyl oxidase like-2 levels and idiopathic pulmonary fibrosis disease progression. *Eur Respir J* 2014; 43: 1430–1438.

55. Akhurst RJ, Hata A. Targeting the TGFβ signalling pathway in disease. *Nat Rev Drug Discov* 2012; 11: 790–811.

56. Horan GS, Wood S, Ona V, *et al.* Partial inhibition of integrin αvβ6 prevents pulmonary fibrosis without exacerbating inflammation. *Am J Respir Crit Care Med* 2008; 177: 56–65.

57. Kulkarni AB, Huh CG, Becker D, *et al.* Transforming growth factor β1 null mutation in mice causes excessive inflammatory response and early death. *Proc Natl Acad Sci USA* 1993; 90: 770–774.

58. Huleihel L, Levine M, Rojas M. The potential of cell-based therapy in lung diseases. *Expert Opin Biol Ther* 2013; 13: 1429–1440.

59. Weiss DJ, Ortiz LA. Cell therapy trials for lung diseases: progress and cautions. *Am J Respir Crit Care Med* 2013; 188: 123–125.

60. Moeller A, Ask K, Warburton D, *et al.* The bleomycin animal model: a useful tool to investigate treatment options for idiopathic pulmonary fibrosis? *IntJ Biochem Cell Biol* 2008; 40: 362–382.

61. McNulty K, Janes SM. Stem cells and pulmonary fibrosis: cause or cure? *Proc Am Thorac Soc* 2012; 9: 164–171.

62. Tzouvelekis A, Paspaliaris V, Koliakos G, *et al.* A prospective, non-randomized, no placebo-controlled, phase Ib clinical trial to study the safety of the adipose derived stromal cells-stromal vascular fraction in idiopathic pulmonary fibrosis. *J Transl Med* 2013; 11: 171.

63. Mora AL, Rojas M. Aging and lung injury repair: a role for bone marrow derived mesenchymal stem cells. *J Cell Biochem* 2008; 105: 641–647.

64. Richeldi L, Costabel U, Selman M, *et al.* Efficacy of a tyrosine kinase inhibitor in idiopathic pulmonary fibrosis. *N Engl J Med* 2011; 365: 1079–1087.

65. Jenkins RG, Simpson JK, Saini G, *et al.* Longitudinal change in collagen degradation biomarkers in idiopathic pulmonary fibrosis: an analysis from the prospective, multicentre PROFILE study. *Lancet Respir Med* 2015; 3: 462–472.

66. Spagnolo P, Tzouvelekis A, Maher TM. Personalized medicine in idiopathic pulmonary fibrosis: facts and promises. *Curr Opin Pulmon Med* 2015; 21: 470–478.

67. Maher TM. Disease stratification in idiopathic pulmonary fibrosis: the dawn of a new era? *Eur Respir J* 2014; 43: 1233–1236.

68. Nathan SD, du Bois RM. Idiopathic pulmonary fibrosis trials: recommendations for the jury. *Eur Respir J* 2011; 38: 1002–1004.

69. Collard HR, Brown KK, Martinez FJ, *et al.* Study design implications of death and hospitalization as end points in idiopathic pulmonary fibrosis. *Chest* 2014; 146: 1256–1262.

70. Ley B, Bradford WZ, Weycker D, *et al.* Unified baseline and longitudinal mortality prediction in idiopathic pulmonary fibrosis. *Eur Respir J* 2015; 45: 1374–1381.

71. Karimi-Shah BA, Chowdhury BA. Forced vital capacity in idiopathic pulmonary fibrosis – FDA review of pirfenidone and nintedanib. *N Engl J Med* 2015; 372: 1189–1191.

72. du Bois RM, Weycker D, Albera C, *et al.* Ascertainment of individual risk of mortality for patients with idiopathic pulmonary fibrosis. *Am J Respir Crit Care Med* 2011; 184: 459–466.

73. du Bois RM, Albera C, Bradford WZ, *et al.* 6-minute walk distance is an independent predictor of mortality in patients with idiopathic pulmonary fibrosis. *Eur Respir J* 2014; 43: 1421–1429.

74. du Bois RM, Weycker D, Albera C, *et al.* Forced vital capacity in patients with idiopathic pulmonary fibrosis: test properties and minimal clinically important difference. *Am J Respir Crit Care Med* 2011; 184: 1382–1389.

75. Zappala CJ, Latsi PI, Nicholson AG, *et al.* Marginal decline in forced vital capacity is associated with a poor outcome in idiopathic pulmonary fibrosis. *Eur Respir J* 2010; 35: 830–836.

76. Kaul S, Diamond GA. Trial and error. How to avoid commonly encountered limitations of published clinical trials. *J Am Coll Cardiol* 2010; 55: 415–427.

77. Durheim MT, Collard HR, Roberts RS, *et al.* Association of hospital admission and forced vital capacity endpoints with survival in patients with idiopathic pulmonary fibrosis: analysis of a pooled cohort from three clinical trials. *Lancet Respir Med* 2015; 3: 388–396.

78. Raghu G, Collard HR, Anstrom KJ, *et al.* Idiopathic pulmonary fibrosis: clinically meaningful primary endpoints in phase 3 clinical trials. *Am J Respir Crit Care Med* 2012; 185: 1044–1048.

79. King TE Jr, Albera C, Bradford WZ, *et al.* All-cause mortality rate in patients with idiopathic pulmonary fibrosis. Implications for the design and execution of clinical trials. *Am J Respir Crit Care Med* 2014; 189: 825–831.

80. Epstein RM, Street RL Jr. The values and value of patient-centered care. *Ann Fam Med* 2011; 9: 100–103.

81. Barber LA, Hageman MG, King JD, *et al.* The influence of patients' participation in research on their satisfaction. *J Hand Surg Am* 2014; 39: 1591–1594.

82. Russell AM, Sprangers MA, Wibberley S, *et al.* The need for patient-centred clinical research in idiopathic pulmonary fibrosis. *BMC Med* 2015; 13: 240.

83. Swigris JJ, Wilson SR, Green KE, *et al.* Development of the ATAQ-IPF: a tool to assess quality of life in IPF. *Health Qual Life Outcomes* 2010; 8: 77.

84. Yorke J, Jones PW, Swigris JJ. Development and validity testing of an IPF-specific version of the St George's Respiratory Questionnaire. *Thorax* 2010; 65: 921–926.

85. Eakin EG, Resnikoff PM, Prewitt LM, *et al.* Validation of a new dyspnea measure: the UCSD Shortness of Breath Questionnaire. University of California, San Diego. *Chest* 1998; 113: 619–624.

86. Gries KS, Esser D, Wiklund I. Content validity of CASA-Q cough domains and UCSD-SOBQ for use in patients with idiopathic pulmonary fibrosis. *Glob J Health Sci* 2013; 5: 131–141.

87. Noble PW, Albera C, Bradford WZ, *et al.* Pirfenidone in patients with idiopathic pulmonary fibrosis (CAPACITY): two randomised trials. *Lancet* 2011; 377: 1760–1769.

88. Martinez FJ, Safrin S, Weycker D, *et al.* The clinical course of patients with idiopathic pulmonary fibrosis. *Ann Intern Med* 2005; 142: 963–967.

89. Swigris JJ, Kuschner WG, Jacobs SS, *et al.* Health-related quality of life in patients with idiopathic pulmonary fibrosis: a systematic review. *Thorax* 2005; 60: 588–594.

90. Nishiyama O, Taniguchi H, Kondoh Y, *et al.* A simple assessment of dyspnoea as a prognostic indicator in idiopathic pulmonary fibrosis. *Eur Respir J* 2010; 36: 1067–1072.

91. Holland AE, Fiore Jr JF, Bell EC, *et al.* Dyspnoea and comorbidity contribute to anxiety and depression in interstitial lung disease. *Respirology* 2014; 19: 1215–1221.

Support statement: T.M. Maher is supported by an NIHR Clinician Scientist Fellowship (NIHR Ref: CS-2013-13-017).

Disclosures: T.M. Maher has no declarations directly related to this chapter. However, he has received industry/academic research funding from GlaxoSmithKline R&D, UCB, Takeda and Novartis, and in the past 12 months has received consultancy or speaker's fees from AstraZeneca, Bayer, Biogen Idec, Boehringer Ingelheim, Cipla, Dosa, Galapagos, GlaxoSmithKline R&D, Roche, Sanofi-Aventis, Prometic, Lanthio, Intermune and UCB. He is an investigator in an ongoing phase 2b study for Gilead and serves on the clinical trial advisory board of GlaxoSmithKline. P. Spagnolo serves as a consultant for Roche/Genentech and Santhera and has received consulting fees from InterMune, Boehringer Ingelheim and Novartis. His wife is an employee of Novartis.

Other titles in the series

ORDER INFORMATION

Monographs are individually priced.
Visit the European Respiratory Society bookshop
www.ersbookshop.com
For bulk purchases contact the Publications Office directly.
European Respiratory Society Publications Office,
442 Glossop Road, Sheffield, S10 2PX, UK.
Tel: 44 (0)114 267 2860; Fax: 44 (0)114 266 5064; E-mail: sales@ersj.org.uk